Obstetric Ultrasound

For Elsevier

Senior Commissioning Editor: Sarena Wolfaard
Project Development Manager: Dinah Thom
Project Manager: Derek Robertson
Designer: Judith Wright
Illustrations: Hardlines

Obstetric Ultrasound
How, Why and When

THIRD EDITION

Trish Chudleigh PhD DMU

Superintendent Sonographer, Fetal Medicine Unit, St Thomas' Hospital, London, UK

Basky Thilaganathan MD MRCOG

Director of Fetal Medicine, St George's Hospital, London, UK

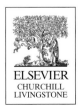

ELSEVIER
CHURCHILL
LIVINGSTONE

EDINBURGH LONDON NEW YORK OXFORD PHILADELPHIA ST LOUIS SYDNEY TORONTO 2004

ELSEVIER
CHURCHILL LIVINGSTONE

An imprint of Elsevier Science Limited

First edition 1986
Second edition 1992
Third edition 2004

ISBN 0 443 054711

British Library Cataloguing in Publication Data
A catalogue record for this book is available from the British Library

Library of Congress Cataloging in Publication Data
A catalog record for this book is available from the Library of Congress

Note
Medical knowledge is constantly changing. As new information becomes available, changes in treatment, procedures, equipment and the use of drugs become necessary. The authors, contributors and publishers have taken care to ensure that the information given in this text is accurate and up to date. However, readers are strongly advised to confirm that the information, especially with regard to drug usage, complies with the latest legislation and standards of practice.

 your source for books, journals and multimedia in the health sciences

www.elsevierhealth.com

The Publisher's policy is to use **paper manufactured from sustainable forests**

Acknowledgements

We are grateful to the members of the Fetal Medicine Unit at St George's Hospital for their support during the preparation of this text. In particular we thank Gill Costello, Anisa Awadh, Sara Coates, Katy Cook, Heather Nash, Shanthi Sairam, Katherine Shirley-Price, Alison Smith and Alison Stock for their constructive criticism and help in providing the images.

To Ben and Ella

Contents

Contributors

Chapters 1 and 15
Tony Evans BSc MSc PhD CEng
Senior Lecturer in Medical Physics, Leeds General
Infirmary, Leeds, UK

Chapters 4 and 5
Dr **Davor Jurkovic** MD MRCOG
Consultant Gynaecologist, Early Pregnancy
and Gynaecology Assessment Unit,
Kings College Hospital, London, UK

Chapter 6
Simon Kelly MB ChB FRANZCOG
Lecturer, University of McGill, Montreal, Quebec,
Canada

Preface

The third edition of this text follows the path of its predecessors in combining the description of best practice with practical advice for all ultrasound practitioners who participate in obstetric imaging programmes. The suggestions we make are derived from our experiences of working for many years in teaching centres of excellence that act both as tertiary referral centres and also as providers of routine screening for their local populations. As in most ultrasound departments, the education and training of others has formed an integral part of what we do. We hope that the combining of the technical expertise of the ultrasound practitioner with the clinical expertise of the obstetrician and our understanding of the challenges of working in a multidisciplinary environment make this text instructive to both the novice and the experienced ultrasound practitioner.

The development of units dedicated to early pregnancy, gynaecological and infertility investigations is encouraging specialization in particular areas of obstetric and gynaecological imaging. In order to gain from the expertise of such specialists this edition incorporates chapters on the imaging and management of early pregnancy, gynaecology and infertility from international experts in these fields. A clear understanding of the principles of ultrasound when applied to 2D imaging or to Doppler examinations is critical to the safe and effective use of ultrasound in clinical practice. Understanding the principles of ultrasound, however, is frequently not synonymous with the skill of being able to impart that knowledge to others. We hope that the reader of this edition will benefit from the clear thinking of, in our opinion, one of the best current teachers of the principles of 2D ultrasound and Doppler ultrasound.

The continuing improvement in resolution of ultrasound systems brings with it both advantages and challenges. While we are able to identify an ever-increasing range of abnormalities in the fetus, this diagnostic sophistication is not without its cost. The interpretation of findings that are not abnormal but may confer an increased risk of a particular condition provide the challenge to us as operators and communicators and to parents as the receivers of our care. The uncertainty surrounding the interpretation of markers of aneuploidy remains an example of such a challenge. This is now further compounded by the introduction of prior screening by nuchal translucency and/or biochemical screening in many departments. The need for the practitioner to understand clearly the purpose of the examination, the information it may provide and how to interpret it has never been greater. This expertise must now be combined with the additional ability to communicate the interpretation of the findings, be they straightforward or complex, to the parents in a way that they can understand. For this reason we have introduced a new chapter into this edition that offers what we consider to be a helpful approach to the communication of 'good' and 'bad' news to parents.

In putting together this third edition it has been our intention to provide a clear, concise and usefully illustrated text that addresses many of the issues that the qualified ultrasound practitioner will face in his or her daily practice. We also hope that it will provide a readable and clinically helpful text for the student sonographer, that it will support them through their training and will ultimately provide a logical foundation on which they base their clinical practice.

Trish Chudleigh and Basky Thilaganathan
London 2004

Chapter **1**

Physics and instrumentation

Ultrasound is very high frequency (high pitch) sound. Human ears can detect sound with frequencies lying between 20 Hz and 20 kHz. Middle C in music has a frequency of about 500 Hz and each octave represents a doubling of that frequency. Although some animals, such as bats and dolphins, can generate and receive sounds at frequencies higher than 20 kHz, this is normally taken to be the limit of sound. Mechanical vibrations at frequencies above 20 kHz are defined as ultrasound.

Medical imaging uses frequencies that are much higher than 20 kHz; the range normally used is from 3 to 15 MHz. These frequencies do not occur in nature and it is only within the last 50 years that the technology has existed to both generate and detect this type of ultrasound wave in a practical way.

WAVE PROPERTIES

When describing a wave, it is not sufficient to say that it has a certain frequency, we must also specify the type of wave and the medium through which it is traveling. Ultrasound waves are longitudinal, compression waves. The material through which they travel experiences cyclical variations in pressure. In other words, within each small region there is a succession of compressions or squeezing, followed shortly afterwards by rarefactions or stretching. The molecules within any material are attracted to each other by binding forces that hold the material together. These same forces are responsible for passing on the pressure variations. It is as though the molecules were joined by springs such that a stretch and release at one end would create a disturbance that traveled across the material to the other side. If the springs are stiff, i.e. require a lot of force to create a small change in length, then the disturbance will travel quickly. Softer or more compressible materials will require more time to respond fully and hence the disturbance or wave will travel slowly. Some examples of sound wave speeds in different materials are given in Table 1.1.

Table 1.1 shows that the stiffer materials are associated with higher sound speeds. It is also noteworthy that the speed of sound in most soft tissues is similar and close to that of water, which is perhaps not surprising in view of their high water content. It turns out that this is critical in the design of ultrasound scanning systems (see 'The pulse echo principle' below). In fact, all ultrasound scanners are set up on the assumption that the speed of sound in all tissues is 1540 m s^{-1}. We can see that this is not strictly true but it is nevertheless a reasonable approximation.

Having chosen to generate a wave at a particular frequency, f, in a particular material with a speed of sound c, the wavelength λ (lambda) is automatically determined. Their relationship is simple:

$$c = f\lambda$$

If we rearrange the above expression, we see that $\lambda = c/f$ and we can calculate the wavelength for an ultrasound wave in soft tissue, assuming a 1540 m s^{-1} speed of sound (see Table 1.2).

Note that the wavelength is always a fraction of a millimetre and that it gets shorter as the fre-

Table 1.2 Values for the wavelength (mm) of ultrasound waves in soft tissue for different frequencies, assuming a sound speed of 1540 m s^{-1}

Frequency (MHz)	Wavelength (mm)
3	0.51
5	0.31
7	0.22
10	0.15

quency rises. This will have an important influence on the quality of the ultrasound images.

THE PULSE ECHO PRINCIPLE

The principle underlying the formation of ultrasound images is the same as that of underwater sonar (**sound navigation and ranging**) used by submarines and fishing boats. It relies on the generation of a short burst of sound and the detection of echoes from reflectors in front of it. The same principle applies when we hear our voices reflected from say, walls, or in tunnels.

If we consider the case in Fig. 1.1, the person P can detect the presence of the wall but can also work out the distance D to the wall by measuring the time it takes for the burst of sound to travel to the wall and back, provided the following assumptions are made:

Table 1.1 Speed of sound in various materials

Material	Speed of sound (m s^{-1})
Air	330
Water	1480
Steel	5000
Blood	1575
Fat	1459
Muscle	1580
Cortical bone	3500

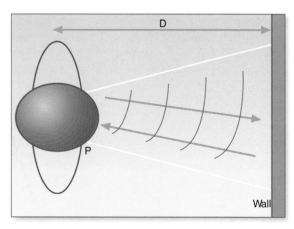

Figure 1.1 Pulse echo principle.

- sound travels in straight lines
- the speed of sound is the same in all materials through which it is traveling; this speed is known
- all echoes received are generated at the interface between the wall and the surrounding medium.

We can then perform the following substitutions:

- sound becomes ultrasound
- the 'person' becomes a device (a transducer) that can send and receive the ultrasound
- the air becomes soft tissue
- the wall becomes a target or interface within the soft tissue.

This creates the situation shown in Fig. 1.2, where echoes are received from a structure inside the body but where the pulse echo principle still applies and the above assumptions are still made.

If there are two or more targets or interfaces behind each other, we can expect to receive echoes from each, although the echoes from the more distant targets will arrive later. In this way, we can build up a kind of one-dimensional (1D) map of

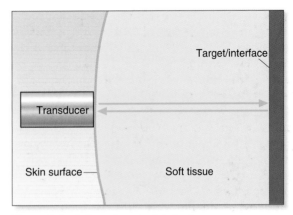

Figure 1.2   Pulse echo principle in tissue.

the positions of reflectors lying along the direction of the sound beam (Fig. 1.3).

TWO-DIMENSIONAL SCANNING

The 1D view in Fig. 1.3 is known as the A-scan. It is difficult to interpret anatomically without detailed prior knowledge or assumptions, and it

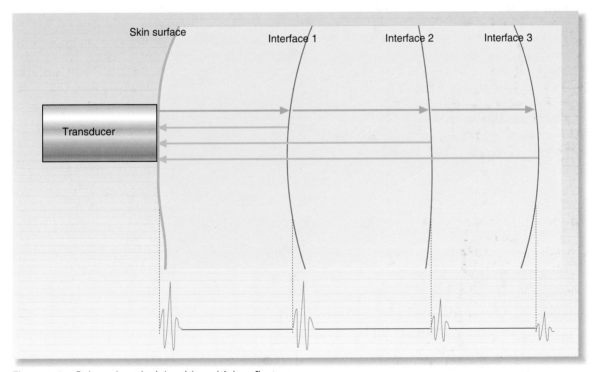

Figure 1.3   Pulse echo principle with multiple reflectors.

is of limited clinical value. To produce a more useful two-dimensional (2D) scan, it is necessary to obtain a series of A-scans and assemble them in a convenient format. This is done either by moving the transducer using a suitable mechanical device or else by having more than one transducer. The latter option is preferred in modern scanners and the 'transducer' that is held by the operator in fact contains a row or array of many transducers (typically 100–200). In this way, a series of A-scans can be obtained in a closely packed regular format. For the purposes of display, the amplitude (height) of each echo is represented by the brightness of a spot at that position. Fig. 1.4 illustrates how the echo amplitudes from the previous section can be turned into spot brightnesses.

This display mode, in which the x and y directions relate to real distances in tissue and the grayscale is used to represent echo strength, is known as the the B-scan (Fig. 1.5).

TIME GAIN COMPENSATION

The echoes shown in Fig. 1.3 show a steady decline in amplitude with increasing depth. This occurs for two reasons. First, each successive reflection removes some energy from the pulse leaving less for the generation of later echoes. Second, tissue absorbs ultrasound strongly, and so there is a steady loss of energy simply because the ultrasound pulse is traveling through tissue. This is generally considered to be a nuisance and attempts are made to correct for it. The amount of amplification or gain given to the incoming signals is made to increase simultaneously with the arrival of echoes from greater depths. The machine control that is used for this is called the time gain compensation (TGC) control and it is fitted to virtually all machines.

Of course, the assumption that all echoes should be made equal is not really valid. We will see later that some structures, e.g. organ boundaries, are much more strongly reflective than others, e.g.

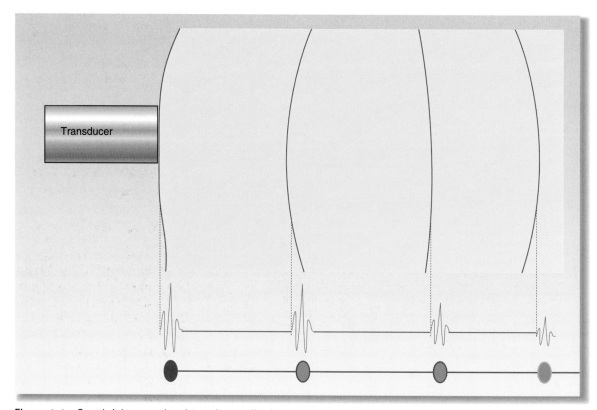

Figure 1.4 Spot brightness related to echo amplitude.

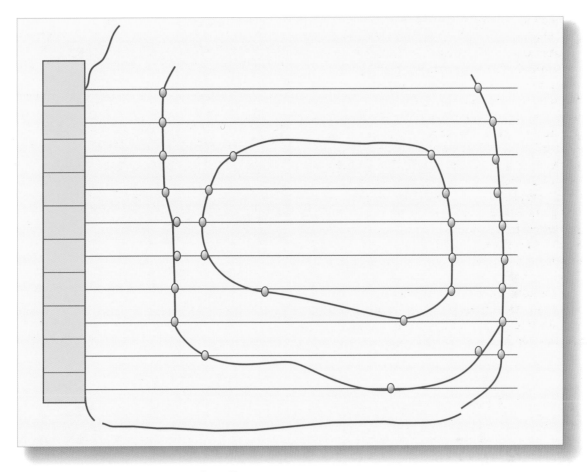

Figure 1.5   Principle of B-scanning using a linear array.

small regions of inhomogeneity within the placenta. The operator needs to use the TGC control with care if misleading images are not to be produced. Providing excessive TGC can turn the normally echo-poor region within a fluid-filled cyst into one that seems to have many small echoes, thereby resembling a tumor. Also, if excessive TGC is used close to the surface, the receiving circuits can be saturated. This can have the effect of causing a blurring of the fine detail and a loss of information. Figure 1.6 shows the same section with both correct and incorrect TGC settings.

The layout of the TGC controls varies from one machine to another. One of the most popular options is a set of slider knobs. Normally, each knob in the slider set controls the gain for a specific depth. It is the task of the operator to set each level

for each patient and often it is necessary to adjust the TGC during a clinical examination when moving from one anatomic region to another.

GENERATION, DETECTION AND DIFFRACTION

The device that both generates the ultrasound and detects the returning echoes is the transducer. Transducers are made from materials that exhibit a property known as piezoelectricity. Piezoelectric behavior is found in many naturally occurring materials, including quartz, but medical transducers are made from a synthetic ceramic material, lead zirconate titanate. This is fired in a kiln just as any other ceramic and can therefore be molded into almost any shape. To establish an electrical

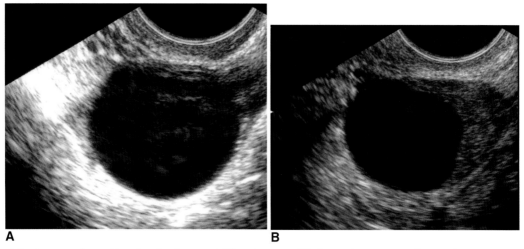

A   **B**

Figure 1.6   Images of a section showing incorrect (A) and correct (B) time gain compensation settings.

connection, thin layers of silver are evaporated onto the surface to form electrodes. This creates a device that will expand and contract when a voltage is applied to it but will also create a voltage when subject to a small pressure such as a returning echo might exert. Obviously the voltages generated when receiving echoes are normally much smaller than those applied to create the ultrasound wave in the first instance. This process is illustrated in Fig. 1.7.

Diffraction is a process that occurs when a wave encounters an obstacle that has dimensions com-

parable to its wavelength. In this case, the transducer itself can be seen as such an obstacle. The diffraction process has a strong influence on the shape of the beam that is generated by ultrasound transducers and, in some respects, this is unexpected. In Fig. 1.5 the 2D image is shown as being assembled from a series of parallel scan lines. The implied assumption made is that each individual scan line or beam is very 'thin' and neither convergent nor divergent. It might be assumed that a thin beam would best be produced by a narrow source, in the same way as a beam of light from a small

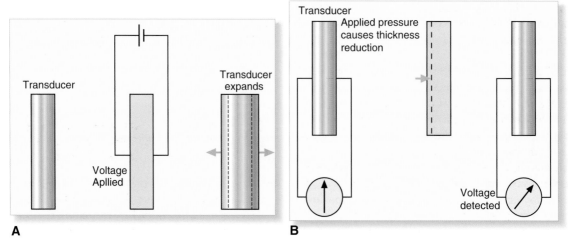

A   **B**

Figure 1.7   A. Generation of ultrasound using piezoelectric devices. B. Detection of ultrasound using piezoelectric devices.

torch would be narrower than that from a larger one. However, for diffractive sources this is not true. Fig. 1.8A shows a simplified version of the beam shape from three transducers of different sizes. In all three cases two different regions can be seen. The first region, closest to the source, roughly approximates to the ideal parallel beam concept. This is known as the *near field*. At some point, this pattern changes into a shape that is divergent and appears to have come from a point at the center of the source; this region is called the *far field*. In Fig. 1.8A, most of the beam is in the near field. Figure 1.8B shows a much smaller source from where it can be seen that the divergent far field dominates; Fig. 1.8C shows an intermediate source. The distance at which the near field pattern changes to the far field pattern clearly depends upon the source diameter. In fact, it turns out that for a circular source, the distance d at which this transition takes place is given by:

$$d = a^2/\lambda$$

where a is the radius of the source and λ is the wavelength. Therefore we have a conflict. If we want a narrow beam, we would normally select a small diameter source, but this will also result in a beam that will diverge readily. If we want a beam that is reluctant to diverge, then this requires a large source and hence does not create a narrow beam. The compromise is to use an intermediate size source and choose the value such that the length of the near field is only just long enough to cover the depth of interest. We can also see that this is aided if the value of λ is low, i.e. if we use high frequencies.

It is possible to reduce the width of the beam to a smaller dimension if focusing techniques are used. Two basic types of focusing can be employed, lenses and mirrors. An ultrasonic lens is similar to the more familiar optical lens except that the surfaces normally curve in the opposite direction. This is because acoustic lenses are normally made of materials with a higher speed of sound than the surroundings which is not true in optics. Figure 1.9 shows how the introduction of a lens has the effect of narrowing the beam at some selected depth F, although it also causes extra divergence at other depths. Thus we trade-off beam width improvements at the focus for beam width degradation else-

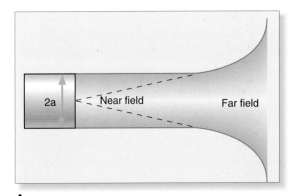

A

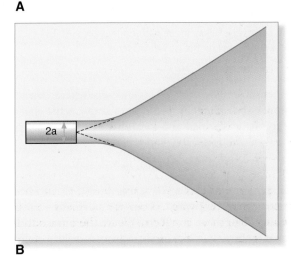

B

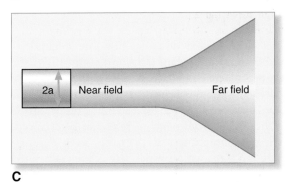

C

Figure 1.8 A. Beam shape with large circular source. The radius of the source is **a**. B. Beam shape with small source. C. Beam shape with intermediate source.

where. Exactly the same focusing effect can be obtained by using a curved front face on the transducer. It is just as if a curved lens was attached to its surface. If the source diameter is increased, the beam width at the focus is reduced further at the

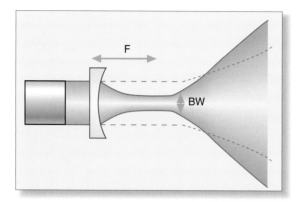

Figure 1.9   Effect of lens focusing. The dotted line represents the beam shape with no lens present. BW, beam width at the focus; F, focal length.

expense of still more divergence elsewhere. For a source of diameter A (sometimes know as the aperture width) focused at a focal distance F, the beam width at the focus BW is given by:

$$BW = F\lambda/A$$

Therefore, the choice of aperture size is another compromise. Improved beam width at one depth means defocusing at others. We shall see later that the same lensing effect can be achieved electronically but the trade-off between beam width and depth range still applies.

The above section describes how the dimensions of the ultrasound beam transmitted into the tissue can be influenced by factors such as the size of the source and the wavelength. However, it should be noted that the same factors also influence the shape of the region from which echoes can be received. When the transducer is operating as a detector there is a zone within which any echoes generated will be detected. The shape of this zone is determined in exactly the same way. Thus focusing applies both on transmission of the beam and during detection of the echoes.

INTERACTIONS OF ULTRASOUND WITH TISSUE

As the ultrasound pulse travels through tissue, it is subject to a number of interactions. The most important of these are:

- reflection
- scatter
- absorption.

Each of these is discussed below.

Reflection in ultrasound is very similar to optical reflection. A wave encountering a large obstacle sends some of its energy back into the medium from which it has arrived. In a true reflection, the law governing the direction of the returning wave states that the angle of incidence, i, must equal the angle of reflection r (see Fig. 1.10). The strength of the reflection from an obstacle is variable and depends on the nature of both the obstacle and the background material. Of particular relevance is a quantity known as the *characteristic acoustic impedance* and normally given the symbol Z. For our purposes we can regard Z as a quantity that is specific to the individual material and dependent upon the density ρ (rho) and the speed of sound in the material c:

$$Z = \rho c$$

The strength of the reflection can be described in terms of a reflection coefficient R, which is defined as a ratio:

$$R = \left| \frac{\text{Energy in the reflected wave}}{\text{Energy in the incident wave}} \right| \times 100\%$$

We can see from this that the maximum value of R is 100% and that this will correspond to a perfect mirror. If we consider the interface between two materials with acoustic impedance values Z_1 and Z_2

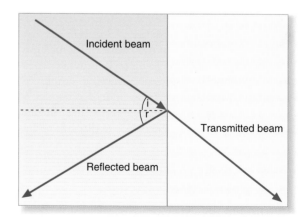

Figure 1.10   Reflection from a large reflector. Note that the angle i equals the angle r and that some of the energy continues beyond the reflecting surface.

then the reflection coefficient for the interface is given by:

$$R = \left(\frac{Z_1 - Z_2}{Z_1 + Z_2}\right)^2 \times 100\%$$

Hence the strength of the reflection depends upon the *difference* in Z values between the two materials that make up the interface. We can expand the data in Table 1.1 to include density and hence calculate the Z values for the materials, as shown in Table 1.3.

It is clear that the Z values of most soft tissues are similar. We would therefore predict that the interface between two soft tissues would result in a small reflection but with most of the energy being transmitted. This is found in practice, which is indeed fortunate because otherwise the idea of getting many echoes along each beam direction (see Fig. 1.4) would not work and only the first reflector encountered would generate a detectable signal. On the other hand, it is equally clear that an interface between any soft tissue and either gas or bone involves a considerable change in acoustic impedance and will create a strong echo. It is quite probable that there would be so little energy transmitted beyond such an interface that no more echoes would be detected, even if there were many targets there. This can be seen, for example, in third-trimester scanning when the large calcified bones of the fetal limbs or skull can create misleading shadows behind them.

As well as this, the strong reflections caused by gas collections have other consequences. First, pockets of bowel gas can make it difficult to visualize anatomy lying posteriorly to them. In obstet-ric ultrasound, for example, this can make it difficult to image certain segments of the uterus. It might be necessary either to scan through a different section, ask the woman to fill her bladder or else consider a transvaginal approach to overcome the problem. Second, it becomes important to use a coupling material between the transducer and woman's skin. A variety of gels and oils are available for this purpose. They need an acoustic impedance value that is intermediate between that of the transducer and the skin. However, acoustically almost any material that displaces air from the transducer–skin interface would work. An important additional feature of couplants is that they act as lubricants, making a smooth scanning action possible.

The reflection model strictly applies only where the interface is large, flat and smooth, and on a scale comparable with the beamwidth. In practice, there are very few such interfaces in the body. Nevertheless, the importance of acoustic impedance matching is valid and provides a useful explanation for many effects observed in routine scanning.

Scattering occurs at the opposite end of the size scale. The theories available here tend to assume that the target is not only very small (much less than a wavelength) but also not influenced by other nearby scatterers. If such a target were to exist in the body, we would expect to see a very weak interaction. In other words, most of the beam energy would pass through with no effect. The small fraction of the energy that interacted would be redistributed in almost all directions including backward, as shown in Fig. 1.11. The closest approximation to this type of scatterer in the body

Table 1.3   Z values of various materials

Material	Speed of sound (m s⁻¹)	Density (kg m⁻³)	Acoustic impedance Z (kg m⁻² s⁻¹) × 10⁻⁶
Air	330	1.2	0.0004
Water	1480	1000	1.48
Steel	5000	7900	39.5
Blood	1575	1057	1.62
Fat	1459	952	1.38
Muscle	1580	1080	1.70
Cortical bone	3500	1912	7.8

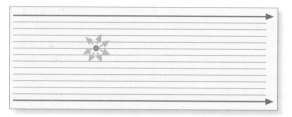

Figure 1.11   Small scatterer (black circle) redistributing energy in all directions.

is the erythrocyte, but even this does not really fit the model because with normal hematocrit levels the distance to the nearest neighbor is too small to achieve independence. Multiple scattering involving many such cells is thought to occur. None the less, this process is critical in the generation of Doppler signals, which is discussed in Chapter 15.

Thus we have two models of interaction; the reflection model and the scattering model, but we are aware that neither is a good descriptor of most interactions. It is interesting to note that this is quite fortunate in one respect. If the anatomy of a particular region was similar to that of a reflector, such as in Fig. 1.10, the returning echo would miss the transducer and not be displayed. Thus, no matter how strong the reflecting surface, it would not be displayed until the angle of incidence was made approximately 90°. When scanning the fetal head, for example to measure the biparietal diameter (BPD), it is often noted that structures such as the the falx cerebri and cavum septum pellucidum and bodies such as the lateral ventricles are best demonstrated clearly when insonated at 90°. This should be remembered when identifying the appropriate section for measurement and/or evaluation.

In practice, most interfaces are somewhat irregular, rough and curved. The interaction of the sound wave with them is complex but has elements of both of the above two descriptions. This means that it is not generally necessary to approach a structure at right angles in order to visualize it and this happy situation makes scanning a much more practical proposition than it would otherwise be.

Absorption, however, has few redeeming features and is generally as undesirable as it is inevitable. It is defined as the direct conversion of the sound energy into heat and it is always present to some extent. In other words, all scanning generates some tissue heating. The extent to which this might constitute a hazard is discussed later (see p. 13). At this stage we should concentrate on two other aspects of absorption. The first is that it follows an exponential law and the loss can be expressed using the same mathematics as used to describe the attenuation of X-rays in tissue. In other words, the fraction of the beam energy lost due to absorption is the same for each centimeter traveled. The second key point is that higher frequencies are absorbed at a greater rate than lower frequencies; this is illustrated in Fig. 1.12.

FRAME RATE

Users of modern ultrasound scanners stress the importance of having machines that operate in real time. Strictly, this means that any real movement in tissue must be immediately associated with a corresponding movement in the displayed image. In practice it is sufficient to satisfy two criteria:

1. The image must appear to be that of a constantly moving object, i.e. there must be no perceptible 'judder' such as can be seen on early cinema movies.
2. The object being imaged must not be able to move excessively between successive views, i.e. it must not be seen to jump.

Satisfying these criteria can be achieved by maintaining a sufficiently high frame rate. This is defined in terms of the rate at which the image is updated or refreshed. To avoid 'judder', the human eye requires that the image be updated at a rate of approximately 25 times a second or higher. If this is achieved, then the image is perceived to be moving continuously

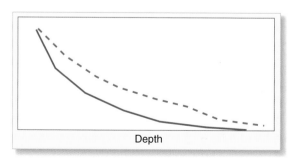

Figure 1.12   Absorption at two frequencies. The dotted line represents a lower frequency.

rather than being a series of still frames. However, if the actual object being scanned is moving slowly, or is still, then it will be sufficient simply to repeat the old frame at this rate without adding any new information. Scanners are equipped with a switch, often labeled frame freeze, to implement precisely this, i.e. the same image is written onto the screen about 25 times a second. In a normal scanning operation, we would normally require an updated image to be displayed at this rate and this imposes some limitations on scanner operation.

If the desired frame rate is 25 frames per second, then it follows that each frame must occupy no more than 1/25 seconds, i.e. 40 ms. During this 40 ms the scanner needs to build up the whole image, as shown in Fig. 1.5. If the image consists of n separate ultrasound lines, then each individual line cannot take more than $40/n$ ms. However, the time taken for each line is not within our control. If we consider that each line requires a pulse to be transmitted to the depth of interest and then that echoes generated at that depth must travel back to the receiving transducer, then it is clear that the time taken by this is determined by the distance traveled and the speed of sound in the tissue. Thus we can say that the time per line, T, is given by:

$$T = (\text{distance travelled})/\text{speed}$$
$$= (2 \times \text{depth})/\text{speed}$$
$$= 2D/c$$

If there are n lines in the image then the time taken for each frame is $2Dn/c$. The corresponding frame rate F_R is 1/(time per frame) and hence:

$$F_R = c/2nD$$

This has a curious consequence. If we substitute reasonable values of a speed of sound of 1540 m s^{-1} and a depth of, say, 15 cm, with a frame rate of 25 frames per second, we find that the maximum number of lines is 205. Limiting the number of lines on display to this kind of value would result in an image that would appear very coarse. We might think of a conventional domestic television that has 625 lines in its display and imagine how poor the image would seem if only one-third of those lines were displayed. In fact, scanner manufacturers avoid this problem by introducing 'manufactured' lines, which are created by assuming

that the values required are intermediate between the adjacent real lines. This technique, called line interpolation, is widely used and results in an image that is more acceptable to the eye while not adding any real information. It does, however, illustrate the difficulties of making the scanner operate in real time. The time constraint limits other aspects of scanner performance as we shall now see.

FOCUSING

As mentioned earlier, it is common to use electronic means to narrow the width of the beam at some depth and so achieve a focusing effect that is similar to that obtained using a lens (Fig. 1.13). This improves the resolution in the plane being imaged. The reduction in beam width at the selected depth in the beam being transmitted is achieved at the expense of degradation in beam width at other depths. Similar methods can be used to achieve focusing of received echoes. The electronic lens can be set up to receive only those echoes originating from a defined region. However, there is an important distinction to be drawn. Whereas a transmitted beam consists of a single pulse traveling through the tissue, the received signal can consist of many echoes originating at a range of depths but separated in time. Thus a single transmitted pulse will normally result in the generation of many echoes. It is possible, when receiving these echoes, to exploit the fact that, at any one time, we know the depth from which the arriving echoes have originated. Echoes from superficial reflectors arrive early whereas those from deeper structures take longer to arrive. The focusing of these received echoes can be altered quickly so that the focal depth always corresponds to the depth of origin. We can say that the focus is swept out simultaneously with the arrival of the echoes. This technique is often called *swept* or *dynamic focusing* and adds to the quality of the image without any penalty apart from an increase in electronic complexity (Fig. 1.13).

It is also possible to consider using similar methods to improve the focusing of the transmitted beam. It was noted earlier (see Fig. 1.9) that we can reduce the beam width at the focus by using a smaller aperture. This can be done for the transmitted beam, resulting in sharper images at the selected

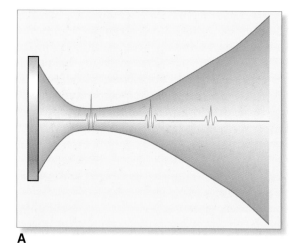

A

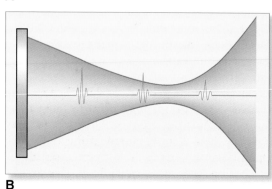

B

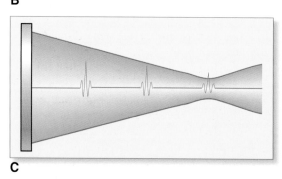

C

Figure 1.13 Focusing on reception. The initial focal depth (A) is set up to focus echoes from superficial depths and the focal depth is swept out synchronously with the returning echoes as in (B) and then (C).

depth. However, it is also clear that this will normally result in poorer images from other depths. One option is to begin by sending out a beam focused at, say, a superficial depth and reject echoes coming back from depths away from that focal region. This can be followed by a second pulse transmitted along the same line but this time focused more deeply. In this case early echoes would be rejected as well as very late ones. A third pulse can then be transmitted focused at greater depths and now all early echoes would be rejected, and so on. In this way a composite image would be built up from the superposition of data from all the depths, resulting in improved resolution throughout. However, in this case, unlike the dynamic focusing on reception, there is a penalty. Each scan line now requires three or more transmissions for its acquisition and this delays the formation of each image frame.

Thus the operator might well have to choose between high frame rates and high resolution. Many machines allow switching between different modes to allow the operator to select the optimal set-up for that particular examination. Indeed, there is nothing to stop the operator from swapping between a high resolution and a high frame rate mode during an examination.

ARTIFACTS

Artifact can be defined as misleading or incorrect information appearing on the display, e.g. a bright dot suggesting the presence of a structure that in fact does not exist. Ultrasound imaging is susceptible to a wide range of artifacts and it is not appropriate to discuss them all in detail in this context. However, they can be divided into the following:

- caused by the nature of the tissue
- caused by the operator
- caused by equipment malfunction.

In many cases, the problem is caused by a violation of one or more assumptions that underpin 2D scanning. These include:

- the beam being infinitely thin
- propagation being in a straight line
- the speed of sound being exactly 1540 m s^{-1}
- the brightness of the echo being directly related to the reflectivity of the target.

Two common examples of such violations are 'acoustic shadowing' and its opposite, 'flaring'. In Fig. 1.14 there appears to be a break in the outline of the

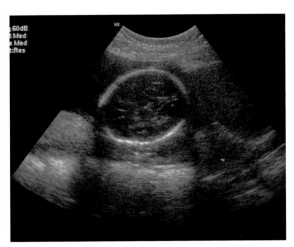

Figure 1.14 Image showing shadowing from the fetal head.

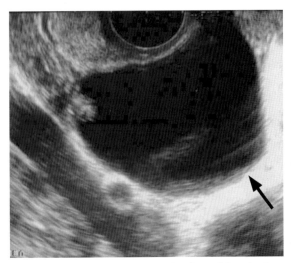

Figure 1.15 Image showing flaring (arrow) in a benign serous cystadenoma.

posterior uterine wall where it lies posterior to the fetal head. In fact, the head structures are the cause of the appearance because they reflect and absorb more of the sound energy than their surroundings. This means that any pulses that would have impacted on the uterine wall and which traveled through the fetal head *en route*, suffer an unexpectedly large loss, and this is repeated on the return journey made by the echoes from this region. The consequence is that the signal strength reaching the receiving transducer from this part of the uterine wall is relatively weak and gives a misleading appearance. The fetal head can be correctly stated to be the cause of acoustic shadowing.

The opposite is true in Fig. 1.15, in which the posterior wall of an ovarian cyst appears to be very bright. In this case, the problem is that the path traveled by the pulse and its corresponding echoes is largely through amniotic fluid, which absorbs very little of the beam energy. This is an example of 'flaring' or 'enhancement'. If the effect is sufficiently marked it can result in saturation of the display at this point and hence a loss of diagnostic information.

However, these artifacts can be used to diagnostic advantage. Some solid masses are quite homogeneous and their image can be devoid of internal echoes. Such an appearance is termed hypoechoic. In this case there is potential for the solid mass to be confused with a cyst of the same dimensions, which would also be expected to be hypoechoic (see Fig. 1.15). However, the solid mass is much more likely to be absorptive than the cyst and hence

the two can normally be distinguished by the presence or absence of flaring or shadowing posteriorly.

The possibility of an operator-induced error also merits attention. The correct use of the TGC control, for example, is critical if the various structures are to be displayed with meaningful gray levels. Too much TGC can incorrectly create filled-in (hyperechoic) regions whereas too little can make solid inhomogeneous regions appear clear. Similarly, the simple error of not using sufficient coupling gel can have dramatic consequences.

For further information of artifacts and their appearances the reader is referred to one of the standard ultrasound texts (Hedrick et al 1995).

SAFETY

The question of whether an ultrasound examination carries risks to the patient and/or operator has been the subject of considerable research for many decades and is ongoing. It remains true that no-one has ever been shown to have been damaged as a result of the physical effect of a diagnostic ultrasound examination. Of course, this is not true of the consequences of a misdiagnosis due to operator or equipment error.

It is well accepted that high levels of ultrasound are capable of producing biological damage. This includes, for example, the use of ultrasound for cell disintegration in cytology laboratories and oncological applications of ultrasound in which tumors are selectively killed. The issue for the diagnostic user is how to operate safely while still optimizing the diagnostic potential of the tool. The modern machine provides some assistance to the operator here but the user needs to understand something of the interaction mechanisms in order to interpret the information supplied.

There are at least three ways in which ultrasound can produce biological effects:

1. cavitation
2. microstreaming
3. heating.

As there are still gaps in our scientific knowledge in this area, the possibility of other mechanisms also being involved cannot be excluded but we will deal only with the above three here.

Cavitation is the growth, oscillation and decay of small gas bubbles under the influence of an ultrasound wave. Small bubble nuclei are present in many tissues. When subject to ultrasound these bubbles can be 'pumped up'. Although their detailed behavior is complex, they often grow to some limiting size and continue to vibrate at the ultrasound frequency. Laboratory studies have shown that cells and intact tissues can be influenced by such local bubble oscillation. However, the results are difficult to predict and to reproduce, and they might not necessarily be harmful. For example, under some conditions, cell growth can be enhanced. This relatively benign situation changes if the bubble oscillation becomes unstable and, under some circumstances, the bubbles can collapse. If this occurs, very high and damaging temperatures and pressures can be generated. It is thought that part of the reason why kidney stones can be broken by ultrasonic lithotripters is because the conditions are such as to encourage collapse cavitation. Although such dramatic events are dangerous, they are confined to a small region and will be over quickly. Cavitation is encouraged by low frequencies, long pulses, high negative pressures and the presence of bubble nuclei. If follows that, if we wish to minimize the risk of cavitation damage, we would favor the opposite of the above conditions.

Microstreaming is the formation of small local fluid circulations and can be either intra- or extracellular. It is an inevitable consequence of the fact the ultrasound is a mechanical wave that will always exert some mechanical forces on the medium through which it travels. Inhomogeneities such as organ boundaries are likely to be areas where such effects are predominantly noticed. However, it is often difficult to separate bioeffects due to microstreaming from those caused by cavitation.

Heating is a consequence of the absorption of the ultrasound wave by tissue. All ultrasound tissue exposures produce heating. The task is to identify where and if it is significant. As absorption increases with increasing frequency, we would expect more heating from higher-frequency probes and, generally, this is true. However, the temperature rise caused by an ultrasound beam is dependent on many factors, including:

- beam intensity and output power
- focusing/beam size
- depth
- tissue absorption coefficient
- tissue-specific heat and thermal conductivity
- time
- blood supply.

There has been considerable research into the prediction of temperature increases as a result of ultrasonic exposures and complex mathematical models have been proposed. These attempt to predict the worst case, i.e. with the specified exposure, what is the greatest temperature rise that could occur? The guidance from the World Federation of Ultrasound in Medicine and Biology (WFUMB) 1989 is:

> *Based solely on a thermal criterion a diagnostic exposure that produces a temperature of 1.5°C above normal physiological levels may be used without reservation in clinical examinations.*

The task, then, is to let the operator know what temperature rise might be involved for each examination so that an informed decision can be made. The system now in place to facilitate this was suggested by the American Institute for Ultrasound in Medicine (AIUM) and National Equipment Manufacturers Association (NEMA), and involves onscreen labeling.

The onscreen labeling scheme, which effectively is now universal on all new machines, involves the display of two numbers on the screen in real time. These are the thermal index (TI) and the mechanical index (MI). As their names imply, the purpose of the TI is to give the operator a real-time indication of the possible thermal implications of the current examination and similarly, the MI is designed to indicate the relative likelihood of mechanical hazard. The displayed numbers are based on real-time calculations, which take into account the transducer in use, its clinical application, the mode of operation and the machine settings.

In simple terms, the TI is defined as:

$$TI = W'/W_{deg}$$

where W' is the machine's current output power and W_{deg} is the power required to increase the temperature by one degree. Thus a TI value of 2.0 suggests that the machine temperature rise that might be induced under the current exposure conditions is 2°C. If the value falls below 0.4 it need not be displayed, but any scanner that is capable of producing a value in excess of 1.0 must display the TI value. The calculation of W_{deg} is complex and depends on the organ being scanned. This has led to the introduction of three different TI indices. TIS (thermal index for soft tissue) is to be used for upper abdominal and other similar applications. TIB (thermal index for bone) is used when exposure to bone interfaces is likely, which is the normal expectation for obstetric and neonatal applications, and TIC (thermal index for cranial bone) is for pediatric and adult brain examinations.

The MI is the counterpart for mechanical effects. These are known to be enhanced by large negative pressure values and low frequencies and therefore it is unsurprising that the definition is:

$$MI = p_-/\sqrt{f}$$

where p_- is the maximum negative pressure in MPa (megaPascals) generated in tissue and f is the fre-

quency in MHz. As in the TI case, the implication is that an MI value of less than 1.0 should be considered safe.

The clinical use of MI and TI merits further discussion. It is not true that scanning under conditions that have either TI or MI in excess of 1.0 is hazardous, and this is not the implication of the scheme. The purpose of the display of the index is to move the responsibility for decision-making back to the operator. If the diagnostic information obtained can be acquired using lower TI and MI values, then this is the preferred option. Often, the same image can be obtained by using better gain settings rather than increased output levels. However, if the operator concludes that the only way to reach the necessary diagnostic outcome is to use levels in excess on 1.0, then this is not contraindicated by this scheme. It should also be noted that the highest values of TI are usually recorded when using the machine in pulsed Doppler mode. For this reason, some authors have been specifically concerned with the use of Doppler ultrasound in early pregnancy. This subject is extensively discussed by the Safety Watchdog Committee of the European Federation of Societies for Ultrasound in Medicine and Biology (EFSUMB), whose regular updates can be found in the European Journal of Ultrasound.

Power output when using Doppler is discussed in detail in Chapter 15.

REFERENCES AND FURTHER READING

Hedrick W R, Hykes D L, Starchman D E 1995 Ultrasound physics and instrumentation, 3rd edn. Mosby Year Book Inc, St Louis, MO

WFUMB 1989 Second World Federation of Ultrasound in Medicine and Biology symposium on safety and standardization in medicinal ultrasound. Ultrasound in Medicine and Biology 15: S1

Chapter 2

Preparing to scan

To obtain maximum information from any obstetric ultrasound examination, the following three points should be observed:

1. the ultrasound equipment should be suited to the required examination and should be functioning correctly
2. the woman should be properly prepared
3. you, as the operator, should be confident in your abilities to perform the examination.

THE ULTRASOUND EQUIPMENT: COMPONENTS AND THEIR USES

The production of ultrasound images is discussed fully in Chapter 1; a further brief explanation only is given here.

Real-time equipment currently available varies greatly in size, shape and complexity, but will contain five basic components:

1. the probe, in which the transducer is housed
2. the control panel
3. the freeze frame
4. measuring facilities
5. a means of storing images.

Current equipment provides 2D or three-dimensional (3D) information. Three-dimensional imaging in real time, known as four-dimensional (4D) imaging, is now becoming available. As almost all obstetric ultrasound examinations and the vast majority of gynecological ultrasound examinations are performed at the present time using 2D imaging; this book addresses in detail the technique of 2D imaging.

The probe

This refers to the piece of equipment in which the transducer (or transducers) is mounted. The transducer is a piezoelectric crystal that, when activated electronically, produces pulses of sound at very high frequencies – this is known as ultrasound. The crystal can also work in reverse in that it can convert the echoes returning from the body into electrical signals from which the ultrasound images are made up. In practise, however, the terms 'probe' and 'transducer' are used interchangeably. The probe can either be a conventional type used externally or an intracavity type, such as that used transvaginally. There are two broad types of transducer: linear and sector. These terms refer to the way in which the crystal or crystals are arranged and manipulated to produce an image. The image field produced by the flat-faced linear transducer is rectangular whereas all the others are sector in shape.

Irrespective of its type, the probe is one of the most expensive and delicate parts of the equipment. It is easily damaged if knocked or dropped and so should always be replaced in its housing when not in use. A damaged probe often causes crystal 'drop out'. This means that the signals from a small part of the probe surface are lost, which in turn produces a vertical area of fallout in the image. A similar appearance is produced if contact is lost between the probe surface and the maternal skin surface. This is most commonly seen when scanning over the umbilicus, or with a hirsute woman, when small amounts of air become trapped in the body hair (Fig. 2.1).

The left–right display of information on the ultrasound monitor is determined by the probe. Providing the invert control is not activated one side of the probe (see point A in Fig. 2.2) always relates to one side of the ultrasound monitor. This relationship is constant however the probe is positioned. When performing longitudinal scans of the pelvis using the abdominal method, as opposed to the transvaginal method, the bladder is conventionally shown on the right of the image

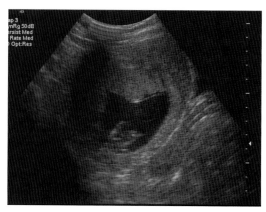

Figure 2.1 Loss of vertical information within the area of interest due to loss of contact over the umbilicus. This can be rectified either by filling the umbilicus with coupling medium to restore contact or moving the probe away (slightly) from the umbilical area and angling the probe back onto the area of interest.

on the ultrasound monitor (Fig. 2.2). There is no convention in the United Kingdom for left–right orientation when performing transverse scans. Some departments adopt the radiological convention, i.e. the patient's left displayed on the right of the screen. Operators performing invasive techniques such as chorion villus sampling and amniocentesis have adopted the converse method and prefer to display the maternal left on the left side of the monitor. It is important that the operator adhers *strictly* to a consistent orientation.

Most machines will display a mark (typically the manufacturer's logo) on the left or right side of the monitor. Its position is determined by the left–right invert control.

The symmetric shape and/or small size of many transabdominal probes, and the symmetric shape of the handle of some transvaginal probes, can make orientation difficult initially. Most transabdominal probes have a raised mark, groove, colored spot or light at one end. Similarly, all transvaginal probes have some distinguishing mark or feature on some part of the handle. This is useful in distinguishing the longitudinal from the transverse axis of the probe before experience takes over. It also provides a reference point that you can use to ensure you

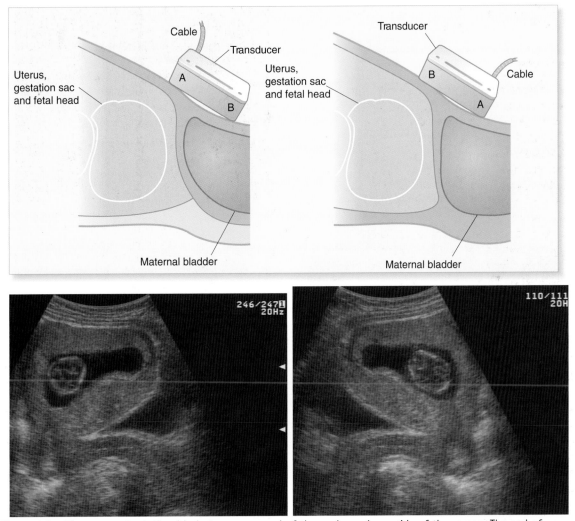

Figure 2.2 The constant relationship between one end of the probe and one side of the screen. The end of probe 'A' relates to the left side of the screen regardless of the orientation on the maternal abdomen. Note that this relationship remains constant providing the image invert control is not activated.

always place the probe on the abdomen or into the vagina using the same orientation. Failure to understand these principles can easily lead to confusion when, for example, localizing the placenta, diagnosing fetal lie or reporting a pelvic mass. An innocuous fundal placenta can be diagnosed as placenta previa, a cephalic presentation might be mistaken for a breech and a right-sided mass reported as left-sided if orientation of the probe is not appreciated. When performing obstetric examinations it is also important to remember that orientation of the maternal anatomy on the screen is unrelated to orientation of the fetal anatomy on the screen.

When scanning in transverse or oblique planes, the relationship between one end of the transducer (point A) and one side of the screen remains. A rather unscientific, but easy method of confirming left and right is to run a finger under one end of the transducer. The shadow seen on the monitor relates to the position of the finger (Fig. 2.3).

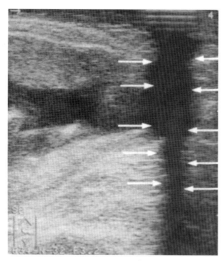

Figure 2.3 An acoustic shadow (arrowed) produced by a finger introduced under one end of the probe can help to orientate the scan.

frequency of the probe, the better the resolution of the image but the shallower the depth of tissue that can be examined. Transvaginal imaging can utilize higher probe frequencies because the area of interest, e.g. the ovary, the cervical canal and internal os, non-pregnant or early pregnant uterus, is much closer to the transducer – and therefore the sound source – than with a transabdominal probe.

The control panel

Sound, be it audible or ultrasound, can be regulated by a volume control that, in the case of ultrasound, is known as a gain control. The amount of sound produced by the transducer and transmitted into the patient by the machine is determined by the overall gain control. The information obtained from the echoes returning to the transducer from the patient and received by the transducer is manipulated by the receiver gain and the time gain compensation controls.

As acoustic exposure is determined by the amount of sound transmitted into the patient the overall gain control should be kept as low as possible. The current safety guidelines relating to the thermal index (TI) and the mechanical index (MI) should be followed. These apply for both imaging and spectral Doppler examinations. It is the user's responsibility to ensure that these safety limits are not exceeded unless clinically indicated. The safe use of ultrasound is discussed in greater detail in Chapters 1 and 15.

The amplification of the returning echoes is known as time gain compensation (TGC). In most machines, TGC is manipulated by a series of sliders that control slices (of, typically, 2 cm in depth) of the image. The receiver gain control or TGC settings are crucial in the quality of the image displayed. Too little gain produces a very dark image (Fig. 2.4A) whereas too much gain produces too bright an image (Fig. 2.4B). Inappropriate settings of the TGC will produce dark and/or light bands within the image (Fig. 2.4C). The correct gain settings produce the image shown in Fig. 2.5.

Structures can be identified more easily and the margin of error in measurement is less when a large image size is used. It is good practice always to scan and record images using as large an image as is comfortably possible.

The left–right invert control, as its name suggests, reverses this carefully elucidated orientation. Unless you are really familiar with ultrasound orientation you should always scan with this control in one position.

At the present time there are no conventions for orientation when using transvaginal imaging. Some operators display the transvaginal sector image with the apex at the bottom of the screen but others prefer the apex at the top (Fig. 4.4). Confusingly, many machines reverse the left–right orientation when switching from the abdominal probe to the transvaginal probe.

Ultrasound frequency

Transducers transmit ultrasound over a range of frequencies but all will have a central frequency (or band of frequencies) that defines the frequency of that probe. Frequency is measured in cycles per second or hertz (Hz). Ultrasound frequencies are described in megaherz (MHz). Transabdominal probes used in obstetrics typically have frequencies of 3.5 MHz or 5 MHz, whereas transvaginal probes can utilize higher frequencies of 7.0 MHz or 8.0 MHz. The important principle to remember is that frequency is related to image resolution but inversely related to penetration of the sound beam into the tissue being insonated. Thus the higher the

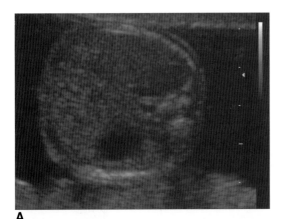

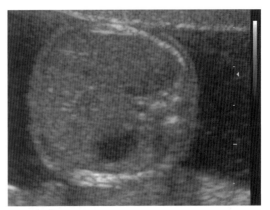

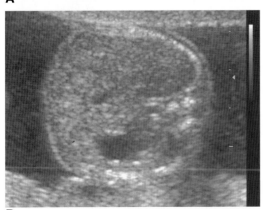

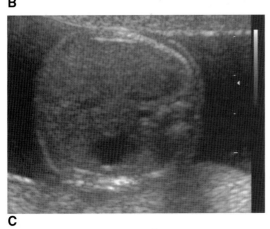

Figure 2.5   Correct gain control settings. Notice how much more detail is seen from the structures within the fetal abdomen compared with Fig. 2.4. The TI value is 0.3 and the MI value is 1.1 in this image.

Figure 2.4   Incorrect receiver gain settings. A. Too little gain. B. Too much gain. C. Incorrect application of TGC, producing a dark band across the image. Compare these with Fig. 2.5, which demonstrates correct gain control settings.

The transmitted and/or received signals can be further manipulated to allow alteration of the pulse repetition frequency (PRF), the dynamic range, frame rate, image persistence and focal zone(s). Different examinations require varying combinations of these controls to maximize the information that can be obtained.

Presets

Transmitted power settings should *always* be set to the lowest possible. Where available, the fetal preset should always be used in obstetric imaging examinations. Similarly, the lowest power settings should always be used when examining the fetus with color, power or spectral Doppler.

Most equipment now has the ability to store specific combinations of machine settings that can be recalled as preset programmes. Some are provided by the manufacturer and others can be determined by the user. Presets for both imaging and spectral Doppler examinations are available. These are very useful time-savers and should be explored and used fully.

Manipulation of specific controls will produce an image that has, for example, more or less contrast, a higher or lower frame rate and/or high or low image persistence. The region of optimal focus can be altered to correspond to the depth of the area of maximum interest. Manipulating the full range of controls available to you is key to your ability to produce optimal images over a range of examinations irrespective of patient habitus.

Typical machine settings for a second trimester obstetric examination might include a dynamic range of 60 dB, medium persistence and a medium frame rate. Such settings produce a 'soft' image, as shown in Fig. 2.5. Note the TIB (thermal index for bone) value of 0.3 and MI value of 1.1. Examining the fetal heart is facilitated by a more contrasted image, as shown in Fig. 2.6. Reducing the dynamic range from 60 to 45 dB increases the contrast of the image, as can be seen on comparison of Fig. 2.5 and Fig. 2.6A. Selecting a cardiac preset will alter not only the dynamic range but also the persistence and frame rate. The fetal cardiac preset shown in Fig. 2.6B includes a dynamic range of 45 dB, low persistence and a high frame rate. Note the slightly higher TIB value of 0.6, due to the

narrower sector width. The MI value is minimally reduced to 0.9.

Freeze-frame control

This is essential for taking measurements and for storing images. The position of the control varies. It can be positioned on the control panel or, most conveniently, as a foot switch. An experienced operator always has a finger within instant striking distance of the control panel freeze-frame control, or a foot resting on the freeze-frame foot switch.

Cine loop

Digital ultrasound machines have the ability to store a specific number of frames of information, which are refreshed in real time. After the freeze frame control is activated this cine-loop facility enables the very last part of the examination to be 'replayed' frame by frame. This facility is invaluable when taking nuchal translucency measurements, examining the fetal heart or evaluating other parts of the fetal anatomy when the fetus is moving vigorously.

Measuring facilities – onscreen measurement

All machines provide facilities for linear, circumference and area measurements. When using spectral Doppler mode, such measurements will relate to indices such as peak systolic velocity (PSV), pulsatility index (PI), resistance index (RI) and time-averaged maximum velocity (TAMXV). Measurements can be displayed alone or together with an interpretation of, for example, gestational age or fetal weight when an obstetric calculation preset program is selected. The gestational age given will vary depending upon the charts programmed into the machine. We recommend that sonographers interpret the measurements from each examination themselves, rather than relying on the information produced by the machine. For example, interpreting measurements made in late pregnancy in terms of gestational age is wrong because such measurements should be used only to evaluate the pattern of fetal growth based on a previously assigned expected date of delivery.

The majority of caliper systems are of the rollerball or joystick types. As with all techniques,

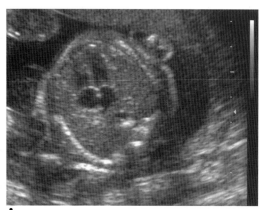

A

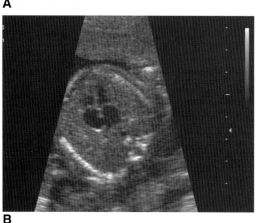

B

Figure 2.6   Correct gain control settings, A. Using a preset designed for imaging the anatomy of the second trimester fetus. The TI value is 0.2 and the MI value is 1.0 in this image. B. A preset designed for imaging the second trimester fetal heart. The TI value has increased to 0.6 in this image, due to the narrower sector width than that used in A.

onscreen measuring requires expertise and it is therefore good practice to take several (we suggest three) measurements of any parameter to ensure accuracy. Linear measurements should be reproducible to within 1 mm, and circumference measurements to within 3 mm. In addition to manual measurement of spectral Doppler traces automatic, continuous measurement is also available on some equipment. We recommend that the automatic readout from a consistent trace is observed for several seconds to ensure that the values recorded are representative of the examination.

The monitor

Ideally, there should be two monitors: a monitor for the operator and a second monitor for the parents or patient. Separate monitors allow both parties to view the examination comfortably and reduces considerably the risk to the operator of ergonomic-related repetitive strain injury. If only one monitor is available, this should be positioned directly in front of the operator and not angled towards the woman, which would necessitate the operator straining his or her neck to view the screen.

Storing the images – recording systems

Digital storage and/or videotape recording are the preferred methods for making a permanent record of interesting or abnormal images.

A thermal imager is ideal for producing memento images for the parents during obstetric examinations. The sensitivity of thermal paper is such that small alterations of the brightness or contrast controls will produce large differences in the quality of the image. Ideally, the controls should be set when the machine is installed. Once ideal settings have been obtained it is advisable to actively discourage overkeen colleagues from fiddling with them. Apparent deterioration in the quality of the images taken is usually due to poor gain settings, insufficient coupling gel, or dirt becoming trapped in the rollers of the thermal imaging apparatus.

THE WOMAN

Privacy is essential during all ultrasound examinations and is a prerequisite for all transvaginal examinations. Ideally, the woman should be given the opportunity to change into a gown before being scanned, to avoid the inconvenience and embarrassment of gel-stained clothing. In the majority of situations this is impractical, so sufficient disposable paper must be used to protect her outer clothing and underwear. Many women feel embarrassed and vulnerable when expected to undress and/or expose their abdomen to a stranger, be that stranger male or female. An operator who covers the woman's legs with a clean sheet can help to alleviate some of this discomfort. This is equally important when performing vaginal examinations or abdominal examinations. When performing an abdominal scan the woman should be uncovered just sufficiently to allow the examination to be performed. This will always include the first few centimeters of the area covered by her pubic hair and will extend far enough upwards to allow the fundus of the uterus to be visualized. A *double* layer of disposable paper towels should be tucked both into the top of her knickers and over her upper clothing.

It is important to consider both the wish of the woman, normally, to see the ultrasound image on the screen and the ergonomic needs of the sonographer performing the examination. These needs are best served by providing a second monitor, which is positioned correctly for the woman's use. The woman should lie on the examination couch in a position such that she is able to see the monitor easily. Most transabdominal scans are performed with the woman supine or with her head slightly raised. However, in later pregnancy many women feel dizzy in this position (the supine hypotension syndrome) and it might be necessary for her to be tilted to one side. This is easily achieved by placing a pillow under one of her buttocks.

Scanning transvaginally naturally requires the woman to remove all her lower clothing. Ideally, she should be positioned on a gynecological couch, with her legs supported by low stirrups, thus allowing maximum ease of access to the pelvic organs. This is especially important when examining the ovaries and adnexae. However, an adequate improvization is to place a chair at one end of the examination couch. The woman lies on the couch with her bottom as near to the end of the couch as possible and rests her feet on the chair.

When scanning transvaginally, an empty bladder is a prerequisite. Send the woman to the toilet before beginning a transvaginal examination as even a small amount of urine in the bladder can displace the organs of interest out of the field of view.

We suggest the following regime when preparing the transvaginal transducer:

1. Apply a small amount of gel to the transducer tip and cover the tip and shaft of the probe with a (non-spermicidal) condom.
2. Apply a small amount of gel, or KY jelly, to the covered probe to allow easier insertion into the vagina.

A woman should only be asked to attend with a full bladder if transvaginal imaging is not available. A full bladder is only necessary in non-pregnant women, those of less than 8 weeks gestation or in women in whom a low-lying placenta is suspected. The woman attending for a transabdominal gynecological or early pregnancy examination should be asked to drink two pints of water or squash 1 h before attending the department. She should not empty her bladder until after the scan is completed. She should be made to understand that one cup of coffee on the way to the department is inadequate and will result in a long wait. When the bladder is overfull and the woman is in obvious discomfort, partial bladder emptying is the best solution. Sufficient urine will usually be retained to make a successful examination possible. Women attending for placental localization in the third trimester should be asked to drink one pint of water or squash half an hour before attending the department.

Any probe should be cleaned before and after use. Individual soap-impregnated wipes and/or hard surface disinfectant spray are commonly employed for this purpose. It is important that advice is sought from the probe's manufacturer because some liquid preparations can adversely affect the transducer covering, making its use unsafe.

THE OPERATOR

It is immaterial whether you are normally left- or right-handed as to which hand is 'better' for holding the probe. It is important that the probe is always held in the hand nearer the woman, as this prevents you tying yourself in knots as you scan or, more importantly, dropping it. It is a matter of individual or departmental preference as to whether the ultrasound machine is positioned to the left or the right of the examination couch. However, the majority of manufacturers work on the right-handed scanning technique and position the probe housing and cabling accordingly.

Transvaginal scanning generally requires a different arrangement of operator and machine. Ensure you are positioned in front of the perineum with the ultrasound machine close enough to operate the controls easily with your non-scanning hand. If the machine is too far away you will jar the vagina with the probe as you stretch forward or sideways to reach the controls. Ensure the woman can see the monitor easily when you are scanning her transvaginally. Initially, many women find this method of examination embarrassing. Being able to watch the images on the monitor will often help her to relax and distract her from what you are doing to her.

Manual dexterity with either technique will be lacking initially, but improves rapidly with practice. Ensure that you are sitting comfortably and at the right height relative to the woman's abdomen when scanning transabdominally, or to the perineum when scanning transvaginally. If your seat is too low, you will quickly develop an aching shoulder; if too high, your arm will ache from continuously stretching downward. Try to think of the probe as an extension of your arm rather than a foreign object, and do not grip it fiercely because this will also produce a painful arm and shoulder.

It is important that you have *instant* access to the freeze-frame control. If this is operated from the control panel you should develop a technique that keeps one non-scanning finger continuously poised over the button. Conversely, if the freeze-frame is operated via a foot switch, always keep your foot resting on the switch so that you can instantly freeze an image if necessary. You will lose many potentially 'perfect' images if you cannot freeze the image as soon as your brain receives the message to do so.

The cine loop is a useful tool but you should learn to freeze optimal images rather than relying on the cine loop, because your finger or foot is too slow.

THE ERGONOMICS OF SAFE SCANNING

The number of reported cases of repetitive strain injury related to ultrasound practice is increasing as the number of operators who have been scanning regularly for many years increases. It is important that the issues of operator strain, fatigue and/or injury are taken seriously, both by the individual concerned and the employing department. Ideally, the height of the examination couch, ultrasound machine console and any other equipment, such as a computer keyboard and mouse for data entry, should be adjustable and should be placed within an arc of less than 60° from your scanning position. Most people sit to scan but you will be just as effective if you discover that you prefer to stand up to scan.

When scanning transabdominally, the machine console, computer keyboard, mouse and the woman's abdomen should all be at the same height. Such positioning, together with correct height selection of your seat, should enable you to access everything required during the scan without twisting, stretching or leaning. An ergonomically designed rotating chair with adjustable back support, partial, adjustable arm rests and a foot-rest should be used in preference to a stool or conventional 'office' chair. The same rules should be applied when scanning transvaginally.

The scanning room should have access to daylight and fresh air. Ideally, it should be air conditioned because the ultrasound machine produces a significant amount of heat, which, over time, is extremely debilitating for the operator, the woman and the machine's performance. If this is not possible, an electric fan and adequate ventilation are essential.

Curtains or blinds over the windows are essential to provide dark (but not pitch black) ambient lighting levels. Scanning in either a very dark or in a room that is too light and/or with an incorrectly adjusted viewing monitor will quickly cause operator eye strain. This can be kept to a minimum by ensuring that the brightness and contrast controls of the viewing monitor are appropriate for the preferred amount of lighting. Controlled daylight, adjustable electric lighting of the room and/or the use of desk lamps, positioned to avoid reflective glare on the monitor(s), will ensure you – the operator – and the woman can see each other sufficiently well to communicate effectively during the examination.

THE COUPLING MEDIUM

There are many proprietary brands of coupling medium available, the variations being in viscosity, color and price. All fulfill the same function of providing an air-free interface between the transducer and the body. Ultrasound gel at room temperature feels very cold so try to ensure the gel is warmed before starting an examination. Electric bottle warmers designed specifically for the ultrasound market are now available. A baby's bottle warmer or a bowl of hot water, regularly replenished, are cheaper, although potentially more dangerous, alternatives. Apply the gel sparingly but remember that you will need more gel in the areas of skin covered with hair.

PROBE MOVEMENTS

There are only a limited number of ways in which a probe can be manipulated. If you understand what each of these movements achieves you will quickly learn how to obtain the correct ultrasound sections. You will also understand how to move from a less than ideal section to the perfect section and when this is difficult, for example due to fetal position, you will not waste time trying to achieve the impossible. Transvaginal scanning involves different movements from those used abdominally.

The abdominal probe

There are four possible movements of this probe (Fig. 2.7).

Sliding

By holding the probe longitudinally and sliding it from side to side across the abdomen, you change the position of the sagittal section relative to the midline of the abdomen. With the probe still held longitudinally it can be slid up and down the woman's abdomen from the symphysis pubis to the umbilicus (Fig 2.7A), or vice versa, a maneuver that is useful for keeping a structure that is being examined in the centre of the screen.

If the probe is held transversely and slid up and down the abdomen from the symphysis pubis to the umbilicus, the level of the transverse section

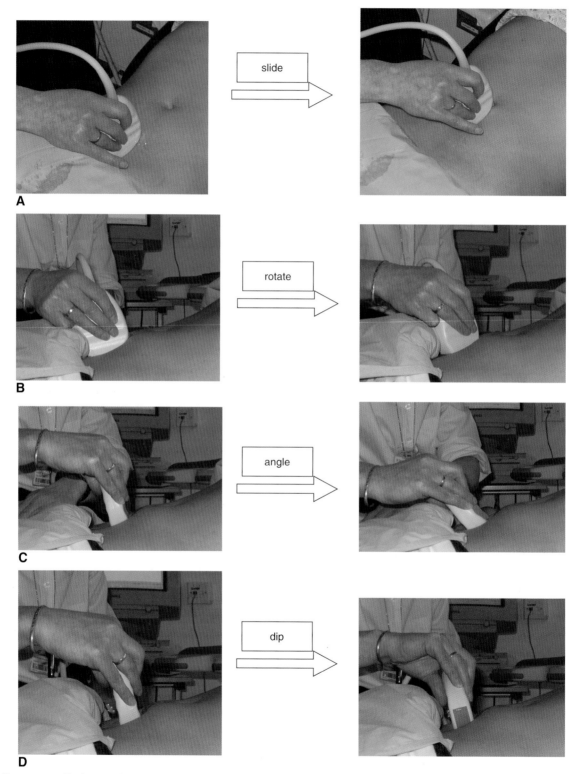

Figure 2.7 Basic scanning movements with the transabdominal probe. (A) Sliding; (B) rotation; (C) angling; (D) dipping.

obtained is altered. With the probe still held transversely it can be slid across the woman's abdomen from her left side to her right side, or vice versa, a manouver that is useful for keeping a structure that is being examined in the center of the screen.

Many beginners make the mistake of changing the angle of the probe when they think they are only sliding the probe. It is very important that you learn, as early as possible, to feel the difference between sliding, angling and a combination of the two. An inability to appreciate the difference between sliding and angling can be a cause of great confusion to a novice sonographer.

Rotating

This term describes rotation of the probe about a fixed point (Fig 2.7B). Its main use is that it allows a longitudinal section to be obtained from a transverse section of an organ (or vice versa) while keeping the organ in view.

Angling

This describes an alteration of the angle of the complete probe surface relative to the woman's skin surface (Fig 2.7C). Its main use is for obtaining correct sections from slightly oblique views.

Many beginners make the mistake of changing the angle of the probe when they are setting out to perform one of the other three probe movements. It is very important that you learn, as early as possible, to feel the difference between angling and any of the other three movements. An appreciation of what the movement feels like and the affect of angling on the image is critical if you intend to develop optimal scanning skills. Most suboptimal views of the intracranial anatomy, for example, are produced because of incorrect angling of the probe.

Dipping

This describes pushing one end of the transducer into the woman's abdomen (Fig 2.7D). It can be uncomfortable, so should be done as gently as possible. Its main use is to bring structures of interest to lie at right angles to the sound beam.

The vaginal probe

The first skill required in transvaginal scanning is to learn how to insert the probe into the vagina and, having done so, to obtain a true sagittal section of the uterus. As with the abdominal probe, four movements are possible with the transvaginal probe (Fig. 2.8), but they are limited by the available space within the vagina. All movements of transvaginal probes should be carried out slowly and gently.

Sliding

This describes the movement of the probe along the length of the vagina (Fig 2.8A). As vaginal probes have a small field of view, sliding up and down the vagina might be necessary to image the whole pelvis.

Rotating

This describes a circular movement of the handle of the probe (Fig 2.8B). Rotating the probe through 90° from the position required for a true sagittal section gives a coronal view of the pelvis. Note that this plane is *not* equivalent to the transverse section of the pelvis or abdomen obtained by rotating the abdominal probe through 90° from the longitudinal plane. Other degrees of rotation are usually necessary to image the pelvic organs adequately.

Rocking

This describes movement of the handle of the probe in an anteroposterior plane such that the tip of the probe moves in the opposite direction. This moves the field of view through a maximum arc of 60°. Further movement is limited by the woman's perineum posteriorly and her urethra anteriorly. This movement is used to image the true longitudinal section of the uterus when its position is not axial. It is also used to obtain true transverse sections of the uterus when the uterus is anteverted.

Panning

This is a photographic term that is borrowed to describe movement of the handle of the probe in

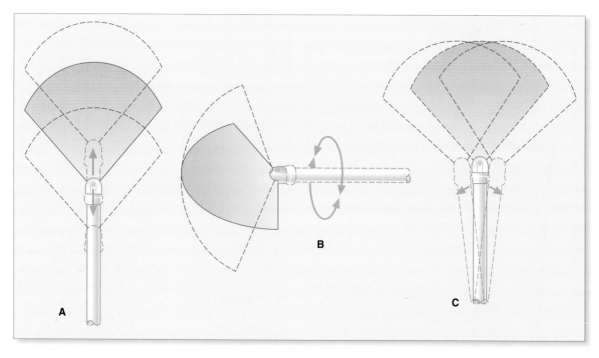

Figure 2.8 Basic scanning movements with the transvaginal probe. A. Sliding; B. rotation; C. panning.

a horizontal plane such that the tip of the probe moves in an opposite direction (Fig 2.8C). This moves the field of view through a maximum arc of about 130°. This movement is used to image structures that lie lateral to the uterus.

A gentle touch is well worth developing whether scanning abdominally or transvaginally. The lightest pressure of the probe on the abdomen is sufficient to produce the majority of images. Digging the probe into the woman rarely improves the image quality and only causes unnecessary discomfort, especially if the woman is in pain or has a full bladder.

Finally, a relaxed and informal atmosphere will give the woman confidence not only in your scanning abilities but also to ask any questions that she might feel are important. The majority of obstetric examinations should be enjoyable, painless and reassuring to the woman. The majority of gyneco-logical examinations might not be enjoyable but should still be painless and reassuring when the findings are normal. The benefits of such examinations, be they medical or emotional, are directly dependent on the quality of operator input.

REFERENCES AND FURTHER READING

Gregory V 2001 Guidelines for reducing injuries to sonographers/sonologists. Online. Available: www.asum.com.au/policies

Royal College of Obstetricians and Gynaecologists 1997 Intimate examinations: report of a working party. The Royal College of Obstetricians and Gynaecologists. RCOG Press, London

United Kingdom Association of Sonographers 2001 Guidelines for professional working standards – ultrasound practice. United Kingdom Association of Sonographers, London

www.soundergonomics.com

Chapter 3

First trimester ultrasound

Although many students start their training scanning second trimester pregnancies, we suggest that it is easier to understand the basic principles involved, how these link to the four probe movements and how these interrelate to produce the required section, if they are applied to the static target of the non-pregnant or early pregnant uterus. For this reason, examination of the uterus using both the transvaginal and abdominal routes is explained in some detail. This chapter also addresses the practical problems of how to find a first trimester pregnancy within the uterus and how to assign the gestational age once this has been achieved.

The most accurate way to calculate the length of pregnancy is by knowing the date of conception. Delivery would then be expected to occur 38 weeks (266 days) later. However, as most women are unaware of the date of conception, the first day of the last menstrual period (LMP) is used to calculate the expected date of delivery (EDD). This is done by applying Naegele's formula to the LMP as follows:

1. add 7 to the days
2. subtract 3 from the months
3. add 1 to the years.

For example, if the LMP is 13.4.04 then the EDD is (13 + 7). (4 − 3). (04 + 1), that is 20.1.05.

Table 3.1 The different ultrasound parameters used to estimate gestational age

Gestational age (weeks)	Parameter
4+ to 6+*	Mean sac diameter
4+ to 6+*	Gestation sac volume
6+ to 12*	Crown–rump length
12 to 15	Defer measurement
15 to 24	Biparietal diameter, femur length and circumference measurements
24 weeks onward	Gestational age cannot be accurately determined by ultrasound

*Recognition of a gestation sac from 4+ weeks and a fetal pole from 6+ weeks will normally be achieved only with a transvaginal probe.

This means that pregnancy is 40 weeks (280 days) long and assumes that conception occurs 2 weeks after the LMP.

The LMP is unreliable (and therefore Naegele's formula cannot be used) if the:

- date of the LMP is not accurately known
- menstrual cycle is not 28 days long
- menstrual cycle is irregular
- woman has only stopped taking the combined oral contraceptive pill ('the pill') within the last 3 months
- woman has bled in early pregnancy
- woman is breast feeding or has been pregnant in the preceding 3–6 months.

This had led to the use of two terms:

1. Gestational age: this is the length of pregnancy based upon a reliable LMP, assuming that conception occurs 14 days later.
2. Postmenstrual age: this is the length of the pregnancy based upon the LMP, irrespective of its reliability.

It should be remembered that embryological or postconception age are calculated from the (assumed) date of conception and are therefore numerically 14 days, or 2 weeks, *less* than the gestational age. The expected date of delivery (EDD) as calculated from both methods will be the same.

Please note that all reference made to weeks of gestation in this text is based on gestational age and not conceptual or embryological age, unless otherwise stated.

Several ultrasound parameters have been used to estimate gestational age. The most commonly used are:

- mean sac diameter
- gestation sac volume
- crown–rump length (CRL)
- biparietal diameter (BPD; see Chapter 7)
- femur length (see Chapter 7).

Use of these is shown in Table 3.1.

FINDING THE UTERUS

The transvaginal probe can utilize ultrasound frequencies of 7.0–8.0 MHz because the probe can be placed in close proximity to the organ of interest, namely the uterus. It is therefore the preferred method of pregnancy assessment in the first 9 weeks of gestation. The gestation at which an intrauterine pregnancy can be confirmed is dependent on the position of the uterus and/or the presence of fibroids. A sharply retroverted uterus or the presence of fibroids might delay the ability to confirm a pregnancy for a further 7–10 days.

The uterus lies centrally within the pelvis, posterior to the bladder and cephalad to the vagina (Fig. 3.1). It is usually anteverted and rotated slightly to the right (dextrorotated). The first aim of any obstetric ultrasound examination is to find the uterus. Scanning the non-pregnant or early pregnant pelvis can be performed using transvaginal or abdominal probes, with the former being the method of choice. Unfortunately, for the beginner, the two techniques are very different. This simple fact can leave even the most experienced transabdominal operator very disillusioned when attempting a transvaginal examination for the first time. Irrespective of the method, once you have learnt how to orientate the probe to obtain longitudinal (sagittal) and cross-sectional views of the pelvis, the examination becomes straightforward.

Transvaginal method

This is the preferred method for imaging the non-pregnant or early pregnant uterus. The prepara-

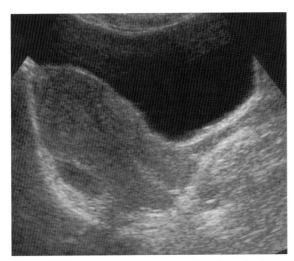

Figure 3.1 Longitudinal midline section through the normal pelvis demonstrating the bladder, vagina and non-pregnant uterus using the transabdominal method. Note the image is oriented such that the maternal bladder can be seen on the right side of the screen and the uterine fundus on the left side of the screen.

tions required for a transvaginal examination are described in Chapter 2 but are briefly summarized again here:

- When scanning transvaginally an empty bladder is a prerequisite. Send the woman to the toilet before beginning a transvaginal examination because even a small amount of urine in the bladder can displace the organs of interest out of the field of view.
- Apply a small amount of gel to the transducer tip and cover the tip and shaft of the probe with a (non-spermicidal) condom.
- Apply a small amount of gel, or KY jelly, to the covered probe to allow easier insertion into the vagina.

Check that the left–right and top–bottom invert controls are activated such that the sector image on the monitor is orientated to your preference before you begin. Ensure that the selected image size is appropriate and that the zoom control is not activated. Hold the prepared probe with the mark or guide positioned to produce a longitudinal view of the pelvis. This usually means having the mark uppermost. Insert the probe gently into the vagina. The uterus will usually be visualized by panning the tip of the probe slightly towards the woman's right shoulder (to compensate for dextrorotation) and

then rocking the handle posteriorly towards the perineum. If you cannot find the uterus you might need to gently slide the probe further into the vagina. By gently panning the probe to left and right, the optimal longitudinal view of the uterine cavity, endometrium and 'cavity line' will be obtained (Fig. 3.2). Do not rotate the probe simultaneously with panning because this will alter your orientation. To ensure that the view is truly longitudinal the entire length of the cavity line should be visualized. The ultrasound appearance of the endometrium will vary depending on the stage of the menstrual cycle.

The cervical canal, internal os and external os are often best seen by withdrawing the probe slightly from the position that demonstrates the optimal longitudinal section of the uterus. If the uterus is anteflexed it might be necessary to rock the tip of the probe posteriorly slightly to best image the cervical canal and internal os (Fig. 3.3).

It is important to appreciate that, first, the position and the degree of flexion of the uterus relative to the vagina and, second, the degree of rocking that can be performed determine the views obtained when the probe (or the beam) is rotated away from a sagittal plane. The section of the uterus that is obtained by rotating the probe through 90° from the sagittal plane might be a coronal section

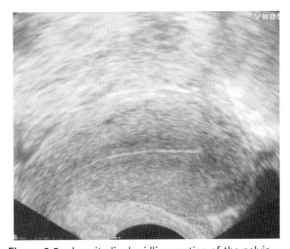

Figure 3.2 Longitudinal midline section of the pelvis demonstrating the non-pregnant uterus using the transvaginal method. Note the absence of the maternal bladder as a landmark. The uterine fundus can be seen on the right side of the screen.

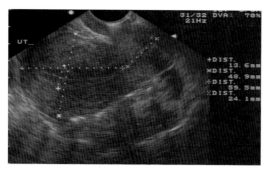

Figure 3.3 Longitudinal midline section of the lower uterus demonstrating the cervical canal (⋅⋅⋅⋅⋅⋅⋅⋅⋅⋅, distance 24.1mm) and internal os using the transvaginal method. Measurement of the endometrial thickness (13.6mm) and uterine length (59.5mm) are also shown.

of the uterus, a true transverse section or an oblique section somewhere between these two planes. For this reason, cross-sectional views obtained by means of a transvaginal probe are not comparable with those obtained abdominally. This fact should be remembered when estimating gestational age from transvaginal images (see p. 34).

The transvaginal probe should be cleaned before and after use. Individual soap-impregnated wipes and/or hard surface disinfectant spray are often used for this and it is important to use the product recommended by the manufacturer of the probe. Some liquid preparations can adversely affect a specific transducer covering, making its use unsafe.

Problems

- Transvaginal examination is obviously inappropriate in girls or women who have never had sexual intercourse.
- There is no evidence that gentle transvaginal scanning is at all harmful but in certain situations the woman or her doctor might want you to carry out an abdominal scan.
- Poor positioning of the woman can reduce the maneuverability of the probe within the vagina, particularly rocking or panning movements. Bringing the woman's bottom right to the end of the couch will improve access for rocking the probe. Opening or relaxing the woman's legs more will improve access for panning movements.

- Visualizing a retroverted uterus can be difficult because the vaginal diameter might limit posterior rocking movements so as to prevent visualization of the fundus in a steeply retroverted uterus. Lack of sound penetration, due to the high frequency of the transducer and/or bowel gas, can also be limiting factors.
- Large and/or multiple fibroids will affect the quality of transvaginal images for two reasons: first, fibroids situated between the probe and the endometrium or gestation sac might displace the area of interest beyond the range of insonation of the high frequency transducer; second, if the area of interest remains within the field of insonation, the sound beam might be attenuated or absorbed by a smaller fibroid such that the organs further from the probe cannot be imaged adequately.

Abdominal method

To perform a pelvic ultrasound examination using the abdominal route, the woman must have a full bladder. This has three effects: first, it pushes the uterus out of the pelvis, thus removing it from the acoustic shadow caused by the symphysis pubis; second, it provides an acoustic window through which the pelvic organs can be visualized; third, it displaces the bowel superiorly, so preventing gas from the bowel scattering the ultrasound beam.

To examine the pelvis adequately, a probe with a small area of contact or 'footprint' is needed. This is most commonly of the sector type, but phased array, annular array and small curvilinear probes are also appropriate. Although images of the pelvis can be obtained with the linear and larger curvilinear probes designed for obstetric use, their size makes a complete examination of the pelvis difficult and they are more likely to produce lateral artifacts (see p. 11).

Before you begin, check that you are holding the probe and/or that the left–right control is activated such that the sector image on the monitor will display the maternal bladder on the right of the screen and the uterine fundus on the left. Place the probe on the abdomen in the midline, immediately superior to the symphysis pubis to obtain a longitudinal section of the pelvis. The bladder should be seen on the right of the screen. The vagina is usually immediately visualized as three bright parallel lines posterior to the bladder (see Fig. 3.1). If only the lower part of the uterus is seen, rotate the probe slightly towards the right side of the woman, to compensate for the dextro-rotation of the uterus. The section should clearly demonstrate the uterine fundus. If the uterine fundus cannot be adequately seen because the bladder is insufficiently filled, the examination should be postponed until this situation is rectified.

The ultrasound appearances of the uterus obtained transabdominally are comparable to those obtained transvaginally (see Fig. 3.2). The cervical canal can be difficult to define in non-pregnant women because of the angle at which it lies relative to the sound beam. This remains a problem irrespective of whether the uterus is anteverted or retroverted. The position of the internal os can be gauged as it lies directly beneath the point at which the posterior wall of the bladder appears to change direction (see Fig. 3.1). This change in direction occurs because the lower part of the bladder (the trigone) is fixed to the cervix and cannot change position as the bladder fills. The external os is not seen transabdominally.

Cross-sectional views of the uterus are obtained by rotating the probe through 90° while keeping the cavity line in view. Sliding the probe up and down the abdomen will produce transverse sections of the uterus from fundus to cervix. Oblique sections of the uterus, rather than transverse sections, will be obtained if the angle of the probe on the woman's abdomen is not at 90° to the longitudinal axis of the uterus or is altered during the examination.

Problems

- The fundus of the uterus will not be visualized unless the bladder is filled sufficiently to cover it.
- A retroverted uterus occurs in about one-third of women and is more common after pregnancy. The uterine fundus and the upper part of the uterine body might not be visualized in this situation because it is impossible to direct the ultrasound beam at right angles to them. Further filling of the bladder is of little help except to displace the bowel that lies between the bladder

and the uterus. If transvaginal scanning is not an option then little can be done in this situation, except to review the findings at a later date. In such situations clinical management must be decided without the benefit of an ultrasound examination.

THE GESTATION SAC

Demonstration of a gestation sac within the uterus is the earliest ultrasonic confirmation of an intrauterine pregnancy. Thickening of the endometrium might be recognized prior to this but cannot be taken as diagnostic of pregnancy. Thickening of the endometrium can be seen in the following situations:

- the late luteal phase of the menstrual cycle
- in a very early intrauterine pregnancy, i.e. before the gestation sac can be resolved
- as a decidual reaction in association with ectopic pregnancy.

In addition, thickening of the endometrium can be confused with retained products of conception within the uterine cavity.

The gestation sac is the first pregnancy structure that can be detected by ultrasound. It is usually visualized from 31 days or 4^{+3} weeks of gestation using the transvaginal method, when it measures 2–3 mm in diameter (Fig. 3.4). It can be identified

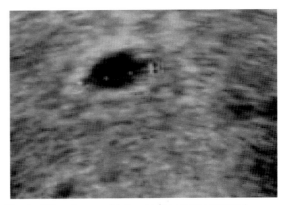

Figure 3.4 A normal intrauterine pregnancy at 4 weeks' gestation imaged using the transvaginal method. The gestational sac measures 3 mm. The yolk sac and embryo are visible at this early stage. Note the echogenic appearance and the thickness of the wall of the sac.

about a week later, i.e. 5⁺³ weeks of gestation, using the abdominal route (Fig. 3.5). The early gestation sac appears as a circular transonic area surrounded by a thick bright ring. It usually lies at the uterine fundus and is eccentrically placed. The ring and the eccentric position of the gestation sac are important markers for confirming an intra-uterine pregnancy. The shape of the sac can be distorted by uterine contractions, fibroids, a full bladder when scanning transabdominally or the pressure of the transvaginal probe. The gestation sac grows approximately 1 mm in diameter per day. The normal sac loses its circular shape and becomes more elliptical when its diameter exceeds 1 cm.

The thick, bright ring of the early gestation sac corresponds to a rim of invading chorionic villi and the underlying decidual reaction. The circular tran-

sonic area of the gestation sac corresponds to two separate fluid-filled compartments, the inner amni-otic cavity and the outer chorionic (or exocelomic) cavity (Table 3.2). In very early pregnancy the chori-onic cavity predominates. From 8 weeks, the amni-otic cavity expands rapidly within the chorionic cavity such that it soon occupies most of the gestation sac volume. By the end of the first trimester the amniotic and chorionic membranes become fused, resulting in complete obliteration of the chorionic cavity.

Normal ranges for gestation sac and amniotic sac sizes in early pregnancy have been recently established (Figs 3.6 and 3.7). An abnormally large amniotic cavity in early pregnancy might indicate embryonic death, whereas oligohydramnios in early pregnancy is often associated with fetal mal-formations.

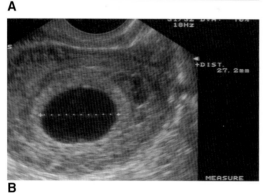

A

B

Figure 3.5   A. Longitudinal section of the uterus demonstrating the maximum longitudinal diameter (L) of the gestation sac. B. Transverse section of the uterus demonstrating the maximum transverse (T) diameter of the gestation sac. Note that the AP diameter is common to both views. The mean gestation sac volume is equivalent to a gestational age of 5 weeks 4 days. Note the echogenic appearance and the thickness of the wall of the sac.

FINDING THE GESTATION SAC

Transvaginal method

First, a true longitudinal (sagittal) view of the uterus should be obtained. If the gestation sac is not immediately visible, pan the transducer gently from side to side until the whole of the uterus has been examined and the maximum length of the gestation sac is displayed. Freeze the image and measure the maximum longitudinal diameter (L) together with the maximum anteroposterior diameter (AP) (Fig. 3.8; Table 3.2).

Rotate the transducer through 90° (keeping the gestation sac in view) to obtain a cross-section of the sac. It is important to appreciate that this might not be equivalent to the transverse section obtained by means of the abdominal method. Pan the probe across the width of the vagina until the gestation sac is visualized and then rock the handle of the probe until the maximum diameter of the sac is obtained in this plane. Freeze the image and measure the maximum transverse diameter (T) (Fig. 3.9). It is also good practice to measure the longitudinal diameter, and this should correspond to that measured in the longitudinal (sagittal) sec-tion (see Fig. 3.8).

If the uterus is very anteflexed or retroverted it might not be possible to rock the transducer suffi-ciently to obtain a true transverse section of the gestation sac (Fig. 3.10). If this is not appreciated,

Table 3.2 Diagrammatic representation of landmarks of early pregnancy, and their measurement

Gestational (chorionic) sac – Measurements should be performed from the inner edges of trophoblast in three planes. The diameters measured correspond to those of the chorionic cavity. The maximum and mean diameters should be recorded. The volume may also be calculated using formula for ellipsoid $V = A \times B \times C \times 0.523$.	
Amniotic sac – The three perpendicular diameters should be measured and the mean diameter calculated. As the amnion is very thin the measurements should be taken from the centre of the membrane.	
Yolk sac – Three diameters are measured from the outer wall of the yolk sac.	
Crown-rump length – In early pregnancy this is the greatest length of the embryo as the crown and rump cannot be distinguished. From 7 weeks onwards the measurement should be taken in the sagittal section, with care taken not to include the yolk sac.	

Heart rate – in the first trimester the measurement of heart rate should be performed using turnover M-mode. The heart rate increases rapidly from six to eight weeks and then remains relatively stable afterwards

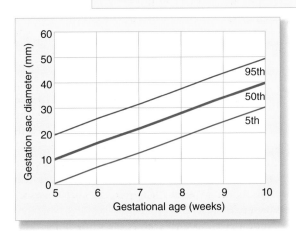

Figure 3.6 Fitted 5th, 50th and 95th centiles of the mean diameter of the gestation sac by gestational age (from Grisolia et al 1993).

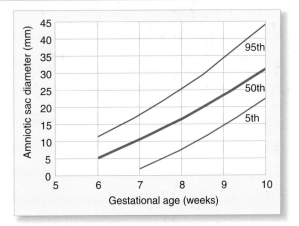

Figure 3.7 Fitted 5th, 50th and 95th centiles of the mean diameter of the amniotic sac by gestational age (from Grisolia et al 1993).

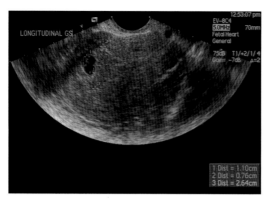

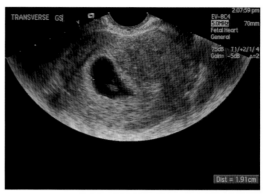

Figure 3.8 Longitudinal section of the uterus with the cursors demonstrating the maximum longitudinal (2...2) and maximum anteroposterior (1...1) diameters of the gestation sac using the transvaginal method.

Figure 3.9 Transverse section of the uterus with the cursors demonstrating the maximum transverse (+...+) diameter of the gestation sac using the transvaginal method.

measurements of the transverse diameter taken from this oblique view will be an overestimate. This is important if it is necessary to estimate gestational age from the mean sac diameter or when serial measurements of gestation sac size are being used to determine whether the pregnancy is ongoing.

Estimation of gestational age from mean sac diameter

This measurement should only be used to date the early pregnancy before the embryo is visible, i.e. between 4+ and 6+ weeks of gestation. Mean sac diameter is calculated from the following:

$$\text{Mean sac diameter (cm)} = [\text{L (cm)} + \text{AP (cm)} + \text{T (cm)}]/3$$

Mean sac diameter is used to estimate gestational age by reference to Table 3.3.

Abdominal method

The bladder must be sufficiently full to cover the uterine fundus when attempting to visualize and measure a gestation sac abdominally. Locate the longitudinal axis of the uterus as described previously. The gestation sac should be visualized towards the uterine fundus (see Fig. 3.5A). By sliding the probe and/or rotating slightly to either side, the maximum longitudinal axis (L) of the sac will be obtained.

Rotate the transducer through 90°. If the sac has now disappeared, slide the probe either up or down the abdomen until you find it again. Obtain the section demonstrating the maximum transverse diameter (T) of the sac. Remember to maintain the correct angle of the probe to the maternal abdomen. Freeze the image and measure the maximum transverse diameter (T) of the sac. The maximum anteroposterior diameter (AP) can be measured from either the longitudinal or transverse section because it is common to both views (see Fig. 3.5B).

Estimation of gestational age from gestation sac volume

This measurement should only be used to date the early pregnancy before the embryo is visible, i.e. between 4+ and 6+ weeks of gestation. Gestation sac volume is calculated from the following:

$$\text{Volume of a sphere (ml)} = 4/3\ \pi r^3$$
$$= 0.5233 \times d_1 \times d_2 \times d_3$$

$$\text{Gestation sac volume (ml)} = \text{L(cm)} \times \text{T(cm)} \times \text{AP(cm)} \times 0.5233$$

Gestation sac volume is used to estimate gestational age by reference to Table 3.4.

As gestation advances, the gestation sac becomes less spherical in shape making gestational age estimates using it less reliable. Once the embryo can be identified within the gestation sac, a crown–rump

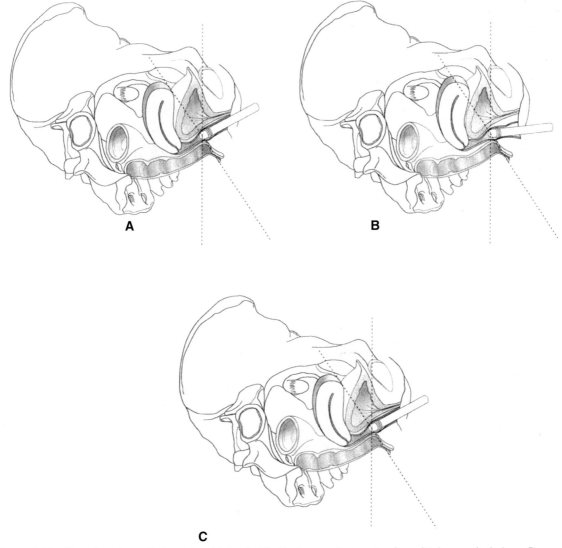

Figure 3.10   Scanning planes that can be obtained with the transvaginal probe. A. sagittal or vertical plane; B. coronal or horizontal plane; C. with a very anteverted uterus the perineum prevents downward depression of the probe, thus an oblique plane of the pelvis is obtained.

length measurement should always be taken in preference to sac measurements.

Uses of gestation sac measurements

- Confirmation of an intrauterine pregnancy.
- Calculation of gestational age before the embryo is visible.
- Diagnosis of miscarriage.

ON-GOING PREGNANCY

The pregnancy can only be said to be ongoing when cardiac pulsations from the embryo can be demonstrated within the gestation sac. Care should be taken when confirming cardiac activity in the very early stages of pregnancy because movement caused by the maternal pulse can be falsely identified as pulsations from the embryo's heart.

Table 3.3 Mean gestation sac diameter* as an estimate of gestational age by transvaginal sonography. After Grisolia et al (1993).

Gestational age (weeks)	5th centile	50th centile	95th centile
5	–	10	20
6	6	16	26
7	13	23	33
8	19	29	39
9	25	35	45
10	30	40	50

*The mean sac diameter was obtained by averaging three perpendicular diameters, one of which was the maximum diameter using the technique described by Levi et al (1988).

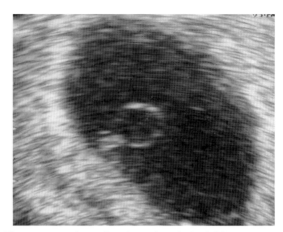

Figure 3.11 A small embryonic pole is visible adjacent to the yolk sac at 6 weeks' gestation imaged using the transvaginal method.

Table 3.4 Gestation sac volume by transabdominal sonography. After Robinson (1975).

Gestational age (days)	Mean gestation sac volume (ml)		
	Mean	+2SD	–2SD
35–37	0.2	1.1	0.04
38–40	0.5	1.1	0.2
41–43	1.0	1.7	0.5
44–46	1.8	6.5	0.5
47–49	2.3	6.6	0.8
50–52	4.5	13.2	1.5
53–55	5.9	18.6	1.9
56–58	11.2	23.4	3.8
59–61	12.0	29.5	4.9
62–64	17.8	38.0	8.3
65–67	22.4	51.3	9.8
68–70	29.5	51.3	17.0

THE EMBRYO

Embryologically, the period from conception to the end of the ninth postmenstrual week is known as the 'embryonic period'. The remaining 30 weeks of pregnancy comprise the 'fetal period'. Before 10 weeks, therefore, the correct terminology for the conceptus is 'embryo' and after 10 weeks is 'fetus'. In clinical medicine, however, the term 'fetus' is frequently used, incorrectly, throughout pregnancy.

The embryo can be visualized from about 37 days using the transvaginal route and is first seen as a bright linear echo, adjacent to the yolk sac and close to the connecting stalk (Fig. 3.11; Table 3.5). At this stage, the crown–rump length (CRL) measures around 2 mm. Cardiac activity can be identified. When the embryo reaches 5 mm in length, equivalent to 6^{+3} weeks' gestation and a mean sac diameter of 15–20 mm, it can be consistently seen separate from the yolk sac. The embryo grows at around 1 mm per day.

All embryos of CRL ≥ 7 mm in length should demonstrate visible cardiac activity. Once an embryo with visible heart action is seen, the pregnancy is unlikely to end in miscarriage. For example, in asymptomatic women with an empty sac identified with ultrasound the risk of miscarriage is approximately 12%; the risk of miscarriage decreases to 7% when a live embryo of CRL ≤ 5 mm is seen; the risk decreases further, to 1%, with a live embryo of CRL > 10 mm. Normal ranges for fetal heart rate in pregnancy have been described showing a rapid increase of the mean heart rate between 6 and 9 weeks followed by a slight decline after 10 weeks (Fig. 3.12). It has been shown that a late onset of cardiac activity and a decreased heart rate in the first trimester are associated with a higher rate of spontaneous abortion.

Rapid changes can be observed in the appearance of the embryo after 7 weeks (see Table 3.5).

Table 3.5   Ultrasound in early pregnancy – landmarks for diagnosis

4^{+3} to 5^{+0}	A small gestation sac (2–5 mm) is seen within the endometrium. The sac is spherical, regular in outline and eccentrically situated towards the fundus. It is implanted just below the surface of the endometrium (midline echo) and is surrounded by echogenic trophoblast. In symptomatic women the scan should be repeated in one week when the yolk sac should be visible.
5^{+1} to 5^{+5}	The yolk sac becomes visible within the chorionic cavity. This should be seen in all pregnancies with a mean gestation sac diameter of > 12 mm. If it is not, the diagnosis of anembryonic pregnancy is almost certain. The scan should be repeated in one week to confirm this.
5^{+2} to 6^{+0}	The embryonic pole is visible and measures 2–4 mm in length. Heart action is also detectable. An embryo is usually visible with a mean gestation sac diameter of > 18 mm. If this is not the case then the pregnancy is likely to be abnormal and the scan should be repeated in one week.
6^{+1} to 6^{+6}	The embryo changes from being a straight line at the top of the yolk sac to being kidney-bean-shaped, with the yolk sac separated from the embryo by the vitelline duct. The crown–rump length measures 4 to 10 mm. If the heart rate is not detectable the diagnosis of missed miscarriage is almost certain.
7^{+0} to 7^{+6}	The crown–rump length measures 11 to 16 mm. The rhombencephalon becomes distinguishable as a diamond-shaped cavity, enabling distinction of the cephalad and caudal poles of the embryo. The spine is seen as double echogenic parallel lines. The amniotic membrane becomes visible defining the amniotic cavity from the chorionic cavity. The umbilical cord can also be seen.
8^{+0} to 8^{+6}	Crown–rump length 17–23 mm. Forebrain, midbrain, hindbrain and skull are distinguishable. Limb buds are also visible. Midgut hernia is present. The amniotic cavity expands and the umbilical cord and vitteline duct lengthens.
9^{+0} to 10^{+0}	Crown–rump length 23–32 mm. The limbs lengthen and hands and feet are seen. Embryonic heart rate peaks at 170–180 bpm.

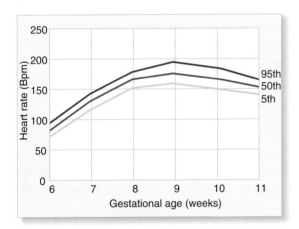

Figure 3.12   Embryonic heart rate in normal pregnancies related to gestational age (5th, 50th and 95th centiles).

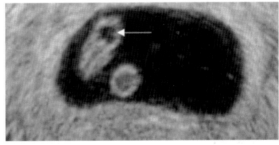

Figure 3.13   A transverse section through the embryonic head at 7 weeks shows a large rhombencephalon (arrow), which is a dominant intracranial structure at this gestation using the transvaginal method.

When it reaches a CRL of 12 mm, equivalent to 7^{+3} weeks, the head can be discriminated from the torso. The differentiation of the nervous system is the dominant phenomenon in the early development of the embryo. Before 7 weeks only the rhomben-cephalic cavity is recognizable using transvaginal ultrasound (Fig. 3.13). The other intracranial structures visible from 7 weeks onwards are the diencephalon with its cavity, the third ventricle, the hemispheres with their cavity, the lateral ventricles and the mesencephalon with the aqueduct of Sylvius. These structures can be routinely visualized using transvaginal ultrasound in all normal pregnancies from 9 weeks.

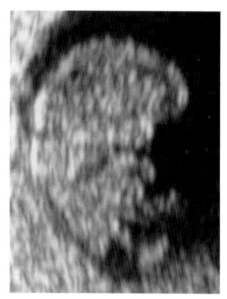

Figure 3.14 A longitudinal section through a 9-week embryo showing well developed limb buds using the transvaginal method.

In a dorsal coronal section of the embryo the spinal canal can be seen as two parallel lines. From 8 weeks, the upper and lower limb buds can be seen more clearly (Fig. 3.14). Prolonged observation will detect the earliest embryonic movements at this time. The site of the definitive placenta is distinguishable and the umbilical cord can be traced to both its placental and embryonic attachments (Fig. 3.15). From about 9 weeks the anterior and posterior contours of the embryo can be evaluated and slight deviations from normal shape, such as nuchal thickening, become apparent.

During its development, the midgut rotates and grows to such an extent so that it can no longer be contained in the abdominal cavity. Room is temporarily found within the umbilical cord, thus forming a physiologic hernia of the midgut. This is visible between 8–10 weeks as a widening of the visibly pulsating umbilical cord close to its abdominal insertion. By 10 weeks the capacity of the abdomen has increased substantially, thus allowing the intestines to begin to return back. Detection or exclusion of abdominal wall defects should therefore not be attempted until after 11 weeks.

THE YOLK SAC

The yolk sac appears as a circular transonic mass within the gestation sac and can first be identified transvaginally at about 35 days, when it measures 3–4 mm in diameter (Fig. 3.16; see Table 3.2). At this stage it is significantly larger than the embryo. It is a prominent landmark to search for within the early gestation sac and, because of its close association with the embryo at this stage, identifying it will automatically lead to the embryo. Care must be taken to ensure that it is not included in the measurement of the crown–rump length. This becomes less likely with the progressive elongation of the yolk stalk with increasing gestation.

The yolk sac grows slowly until it reaches a maximum diameter of 6 mm at 10 weeks (Fig. 3.17). The yolk sac floats freely in the chorionic cavity

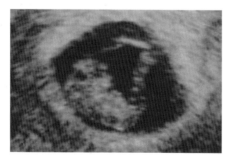

Figure 3.15 A longitudinal section through a 9-week embryo demonstrating the whole length of the umbilical cord including both abdominal and placental insertions using the transvaginal method.

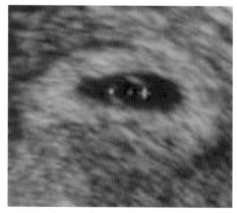

Figure 3.16 A 5-week gestation sac with a clearly visible yolk sac imaged using the transvaginal method. The yolk sac wall appears thin and well defined at this gestation.

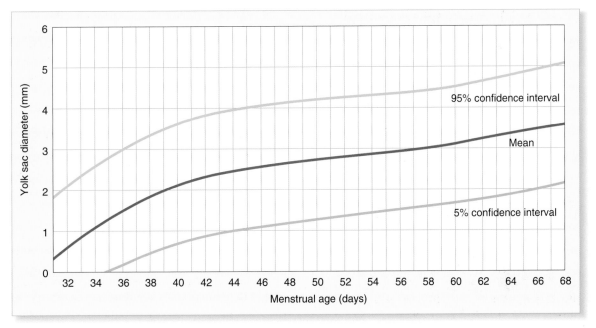

Figure 3.17 Average yolk sac size compared with menstrual age with 95% confidence intervals (Lindsay et al 1992).

until the increasing size of the amniotic sac compresses it against the wall of the chorionic cavity. This factor makes identification of the yolk sac difficult after about 12 weeks.

Correlation between yolk sac morphology and the outcome of pregnancy is not clear. Some studies suggest that the absence of the yolk sac before 8 weeks indicates an abnormal pregnancy even when the embryo is alive. Miscarriage is apparently common in this situation. Furthermore, in cases of missed abortion with a visible embryo, the yolk sac tends to be larger and its wall is thinner than in normal pregnancies. However, other studies have not show any significant correlation between size and shape of the yolk sac and pregnancy outcome.

MEASUREMENT OF CROWN–RUMP LENGTH

Fetal growth can be monitored accurately later in pregnancy only if the exact information about gestational age is available. As less than 50% of women are certain about their menstrual dates, this calculation is not always accurate and every effort should be made to estimate fetal age early in pregnancy when biological variability is minimal.

As soon as the embryo can be seen the gestational age can be estimated by measuring the crown–rump length. Through the advances in in vitro fertilization programs it is now possible to study fetal growth without the uncertainties caused by the irregularities of the menstrual cycle. The biological variability of the crown–rump length is small and growth is very rapid. However, there are still a number of factors that can affect the size of an early embryo, such as measurement errors, differences in growth rates between individuals, fetal sex and maternal conditions such as diabetes mellitus. It has also been shown that the conventional curves constructed using optimal menstrual history tend to underestimate the gestational age by 2–3 days compared to the reference ranges constructed with a known date of conception. A discrepancy between certain menstrual dates and crown–rump length might indicate an early intrauterine growth restriction. The risk of miscarriage is reported to be significantly increased in these cases. In addition, those pregnancies that progress beyond the second trimester are likely to be complicated by preterm labour and intrauterine growth restriction (IUGR).

A correctly performed measurement of CRL is the most accurate means of estimating the gestational age. An optimal CRL image, accurately measured, is thus more accurate than the biparietal diameter in dating a pregnancy. However, accurate crown–rump measurements can be the most difficult measurements to obtain during pregnancy. The ability correctly to establish gestational age by this method depends solely on the operator obtaining a true, unflexed, longitudinal section of the embryo or fetus, with the end-points of the crown and rump clearly defined, and then placing the callipers correctly on these defined end-points. Appreciation of the optimal CRL and correct calliper placement only come with experience. Departmental audit should be employed to evaluate the correlation of gestational age assessment between first and second trimester biometry techniques.

Owing to fetal movement, there can be no standardized technique for obtaining a CRL. First, find a longitudinal section of the uterus and gestation sac. Slide (if scanning abdominally) or pan (if scanning transvaginally) the probe slowly to each side until pulsations from the fetal heart can be seen. Slowly rotate the probe, keeping these pulsations in view, until the long axis of the fetus is obtained. Freeze this image. Measurements are taken from the top of the head (crown) to the end of the trunk (rump) using the onscreen calipers (Fig. 3.18; Appendix 1).

The very early embryo is unflexed. There are two main reasons why CRL measurements taken between 5 and 7 weeks are inaccurate:

1. The full length of the embryo has not been obtained – this will produce an underestimated CRL (Fig. 3.19A).
2. The end-points of the embryo have not been clearly identified as separate from the closely adjacent yolk sac or the wall of the gestation sac and one or both have been included in the measurement – this will produce an overestimated CRL (Fig. 3.19B).

Although it becomes much easier to identify the end-points of the embryo after 7 weeks, it remains just as important to ensure that you are imaging the maximum length of the embryo before taking your measurements. To confirm this, continue to pan, rock or rotate the probe past your intended optimal section. If the selected section is optimal then the subsequent CRLs should reduce in size. Return to the original section, freeze the image and measure the optimal CRL. The CRL should be measured from three different images and the measurements should agree to within 3 mm in the embryo and 5 mm in the fetus.

Once the fetal spine can be easily identified, i.e. from about 9 weeks, this should be used as a guide in assessing true fetal length. The aim is to examine the fetus with the full length of its spine positioned directly anteriorly or posteriorly, thereby enabling you to assess any degree of flexion.

Problems

Any degree of flexion of the fetal spine will produce an underestimate of the CRL when linear calipers are used (Fig. 3.19C). Should the fetal spine be lateral, the degree of flexion can be difficult to estimate. When scanning transabdominally, alteration of the angle of the probe relative to the maternal abdomen might bring the spine into a more anterior, or posterior, position, thus making accurate measurement possible. When the fetus remains obstinately curled, you have four choices:

1. Sit and wait.
2. Measure the flexed length using onscreen nonlinear measuring facilities (Fig. 3.20A).

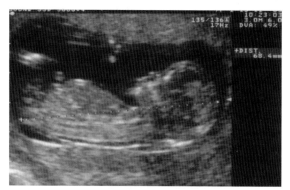

Figure 3.18 The longitudinal axis of the fetus using the transabdominal method. The calipers demonstrate measurement of the crown–rump length.

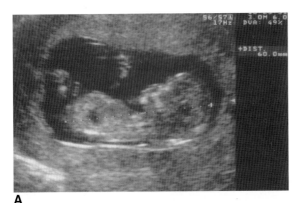

A

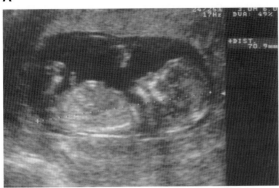

B

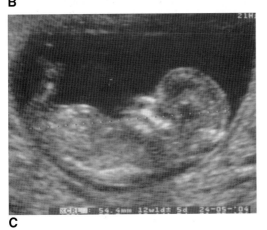

C

Figure 3.19 A. Underestimation of the crown–rump length because the full length of the embryo has not been obtained. B. Overestimation of the crown–rump length because the end-points of the embryo have not been clearly identified. C. Underestimation of the crown–rump length because the fetal spine is flexed and the 'measurement' has been made using the linear calipers.

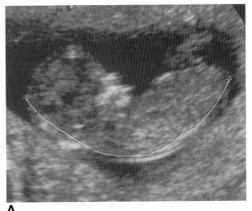

A

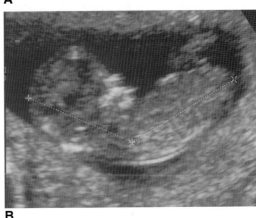

B

Figure 3.20 A. Measurement of the crown–rump length using non-linear calipers along the full length of the flexed fetus. (B) Measurement of the crown–rump length is made by measuring the linear parts of the fetus separately (crown to shoulder, shoulder to rump) and adding the results together.

3. Use the linear calipers to measure the parts of the fetal length that are in straight sections, and then add them together (Fig. 3.20B).
4. Underestimate the CRL by using the linear calipers along the flexed length (see Fig. 3.19C). *This is not to be recommended under any circumstances.*

The accuracy of methods 2 and 3 will depend on your perception of the degree of flexion of the fetus. In theory, method 2 should be the most accurate. However, the caliper system is often very sensitive or obstinate (or both) and you will tend to overestimate the true measurement. Method 3 horrifies all purists (usually quite rightly) but is actually often a better, although less scientific, compromise.

When you have gained sufficient experience compare the three active alternatives on the same fetus. It is a salutary experience to discover how easy it is to produce errors of 10–15 mm simply by measuring a 12–13 week fetus incorrectly.

With increasing gestational age, the fetus is more likely to be found in a flexed position. After 12 weeks this generally makes assessment of the gestational age by CRL inaccurate because inaccuracies of 7–10 days can easily be obtained. At this stage of gestation, measurement of the biparietal diameter and femur can be made. We would recommend that dating the pregnancy is delayed until after 15 weeks, when the biometric data for these two parameters are more reliable.

Transvaginal method

The above problems of flexion are just as relevant using this method. The lack of maneuverability of the probe within the vagina is a major problem when the fetal spine is not optimally placed. The CRL can be measured providing the full length of the fetus can be visualized on the screen. With the transvaginal route this frequently becomes difficult after 13 weeks.

Estimation of gestational age from crown–rump length

The transvaginal route is the method of choice for assessing gestational age by CRL until 9–10 weeks of gestation. After that time the transabdominal route is the preferred method for the reasons stated above.

The CRL measurement can be used to assign a gestational age where the menstrual history is unknown or unreliable or to confirm the post-menstrual age where a reliable menstrual history is known:

- A dating chart should be used to assign the gestational age (see Appendix 2) and the EDD calculated appropriately.
- Where a reliable menstrual history is available, the CRL measurement should be compared to its normal range for the known gestational age. If the

value lies within the normal range then the woman's menstrual dates and the EDD as calculated from those dates are accepted. If the value is outside the normal range the reliability of the menstrual history should be discussed with the woman.

There is now good evidence that dating by ultrasound is more accurate than even a reliable menstrual history in the majority of cases. We therefore recommend that, in cases where the conception date is unknown, the pregnancy should be redated using the CRL measurement, and the EDD should be recalculated, from the ultrasound-assigned gestational age. However, it should be remembered that it is not possible to distinguish between very early growth restriction and incorrect dates. As noted above, the former can be associated with problems later in pregnancy and also with chromosomal abnormalities. Care should therefore be taken if a pregnancy is to be redated in the presence of a reliable menstrual history.

Pregnancies with a reliable menstrual history but that are redated from the CRL should be reviewed in a further 3–4 weeks to confirm normal growth velocity of the embryo or fetus.

Estimation of gestational age in twin pregnancy

The CRL of both fetuses should be measured. The larger CRL should be used for assigning or confirming gestational age as described for the singleton pregnancy. A gestational age equivalent difference between the fetuses of more than one week in the first trimester should be noted and monitored with serial ultrasound scans. Although the discrepancy is often due to constitutional differences, early onset IUGR, structural and/or karyotypic abnormality need to be excluded.

NUCHAL TRANSLUCENCY SCREENING BETWEEN 11 AND 14 WEEKS

This test has arisen from the observation that fetuses with chromosomal abnormalities, and principally trisomy 21, demonstrate an increased collection of subcutaneous fluid or nuchal translucency (NT) behind the neck between 11 and 14 weeks of gestation. Increased NT has also been described in association with a range of structural abnormalities, genetic conditions and cardiac abnormalities. Measuring NT enables a more sensitive estimation of the risk of trisomy 21 than that derived from the maternal age to be made. Risk can be evaluated using a simple numerical cut-off, a numerical cut-off related to gestational age or a computer program that provides an 'adjusted risk' based on the combination of the maternal age related risk, CRL and NT.

Measuring nuchal translucency

Obtain a midsagittal section of the fetus demonstrating the profile anteriorly and the spine posteriorly. The fetal neck should be neither flexed or extended. The strong linear echo from the nuchal skin will be seen and this must be distinguishable from the similar echo pattern obtained from the amnion. If it is not possible to distinguish one from the other you must wait until the fetus moves away from the amnion before freezing the image for measurement (Fig. 3.21). As such fetal movements tend to be both rapid and short lived, employing the cine-loop facility will make capturing the optimal section much easier. The image selected for measurement should be large enough that the fetal head and upper thorax only occupy the screen. Employing the read zoom facility, if available, to

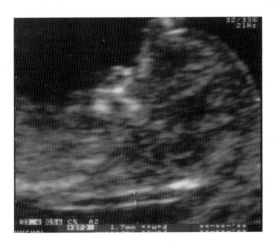

Figure 3.21 Measurement of the nuchal translucency obtained using the transabdominal method. Note the section of the fetus is midsagittal and the fetal neck is neither flexed or extended. The nuchal skin echo can be readily distinguished from the amnion.

the frozen image is helpful. The intersection of the two arms of the callipers are placed on the outer border of the cervical spine and the inner border of the skin lying directly posterior to it respectively, to produce a measurement of the transonic or echo-poor nuchal fluid only. This procedure should be repeated twice more, each from a different image. The largest of the three measurements should be taken to evaluate the adjusted risk.

MULTIPLE PREGNANCY

Zygosity

Twins arise from the ovulation and fertilization of two eggs (dizygotic twins) or a single egg (monozygotic twins). The fertilized egg is termed the zygote. All dyzygotic twin pairs have separate placentas and therefore separate chorionic sacs and separate amniotic sacs. They are always 'diamniotic dichorionic' twins. The single egg of the monozygotic twins can divide into two individuals at different stages resulting in three types of monozygotic twins:

- Dichorionic diamniotic (DCDA) – as in dyzygotic twins but will be of the same sex. Approximately one-third of monozygotic twins are DCDA.
- Monochorionic diamniotic (MCDA) – one placenta, therefore one chorionic cavity. Each twin develops in its own amniotic cavity. Approximately two-thirds of monozygotic twins are MCDA.
- Monochorionic monoamniotic (MCMA) – one placenta, therefore one chorionic cavity. Both twins develop in the same amniotic cavity. Less than 1% of monozygotic twins are MCMA.

All dyzygotic twins are dichorionic. However not all (approximately 60%) monozygotic twins are monochorionic. Dyzygotic twins can be the same sex or different sex; monozygotic twins will be the same sex.

Chorionicity and amnionicity

The assessment of chorionicity and amnionicity is important because monochorionic twin pregnancies are at high risk of developing various pregnancy complications. Later in pregnancy the assessment of chorionicity is much more difficult, thus emphasizing the importance of achieving a correct diagnosis in the first trimester.

Monochorionic diamniotic twin pregnancies carry a 25% risk of twin–twin transfusion syndrome (TTTS) and therefore require more careful antenatal surveillance than dichorionic twin pregnancies, which do not have this risk. Monochorionic monoamniotic twins are not at increased risk of TTTS but have a high risk of cord accidents due to cord entanglement and premature delivery due to severe polyhydramnios. These factors result in a very high fetal loss rate, of 50–75%, in monochorionic monoamniotic twins.

The prevalence of fetal structural defects and IUGR are also increased in twins, particularly in monozygotic pregnancies.

Ultrasound labeling of twins

To ensure consistency of fetal assessment throughout pregnancy it is important that each twin can be correctly identified. The position of the two gestation sacs relative to the cervix remains unchanged with gestation and for this reason we recommend the following method of labeling – the twin in the sac closer to the cervix should be identified as Twin 1 and the twin in the sac further from the cervix as Twin 2. This notation should be strictly applied from the very beginning of pregnancy.

The position of each fetus will change many times during pregnancy, thus attempting to identify each twin by presentation (e.g. cephalic, breech) is fruitless. Identifying each fetus by the position of its placenta (e.g. anterior, posterior, fundal) is of value in a dichorionic pregnancy where the implantation sites of the two placentas can be identified separately but of no value in monochorionic gestations. The relative position of the twins (e.g. left, right or top, bottom) is useful in the majority of cases and we recommend this is recorded as confirmation that the correct labeling has been applied.

It should be noted that none of these parameters can be applied to monoamniotic twins, which are the same gender, share a single placenta and develop within the same sac. Monoamniotic twins can only be distinguished if they demonstrate

differential growth rates or are discordant for a structural abnormality.

A potential discrepancy exists between the pre- and postnatal labeling of twins. The postnatal labeling of the twins relates to the time of their deliveries, the first baby delivered is referred to as Twin 1 and the second as Twin 2.

Ultrasound assessment of multiple pregnancy

The incidence of multiple pregnancy has increased significantly in recent years, primarily due to the widespread use of stimulation of ovulation and other techniques of assisted conception. Ultrasound examination of multiple pregnancy in the first trimester should provide information about the number of fetuses and chorionicity of pregnancy. Multiple gestation sacs can be identified as early as singleton sacs, i.e. from 4+ weeks transvaginally and from 5+ weeks transabdominally. However, the presence of a gestation sac does not indicate an ongoing pregnancy, but merely confirms an intrauterine pregnancy. Unfortunately, not all live twin pregnancies confirmed in the first trimester will go on to deliver twin infants, as the conception rate is approximately double that of the twin delivery rate and the overall loss rate of one embryo or fetus in the first trimester is approximately 30%. These points are important to remember when discussing early ultrasound findings with the parents.

The presence of two separate gestation sacs before 6 weeks is compatible with the diagnosis of a dichorionic pregnancy, which can be either dizygotic or monozygotic. However, both (or any) of the sacs might contain more than one embryo and therefore the number of sacs should not be used as a conclusive indication of the number of future embryos. In addition, apparently empty sacs in a multiple pregnancy might regress spontaneously before the embryo develops. This 'vanishing twin' phenomenon has been reported to affect up to 20% of multiple pregnancies. Although this figure might be an overestimate, the presence of this phenomenon further supports delaying the diagnosis of multiple pregnancy until live embryos can be identified.

After 7 weeks, the presence of more than one embryo within a single gestation sac enables the

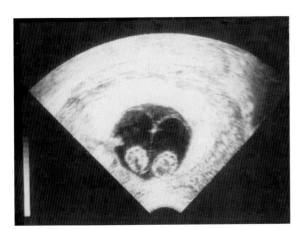

Figure 3.22 A case of twins at 8 weeks imaged transvaginally. Note the single chorionic cavity, which contains two amniotic cavities, confirming this is a case of monochorionic diamniotic twins.

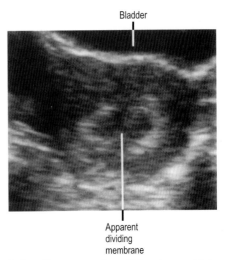

Bladder

Apparent
dividing
membrane

Figure 3.23 Transverse view of the uterus obtained abdominally, demonstrating the lateral artefact that mimics twin gestation sacs.

conclusive diagnosis of a monozygotic monochorionic multiple pregnancy. However, the complete assessment of monochorionic pregnancy includes amnionicity, which cannot be established before 8 weeks (Fig. 3.22). At this time, the amount of amniotic fluid increases and the amniotic membrane separates from the fetus, facilitating its visualization by ultrasound (Table 3.6).

Having diagnosed a twin pregnancy, always make sure you have not missed an elusive triplet. The woman's confidence tends to falter if another fetus is discovered at every ultrasound examination. She will rarely return for a fourth appointment!

Problems

Not all cystic areas within the uterus are gestation sacs and it is important to distinguish between the following:

- A genuine multiple gestation (Fig. 3.22).
- Twin sacs due to artifact (Fig. 3.23). Known as a lateral artifact, this is particularly likely to occur if a linear array probe is used transabdominally in early pregnancy. It is readily recognized because the two apparent sacs are only seen in transverse section.
- An implantation bleed accompanying a singleton pregnancy (Fig. 3.24). The gestation sac does not completely fill the cavity of the uterus until approximately 10 weeks gestation and therefore a space can be visualized between the sac and the cavity line. This space follows the contours of the cavity and does not have the echogenic ring characteristic of the gestation sac.
- A kidney-shaped gestation sac will produce the appearance of twin sacs when viewed in certain sections. If this is a single sac then the two 'sacs' must join up at some point. Careful scanning of the sac(s) in several planes perpendicular to each other will determine if this is truly a multiple gestation.

Table 3.6 Diagnosis of chorionicity and amnionicity in early twin pregnancy

Gestational age (weeks)	Dichorionic diamniotic		Monochorionic diamniotic	Monochorionic monoamniotic
5	○	○	○	○
6	◐	◐	◖◗	◖◗
7	◉	◉	◉◉	◉◉

○ = gestation sac   ◐ = amniotic sac   ▮ = embryo

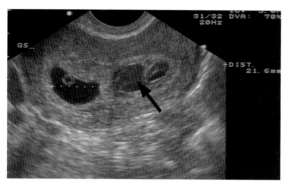

Figure 3.24 Implantation bleed (arrow) associated with a singleton pregnancy obtained using the transabdominal method and mimicking a twin gestation.

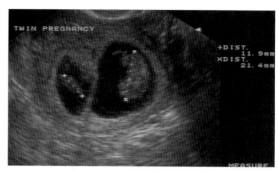

Figure 3.25 A dichorionic twin pregnancy demonstrating one sac containing a live fetus (CRL 21.4mm) and a dead twin (CRL 11.9mm) in the second sac.

After 8 weeks a genuine twin gestation will usually demonstrate fetuses in separate sacs. The sacs are generally adjacent but of differing shape and the fetuses will generally lie in different planes and move independently. Rare exceptions are:

- Monoamniotic twins – both fetuses lie within a single amniotic sac and there is no dividing membrane between them.
- Conjoined twins – both individuals move together, being partially fused. These are also obviously monoamniotic.

As discussed above, multiple sacs will not always contain live fetuses. Identifying a live singleton pregnancy together with an empty second sac, or dead second twin, is therefore common (Fig. 3.25), especially if there has been some vaginal bleeding. Reassurance to the woman as to the live fetus is obviously important but further explanation of the original twin conception must depend upon the individual situation.

ESTABLISHING CHORIONICITY AND AMNIONICITY

The object of this exercise is to distinguish between dichorionic and monochorionic twin pregnancies. As discussed above, the identification of a monochorionic pregnancy is of clinical significance. It should be performed in the first trimester, after 8 weeks. The optimal time to distinguish between dichorionic, monochorionic and monoam-

niotic twin pairs using ultrasound is between 10 and 14 weeks of gestation.

The presence of two separate sacs each with its own placenta is diagnostic of a dichorionic twin pregnancy.

The presence of an apparently single placenta can indicate either a dichorionic pregnancy with adjacent implantation of the two placentas or a monochorionic pregnancy with a single placenta. In such a situation chorionicity should be established. Locate the insertion of the chorional membranes into the placenta, not the uterine insertion. A dichorional placenta will demonstrate the 'delta' or 'lambda' sign (Fig. 3.26). This comprises the amniotic and chorionic membranes surrounding each fetus separated slightly at the insertion site by a tongue of placental tissue (which produces the 'delta' appearance). This type of twinning is therefore dichorionic diamniotic (DCDA).

A monochorional placenta will demonstrate the 'T sign' at the placental insertion of the amniotic membranes (Fig. 3.27). This comprises the fused amniotic membrane surrounding each fetus (both of which lie within a single chorionic cavity) inserting into the shared placenta. This type of twinning is therefore monochorionic diamniotic (MCDA). Care should be taken to distinguish between placental and uterine insertions of the amniotic membrane, as the latter will always demonstrate a pseudo 'T sign'.

If no dividing membrane can be identified between the two fetuses then monochorionic

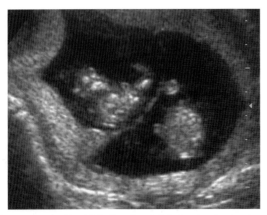

Figure 3.26 The 'delta' or 'lambda' sign is obtained at the point of insertion of the membrane dividing the twin pair into the placenta. This appearance is diagnostic of a dichorionic diamniotic twin pregnancy.

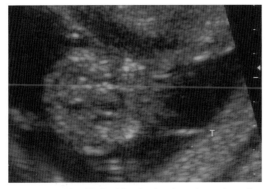

Figure 3.27 The 'T sign' is obtained at the point of insertion of the membrane dividing the twin pair into the placenta. This appearance is diagnostic of a monochorionic diamniotic twin pregnancy.

monoamniotic (MCMA) twins should be suspected. As the dividing membrane between MCDA twins is very thin and mobile it can be difficult to visualize in the first trimester twin pregnancy. Conversely, reverberation artifacts can lead to the incorrect diagnosis of a dividing amniotic membrane in a true monoamniotic twin pregnancy. Confirmation of an MCMA pregnancy should therefore always be made in the second trimester so that the correct advice can be given to the parents. Note that absence of an intertwin dividing membrane in the second trimester or later might be a sign of TTTS. Indeed, the latter problem is far more frequent in MCDA than MCMA pregnancy.

Measuring nuchal translucency in multiple pregnancy

The NT should be measured in each fetus and the adjusted risks calculated. Both adjusted risks should be reported in dichorionic twin pairs. In cases of increased risk in one fetus it is important to report the placental sites and relative positions within the uterus of the two gestations. This aids in further distinguishing between the two fetuses in cases of transient increased NT.

In monochorionic twin pairs, both can be considered to have the same risk of the same chromosomal abnormality. It should be remembered that increased NT has been reported as a marker for cardiac abnormalities and genetic syndromes. It is therefore possible for only one of a monochorionic twin pair to demonstrate an increased NT. Both adjusted risks should therefore be reported. Discrepant NT in MCDA pregnancy increases not only the risk for congenital heart disease but also for TTTS in the remainder of the pregnancy.

REFERENCES AND FURTHER READING

Grisolia G, Milano V, Pilu G et al 1993 Biometry of early pregnancy with transvaginal sonography. Ultrasound in Obstetrics and Gynaecology 3:403–411

Lindsay D J, Lovett I S, Lyons E A et al 1992 Yolk sac diameter and shape at endovaginal US; predictors of outcome. Radiology 183:115–118

Chapter 4

Problems of early pregnancy

Early pregnancy disorders are one of the most common indications for referral to hospital emergency services and they account for approximately three-quarters of acute gynecological admissions. Miscarriage is the most common complication of pregnancy; it has been estimated that the overall miscarriage rate is around 50%. Even though the majority of these losses occur before a missed menstrual period, bleeding complicates 21% of clinically detected pregnancies and 12–15% are lost. Clinical symptoms of miscarriage are often dramatic and include pelvic pain and bleeding. This, compounded by a woman's fear of losing her pregnancy, contributes to the readiness to attend hospital immediately.

In the last few decades a dramatic rise in the incidence of ectopic pregnancy has been reported world-wide. The clinical signs and symptoms of this are very similar to miscarriage and general practitioners feel compelled to refer their patients to hospital to establish a correct diagnosis. In addition, ectopic pregnancy is often portrayed as a life-threatening condition unless diagnosis is made early before serious complications occur. This increases pressure on healthcare providers to investigate early pregnancy problems aggressively, because a delayed or missed diagnosis of ectopic is seen as failure of care and can result in litigation.

Ultrasound is the only method that provides non-invasive diagnosis of early pregnancy complications. Despite this, the implementation of ultrasound in routine clinical practice has been slow, because of the poor diagnostic accuracy of transabdominal ultrasound in early pregnancy, the limited availability of ultrasound equipment and the lack of sonographers trained in early pregnancy diagnosis. However, since the introduction of transvaginal sonography in the late 1980s, decreased costs and wider availability of equipment, ultrasound examination has become the mainstay of early pregnancy diagnosis. As a result, the demand for ultrasound examination has been increasing steadily. To accommodate this, the first dedicated early pregnancy units were opened in the United Kingdom in the early 1990s.

HORMONE MEASUREMENT IN EARLY PREGNANCY

Human chorionic gonadotrophin (hCG)

Most commercially available monoclonal-antibody-based urine pregnancy tests can detect the presence of human chorionic gonadotrophin (hCG) at a level above 25 IU/L, which corresponds to day 24–25 of a regular 28-day cycle. In normal early pregnancies, serum hCG levels double approximately every 2 days. In clinical practice, the measurement of serum hCG is used to diagnose ectopic pregnancy; to help select patients for expectant, medical and surgical management of early pregnancy failure; and to assess the efficacy of treatment at follow-up visits.

Traditionally, an ectopic pregnancy is suspected in women in whom intrauterine pregnancy is not demonstrated on ultrasound. In this situation, many clinicians resort to the assessment of the daily rate of serum hCG levels. An ectopic pregnancy is suspected if the hCG does not double in 2–3 days. Another approach to the diagnosis of ectopic pregnancy is to use a cut-off level above which an intrauterine pregnancy should be seen on ultrasound. With the use of transvaginal sonography this level has been set to the serum hCG level of 1000 IU/L (the first International Standard). However, neither abnormal doubling time nor the cut-off method is sensitive or specific enough to diagnose ectopic pregnancy.

Serum hCG measurement is also used for selection of women for conservative or medical management of ectopic pregnancy. Expectant management of ectopic pregnancy is likely to be successful if the initial hCG is < 1000 IU/L and medical treatment of tubal ectopic is rarely used if the hCG > 15 000 IU/L because the risk of failure and complications is increased.

NORMAL EARLY PREGNANCY

The majority of women referred for early pregnancy assessment have a normal intrauterine pregnancy (Fig. 4.1). However, ultrasound features in early pregnancy change rapidly and a good understanding of these is essential for the detection of abnormalities.

Before starting the scan, the woman should be told that the aim of examination is to confirm an intrauterine pregnancy and to check for fetal cardiac activity. Most women welcome the opportunity to observe the examination on the ultrasound screen and it is important to offer this. Using the transvaginal approach, most normal pregnancies will be detected on the initial scan. A small number of women will attend for a scan between days 24–25 of a regular 28-day cycle, when urine pregnancy tests become positive, and days 29–31, when the gestational sac can be visualized. In order not to miss unusual types of ectopic pregnancy (such as interstitial, cervical or abdominal) it is essential to ensure that the gestational sac is located within the uterus and is completely surrounded by endometrium. A longitudinal section demonstrating continuity between cervical canal, endometrial cavity and gestational sac helps to confirm the diagnosis of a normal intrauterine pregnancy. In women with a history of pelvic pain, the adnexae should be examined for the presence of ovarian and tubal pathology. Every effort should be made to exclude the diagnosis of heterotopic pregnancy in women with persistent pain, or in those who conceived following infertility treatment.

MISCARRIAGE

Approximately 20% of women attending early pregnancy units suffer a miscarriage. Most women will present with a history of vaginal bleeding or abdominal pain, both of which are traditionally

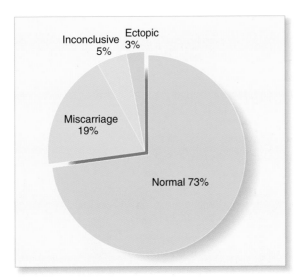

Figure 4.1   Final outcomes in 2114 women with suspected early pregnancy failure referred to the early pregnancy unit at King's College Hospital, London.

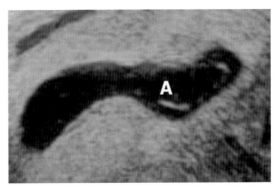

Figure 4.2   A case of missed miscarriage at 8 weeks' gestation. An irregularly shaped gestation sac is seen containing a small amniotic cavity (A) with no fetal pole.

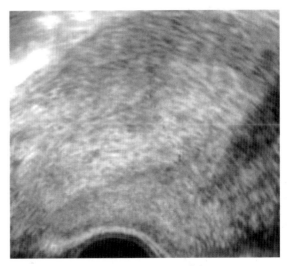

Figure 4.3   A longitudinal section of the uterus showing the uterine cavity, which contains a large amount of irregular echogenic tissue. This is a typical ultrasound finding in incomplete miscarriage.

associated with miscarriage. However, a significant proportion of women will be asymptomatic and will include women with previous pregnancy losses and those who conceived following infertility treatment. As clinical assessment alone is rarely sufficient to establish a correct diagnosis in women with suspected early pregnancy failure, ultrasound examination is used routinely in these cases. The main role of ultrasound is to make the definitive diagnosis of miscarriage to assist in selection between conservative and surgical management options. In addition, a detailed ultrasound examination of potentially viable pregnancies can be used to estimate the risk of miscarriage later in pregnancy.

Ultrasound diagnosis of miscarriage

Miscarriage is classified as threatened, missed (Fig. 4.2), incomplete (Fig. 4.3) and complete (Fig. 4.4) based on the ultrasound findings.

Threatened miscarriage

Threatened miscarriage is usually diagnosed in women with a history of vaginal bleeding and in whom a live embryo can be visualized on the scan.

In 15% of these women the pregnancy will be lost, a significantly higher figure than the 2–7% in pregnancies not complicated by bleeding. The presence of subchorionic hematoma is not associated with poor outcomes.

Missed miscarriage

Missed miscarriage is defined as the retention of a gestational sac within the uterus following

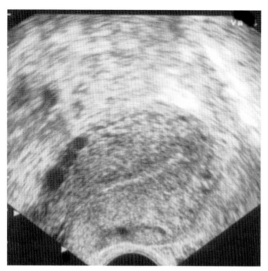

Figure 4.4 A thin endometrial echo in a woman with a positive pregnancy test and a history of heavy bleeding is highly suggestive of complete miscarriage.

embryonic or early fetal death. The diagnosis is usually based on the absence of cardiac activity within the fetal pole. The terms 'blighted ovum' and 'anembryonic pregnancy' have been used to describe a gestational sac without a detectable fetal pole. These terms should be avoided because there is usually histological or biochemical evidence of early embryonic death in nearly all cases. The ultrasound diagnosis of missed miscarriage is straightforward when the embryo is relatively large. However, when the embryonic echoes are very small or non-detectable it is difficult to differentiate between a very early normal pregnancy and a missed miscarriage. Diagnostic errors have been reported in such cases.

The Royal College of Obstetricians and Gynaecologists (RCOG) has proposed a set of guidelines to establish embryonic death by ultrasound. According to these guidelines, the absence of cardiac activity in an embryo of crown–rump length (CRL) > 6 mm, or the absence of a yolk sac or embryo in a gestation sac of mean diameter > 20 mm, enables conclusive diagnosis of a missed miscarriage. In pregnancies in which the embryo and sac are smaller than 6 mm or 20 mm, respectively, a repeat ultrasound examination 1 week later is necessary to clarify the diagnosis (RCOG 1995).

Complete and incomplete miscarriage

The diagnosis of complete and incomplete miscarriage depends even more on the experience and skill of the operator than the diagnosis of missed miscarriage.

Complete miscarriage is usually diagnosed when the endometrium is very thin and regular. The ultrasound appearances are therefore comparable to those of the non-pregnant uterus in the early proliferative phase. The diagnosis of *incomplete miscarriage* is more controversial and diagnostic criteria of endometrial thickness vary between 5 and 15 mm.

The main difficulty with using predefined cut-off levels is the inability to differentiate between blood clots, which are often seen within the uterine cavity at the time of miscarriage and retained products. We therefore favor subjective assessment of the endometrium in preference to quantitative criteria. Retained products are usually seen as a well-defined area of hyperechoic tissue within the uterine cavity as opposed to blood clots that are more irregular. Blood clots will be also seen sliding within the uterine cavity when pressure is applied on the uterus by the transvaginal probe. However, even with a Doppler examination the diagnosis of incomplete miscarriage is difficult and ultrasound should always be combined with clinical and biochemical assessment to rule-out the possibility of an ectopic in these cases.

Management of miscarriage

Surgical evacuation of retained products has become universally accepted as the method of choice for the management of miscarriage. When it was introduced (in the 1960s) the rationale for the use of curettage was a perceived risk of sepsis and hemorrhage associated with spontaneous abortion. It is likely that a number of complicated miscarriages at that time represented retained products following illegal abortions, which contributed to the severity of clinical presentation. Women's general health has improved considerably in the intervening 50 years and most infections can now be treated effectively using antibiotics. Legalisation of abortion has eliminated problems caused by criminal abortion in many developed countries.

However, there is now a growing concern about the unconditional and non-selective use of surgery for the treatment of miscarriage. There is also concern about morbidity caused by surgical and anesthetic complications. Expectant management of incomplete miscarriage is an attractive option in this context. It follows the natural history of the disease, avoids iatrogenic problems associated with both medical and surgical treatment and, as such, is likely to be cost effective. In cases of missed miscarriage, both expectant and medical management are relatively ineffective and are suitable only for individual, highly motivated women or those who have difficulty in accepting the diagnosis of a failed pregnancy and feel unable to make a rapid decision about surgical treatment.

ECTOPIC PREGNANCY

An ectopic pregnancy is defined as implantation of the fertilized ovum outside the uterine cavity. A total of 93% of ectopic pregnancies are tubal (Fig. 4.5). The incidence of ectopic pregnancies in the UK increased from 4.9/1000 in 1970 to 9.6/1000 pregnancies in 1992 (RCOG 2000). Ectopic pregnancies can present with abdominal pain with or without vaginal bleeding. Particular groups of patients are at high risk and include those with previous tubal pathology or surgery, and those with an intrauterine contraceptive

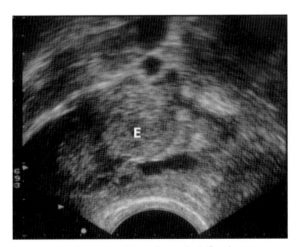

Figure 4.5 A small, echogenic, well-defined mass (E) adjacent to the uterus is a case of tubal miscarriage.

device. The possibility of an ectopic pregnancy should be considered in high-risk patients with a positive pregnancy, even in the absence of symptoms.

Ultrasound findings of ectopic pregnancy

Traditionally, the findings of a positive pregnancy test and an empty uterus seen at the time of ultrasound scan have been synonymous with the presence of an ectopic pregnancy. However, with the use of transvaginal ultrasound around 85% of ectopics can be directly visualized at the initial ultrasound scan.

A pseudosac is visible within the uterus in 10–29% of ectopic pregnancies, and this finding should not be mistaken for an early gestational sac. The pseudosac represents the accumulation of non-clotted blood within the uterine cavity. A single rim of thin endometrium surrounds it and the shape of the sac reflects the shape of the uterine cavity. In longitudinal section, the pseudosac will appear elongated and thin, whereas a gestational sac appears more circular. However, the presence of chorionic tissue, which forms an echogenic rim around the gestation sac, helps to establish the correct diagnosis of intrauterine pregnancy. On Doppler examination, a pseudosac will typically appear avascular, whereas high velocity peritrophoblastic flow surrounds an early gestational sac.

Visualization of the corpus luteum can aid detection of an ectopic pregnancy because around 78% of ectopic pregnancies will be ipsilateral to the corpus luteum. It can sometimes be difficult to differentiate the corpus luteum from the ectopic pregnancy. The 'sliding organs sign' can be used to distinguish a bulging corpus luteum from an ectopic pregnancy. Using this technique, gentle pressure with the tip of the probe is used to observe whether the mass moves separately from the ovary.

The presence of fluid in the pouch of Douglas is associated with 20–25% of ectopic pregnancies. Blood and clots appear as hyperechoeic fluid on ultrasound, the presence of which is suggestive of tubal abortion or a ruptured ectopic. However, blood in the pouch of Douglas can also be seen in a woman with a ruptured corpus luteum cyst.

False-positive diagnosis of an ectopic can result from a static loop of bowel, hydrosalpinx, adhesions or an endometrioma.

Direct ultrasonic visualization of the ectopic pregnancy is essential not only to facilitate diagnosis but also to decide upon the best management option. Morphology of ectopic pregnancies varies and the relative frequency of different morphological features will depend on accessibility of the ultrasound service, quality of the equipment and the experience of the sonographers (Fig. 4.6).

Management of ectopic pregnancy

Expectant management

It is now well recognized that not all ectopic pregnancies require treatment and that some will resolve spontaneously. Expectant management is becoming increasingly important as the ability to detect small ectopic pregnanices and tubal miscarriage increases. Previous studies showed that around a quarter of ectopic pregnancies are suitable for expectant management. The selection criteria for expectant management vary but those ectopic pregnancies with a live fetus or the presence of hemoperitoneum would be considered unsuitable for all but surgical management. The main problem with expectant management is a high failure rate of 40–50%, and many women need additional treatment after prolonged follow-up and a number of visits to hospital.

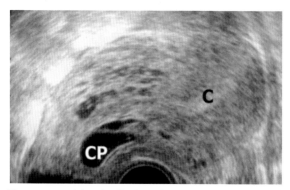

Figure 4.6 A longitudinal section of the uterus showing a cervical pregnancy (CP) and empty uterine cavity above it (C).

Medical treatment

Methotrexate is used in the treatment of ectopic pregnancy to minimize the need for surgical intervention. Methotrexate is a folic acid antagonist, which leads to interference with DNA synthesis and cell multiplication in the conceptus. Methotrexate can be given either intramuscularly or by direct injection into the ectopic pregnancy under laparoscopic/ultrasound guidance. Side-effects include gastritis, stomatitis, alopecia, headaches, nausea and vomiting. Disturbances in hepatic and renal function and leukopenia or thrombocytopenia can also occur. The success rate for treatment of ectopic pregnancy with methotrexate varies between 74 and 94%. Fertility rates following methotrexate therapy are compatible with surgical treatment.

Surgical treatment

Surgical options include salpingectomy or salpingostomy, performed either as an open procedure or laparoscopically. Three randomized trials have shown that laparoscopy is superior to laparotomy in hemodynamically stable patients. In the laparoscopic approach there is less blood loss, less analgesic requirement and a shorter hospital stay. However, persistent trophoblast is a complication, which occurs more often after laparoscopic surgery. Postoperative follow-up with monitoring of weekly serum hCG levels is necessary in all women following salpingostomy and tubal conservation.

Interstitial ectopic pregnancy

An interstitial pregnancy is implanted in the interstitial portion of the fallopian tube (Fig. 4.7). Interstitial pregnancy occurs in 1.1–6.3% of all ectopic pregnancies. Implantation of the fertilized ovum is more likely to occur in the interstitial part of the fallopian tube following in vitro fertilization (IVF) and previous salpingectomy. The ultrasound diagnosis of an interstitial pregnancy is made when the products of conception are seen in the upper lateral aspect of the uterus, outside the uterine cavity and at least partially surrounded by myometrium. The proximal interstitial segment of

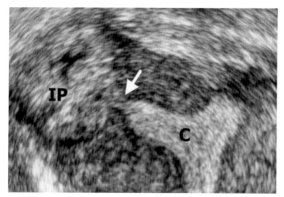

Figure 4.7 A case of right interstitial pregnancy (IP). The interstitial part of fallopian tube (arrow) is seen adjoining the pregnancy and empty uterine cavity (C).

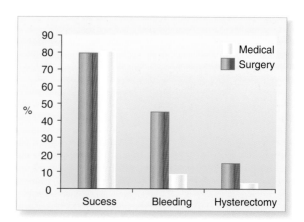

Figure 4.8 A comparison of the results of surgical and medical treatment of cervical pregnancy.

the tube joining the uterus to the ectopic pregnancy can be visualized.

Traditionally, interstitial pregnancies were treated surgically by laparotomy, because diagnosis was usually not made until after rupture. The clinical presentation of ruptured interstitial pregnancy is severe and is often complicated by severe hemorrhage and hysterectomy. However, earlier diagnosis has allowed more conservative management to be used. Methotrexate is effective for the treatment of early interstitial pregnancies.

CERVICAL PREGNANCY

A cervical pregnancy occurs when the conceptus is implanted below the level of the internal os (see Fig. 4.6). The incidence of cervical pregnancy ranges from 1:2400 to 1:50 000 pregnancies and 0.15% of all ectopic pregnancies. The diagnosis of cervical pregnancy can be made using the following ultrasound criteria:

- no evidence of an intrauterine pregnancy
- an hourglass uterine shape with ballooning of the cervical canal
- the presence of a gestation sac or placental tissue within the cervical canal
- a closed internal os.

The internal os can appear open in large cervical pregnancies or in those implanted high in the cervical canal. The diagnosis of a cervical pregnancy can only be made easily if cardiac activity is present. In women with an intrauterine pregnancy that has become detached from the uterine cavity and is temporarily retained within the cervical canal, gentle pressure with the probe will demonstrate sliding between the gestation sac and cervical canal. This sign is absent in true cervical pregnancies.

Management of cervical pregnancy can be surgical with dilatation and curettage, but this carries the risk of uncontrollable hemorrhage and a high rate of hysterectomy. Local injections of methotrexate or potassium chloride would appear to be the most effective way of treating early cervical pregnancies under ultrasound control. Systemic therapy with methotrexate is also effective, although the side-effect profile will be higher (Fig. 4.8).

OVARIAN PREGNANCY

The incidence of ovarian pregnancy ranges from 1:4000 to 1:7000 deliveries. For the pregnancy to be diagnosed as ovarian, the ipsilateral tube must be intact, the gestation sac must be within the ovary, the ovary must be connected to the uterus by the ovarian ligament and ovarian tissue must be within the sac wall. On ultrasound scan, an ovarian pregnancy can be diagnosed when the gestation sac cannot be separated from the ovary (Fig. 4.9). If the gestation sac appears empty it is essential that the corpus luteum is identified separately to the gestation sac to avoid misinterpreting the corpus luteum as an ovarian pregnancy. False-positive diagnosis of ovarian pregnancy can also occur in women with pelvic adhesions fixing the fallopian tube to the ovary. In these cases it is impossible to

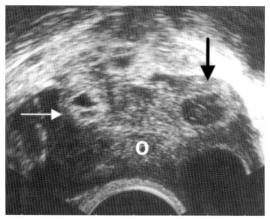

Figure 4.9 A case of ovarian pregnancy at 6 weeks' gestation. The ovary (O) is enlarged and it contains a corpus luteum in its lateral pole (black arrow). A small empty gestation sac is seen implanted into the medial aspect of the ovary (white arrow).

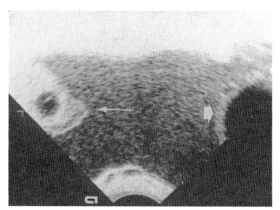

Figure 4.10 A small gestational sac is seen implanted into the pouch of Douglas (thin arrow) and is surrounded by a large amount of echogenic free fluid. A corpus luteum cyst is also seen anteriorly (thick arrow).

separate the gestation sac from the ovary by using pressure applied with the probe.

Ovarian ectopic pregnancies are usually treated by local excision, which can be done laparoscopically. The preoperative ultrasound diagnosis is difficult and there are no reports of expectant or medical treatment of ovarian pregnancy, although it is likely that these treatment options will be safer than surgery in many cases.

ABDOMINAL PREGNANCY

This is rare form of ectopic pregnancy, which occurs in 1:3400 to 1:8000 deliveries. Abdominal pregnancy is defined as an intraperitoneal implantation exclusive of intratubal, ovarian or intraligamentous sites of nidation. To make a first trimester diagnosis, a gestation sac or fetal parts are usually seen behind the uterus in the pouch of Douglas or laterally within the broad ligament (Fig. 4.10).

HETEROTOPIC PREGNANCY

Heterotopic pregnancy is the combination of an intrauterine and an ectopic pregnancy. The incidence of heterotopic pregnancy in the general population is around 1:6000, and is particularly high in women who undergo some form of assisted conception. The diagnosis of a normal intrauterine

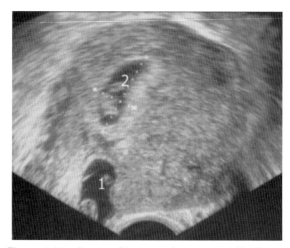

Figure 4.11 A case of heterotopic pregnancy. The lower sac (1) is implanted into the cervix, whereas the upper sac (2) is normally located within the uterine cavity.

pregnancy thus cannot rule out a concomitant ectopic pregnancy, and every effort should be made to exclude this in a symptomatic patient (Fig. 4.11).

PREGNANCES OF UNKNOWN LOCATION

Transvaginal sonography enables conclusive diagnosis of miscarriages and ectopic pregnancies to be made in the majority of cases. It has therefore been increasingly used as the method of choice for the initial assessment of women with suspected early pregnancy abnormalities. However in 8–31% of women with suspected abnormal early pregnancies the diagnosis cannot be made by ultrasound at the initial visit. Studies have shown that only a minority of these pregnancies will require active intervention, as a substantial number of non-visualized pregnancies are failing pregnancies, either intrauterine or ectopic, which will resolve spontaneously (Fig. 4.11). The second most likely diagnosis is a normal very early pregnancy, which cannot yet be visualized on ultrasound. The ability to predict final outcome using serum hCG and progesterone measurements facilitates the use of expectant management in these women without fear of missing a potentially dangerous ectopic pregnancy. Intervention can be almost always avoided in women with a normal intrauterine pregnancy, thus reserving it only for those patients with worsening clinical symptoms or non-declining hCG levels.

TROPHOBLASTIC DISEASE

Trophoblastic disease covers the spectrum from benign hydatidiform mole to malignant choriocarcinoma. Early diagnosis enables appropriate management and counseling to be planned. However, diagnosis in the first trimester is difficult because the clinical presentation, sonographic findings and pathologies are variable.

Complete hydatidiform mole

Complete hydatidiform moles are characterized by generalized swelling of the villous tissue and diffuse trophoblastic hyperplasia in the absence of embryonic or fetal tissue. The diagnosis of a complete hydatidiform mole was first made using bistable static scanning equipment. The typical second trimester ultrasound appearance used to be described as a 'snowstorm'. This description was superseded when the superior resolution of real-time imaging enabled the homogenous distribution of cystic areas within the uterus to be identified. Other common findings were one or several areas of fluid collections, with irregular contours and thin walls. Serum hCG will be high in these women, usually > 2.5 multiples of the median (MoM), and will continue to increase as

the pregnancy advances. Management of complete moles is by surgical evacuation of the pregnancy with follow-up of serial hCG measurements.

Partial hydatidiform mole

Partial moles are characterized by focal swelling of the villous tissue and focal trophoblastic hyperplasia in the presence of embryonic or fetal tissue. Sonolucent areas found within placenta might represent either a partial mole or a twin pregnancy in which one conceptus is normal and the other a complete mole. In the case of a complete mole coexisting with a fetus, the molar placenta will be clearly separated from the normal placenta, whereas in partial moles the molar structures are dispersed inside the placental mass. With triploid partial moles, major fetal abnormalities or severe intrauterine growth restriction are almost always present.

Choriocarcinoma

Choriocarcinomas are highly malignant and the woman usually presents with multiple metastases. The primary tumor is often very small and an extensive search of the placenta is frequently required to find the lesion.

OVARIAN PROBLEMS IN EARLY PREGNANCY

Routine ultrasound examination during pregnancy has increased the number of incidental diagnoses of adnexal masses in asymptomatic pregnant women. The majority of these tumors are ovarian in origin.

Ovarian cysts in pregnancy

Most of the ovarian masses seen are corpus luteum cysts, which normally resolve spontaneously by the end of first trimester. Management is more difficult in women with persistent complex ovarian cysts, and traditionally involves laparotomy and removal of all adnexal masses that persist beyond 16 weeks' gestation. This aggressive approach is based on the traditional teaching that any complex cyst has a potential of being malignant, and should therefore be removed, even if the woman is asymptomatic.

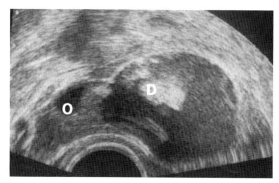

Figure 4.12 A dermoid cyst found accidentally during pregnancy. On the left is normal ovarian tissue (O) with the dermoid cyst protruding laterally (D).

Improved ultrasound imaging and recent developments in operative laparoscopy have provided the possibility of less-invasive management of ovarian cysts (Fig. 4.12). Despite the increasing size of the gravid uterus and alterations in pelvic anatomy during pregnancy, sonography can accurately differentiate between benign and malignant cysts in pregnancy. Thus, a number of smaller benign cysts can be managed expectantly or by laparoscopy. However, laparotomy and oophorectomy remain the method of choice for treatment of a minority of ovarian cysts, which are suspicious of malignancy.

Functional cysts

The cystic corpus luteum can vary greatly in size and appearance. It can appear as a simple cystic mass within the ovary or as a more complex mass with evidence of internal hemorrhage and solid areas. Doppler examination of the cyst will reveal circumferential flow, which is of high velocity and low impedance. Management should be expectant and most functional cysts will resolve spontaneously by the end of first trimester.

Theca-lutein cysts are usually found in association with high levels of circulating hCG. Thus they can be present with molar pregnancy, ovarian hyperstimulation syndrome or be seen with normal intrauterine pregnancies. They are usually multilocular and bilateral, and can be large. As with other functional cysts, they will usually

resolve spontaneously by 16 weeks' gestation, although the mean time for resolution is 8 weeks.

Ovarian masses

Although the risk of malignancy in women of reproductive age is low, any adnexal mass seen on routine sonography must be evaluated fully to exclude malignancy. The most common persistent ovarian masses seen in pregnancy are dermoid cysts, benign cystadenomas and endometriomas.

UTERINE FIBROIDS

Around 1–4% of pregnancies are associated with fibroids. The presence of fibroids can lead to difficulties in obtaining accurate measurements of the gestation sac or fetus. During pregnancy, fibroids usually increase in size due to the high levels of circulating estrogen. Moreover, the location of the fibroid in relation to the uterine cavity appears to be more important than its size and submucous fibroids can increase the miscarriage rate. Fibroids in close proximity to the placenta are often associated with early pregnancy bleeding. Other complications of fibroids in pregnancy include antepartum hemorrhage, abdominal pain due to degeneration, malpresentation, obstructed labor and morbid adherence of the placenta (see also Chapter 5).

PREGNANCY AND AN INTRAUTERINE CONTRACEPTIVE DEVICE

If an intrauterine pregnancy occurs with an intrauterine contraceptive device (IUCD) in situ, removal of the IUCD is the preferred option. Leaving the device in situ is associated with a high rate of miscarriage and an increased risk of hemorrhage, sepsis, preterm delivery and of stillbirth. An ultrasound examination performed as early as possible in pregnancy will usually show that the IUCD is situated below the gestation sac; IUCD malposition is the most common cause of failure (Fig. 4.13). If the threads are visible then the IUCD should be removed. If the threads are lost, or the IUCD appears embedded in the gestation sac, attempts at its removal are likely to cause miscarriage.

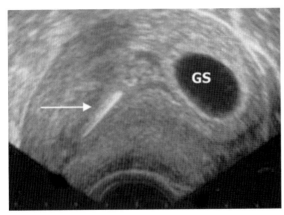

Figure 4.13 A longitudinal section of the uterus showing a 6 week gestation sac (GS) normally implanted within the uterine cavity. A Nova T IUCD (arrow) is also seen displaced into the upper part of the cervical canal.

Should the woman decide to continue with pregnancy she should be informed that there is no evidence that the fetus is at an increased risk of fetal abnormalities, but that the risk of second trimester miscarriage is approximately 50%. Although ectopic pregnancies are more commonly seen when an IUCD is present, IUCDs do not increase the overall risk of an ectopic pregnancy compared with controls not using any contraception. However, an early ultrasound is warranted in every women who conceives with an IUCD in situ to locate the pregnancy.

ORGANIZATION OF EARLY PREGNANCY UNITS

The organization and aims of early pregnancy units vary and there is no agreement which health professionals should be running the unit, what facilities should be available within the units and who takes the overall responsibility for patient care. In many cases, early pregnancy units are run as dedicated sessions within imaging departments, and clinical staff with no skills in ultrasound diagnosis decide on further patients' care. More recently, the role of early pregnancy units has been extended to include not only ultrasound diagnosis but also clinical management of early pregnancy complications. In this way, the unit provides comprehensive care for women with early pregnancy problems, which includes clinical assessment, ultrasound diagnosis, decisions on appropriate treatment options, follow-up, counseling and psychological support (Fig. 4.14).

When organized in this way, and staffed by a multidisciplinary team of health professionals, the early pregnancy unit provides a fast and complete reassurance to women with normal intrauterine pregnancies and minimizes the need for both diagnostic and operative interventions in women with early pregnancy abnormalities. Such a unit might be self-contained or linked to the gynecology ward. However, in all cases the unit has to incorporate certain components to make it effective. An efficient appointments system, with direct access to appointments for primary health care (general practitioners/physicians, nurses, midwives) and other hospital departments (Emergency Room/Accident and Emergency) should be available. Patients with previous problems such as recurrent miscarriage or ectopic pregnancy should be encouraged to self-refer in their next pregnancy. Such a service should be available daily, with extended evening sessions, and all staff should be appropriately trained. A dedicated area should be set aside for counseling and staff trained to provide this. There should be up-to-date ultrasound equipment including transvaginal ultrasound probes in compliance with current recommendations. Good laboratory back-up is essential, with access to serum hCG and progesterone estimations within a few hours.

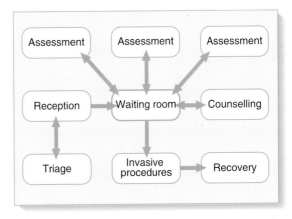

Figure 4.14 Organization of an early pregnancy unit.

REFERENCES AND FURTHER READING

Grudzinskas J G, O'Brien P M S 1997 Problems in early pregnancy: advances in diagnosis and management. RCOG Press, London, p 160–173

Royal College of Obstetricians and Gynaecologists 1995 Guidance on ultrasound procedures in early pregnancy. RCOG Press, London

Royal College of Obstetricians and Gynaecologists 2000 The management of tubal pregnancies. RGOG Press, London

Chapter 5

Scanning the non-pregnant pelvis

The pelvic ultrasound scan has become an essential extension of the clinical examination in gynecology. The investigation of abnormal uterine bleeding has been transformed by the use of transvaginal ultrasound to assess the endometrial cavity, which allows hysteroscopy to be reserved for those patients requiring resection of submucous fibroids or endometrial polyps. In many cases, adnexal masses can be fully characterized using ultrasound, and 3D ultrasound has become the method of choice in the assessment of congenital uterine anomalies.

A successful ultrasound examination of the pelvis cannot be achieved without knowledge of a woman's full clinical history. Throughout the menstrual cycle, the uterus and ovaries are subject to a range of functional changes that are a reflection of the hormonal milieu. The use of contraceptives such as the progesterone-only pill causes an increased incidence of functional ovarian cysts and a thin endometrial echo, whereas tamoxifen increases the endometrial thickness and predisposes towards the development of endometrial polyps. As postmenopausal ovaries no longer undergo cyclical changes, the knowledge of the menopausal status of a woman can avoid an incorrect diagnosis of a functional cyst. Gynecological malignancy is more common in the menopause, the risk increases with age and a family or personal history of breast, ovarian, endometrial or bowel cancer.

EXAMINATION TECHNIQUE

Transvaginal ultrasound scan is the method of choice for the examination of the non-pregnant pelvis (see Chapters 2 and 3). The examination follows the principles of bimanual vaginal examination. A combination of palpation and visual information greatly increases the accuracy of diagnosis. The position of pelvic organs can be modified to optimize the image quality. This also enables assessment of the mobility of pelvic organs and accurate localization of pelvic pain. The close proximity of pelvic organs to the ultrasound probe enables the use of high frequency transducers, which further contributes to the image resolution. Transabdominal ultrasound examination, however, remains the only method for examining virgins and those women who are unable to tolerate vaginal examination. The full bladder technique is necessary in these cases. The transabdominal technique should also be used as an adjunct to a vaginal scan in women with large pelvic masses that cannot be completely assessed transvaginally. However, a full bladder is not necessary in these cases.

The pelvis should be examined systematically, with care taken to identify normal pelvic structures such as the uterus and healthy ovaries. Any abnormalities should then be examined in detail, after noting their origin and relation to the surrounding pelvic anatomy. The mobility and tenderness of the abnormality should be assessed along with the regularity of its border. The structure of the mass should be classified as cystic or solid and the locularity and solid areas of a cystic mass noted. A multilocular cyst (Fig. 5.1) contains septations, which can be thick and irregular in the case of malignant lesions. A septation is incomplete if, in any view, continuity from one cyst wall to the other is not maintained.

Papillary proliferations are defined as solid projections from the wall or septation into the cyst cavity and appear as irregular, cauliflower-like excrescences (Fig. 5.2). Calcified elements are seen in dermoids and in some fibroids and are usually a reassuring sign, although they are occasionally noted in malignant tumors. Spiculations are findings confined to dermoid cysts. They are thin, echogenic linear echoes that represent hair fibers within the cyst.

The fluid within a cystic lesion can be classified according to its echogenicity. Anechoic fluid appears uniformly black irrespective of how the

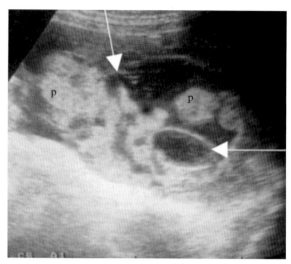

Figure 5.1 A large serous cystadenocarcinoma viewed abdominally demonstrating the typical anechoic fluid and multilocular appearance. Note the thick irregular septations (arrows) and numerous papillary proliferations (p).

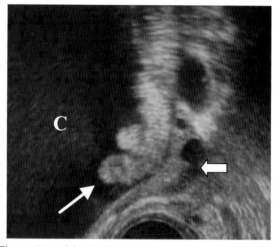

Figure 5.2 A borderline cystadenocarcinoma displaying a lateral rim of healthy ovarian tissue (thick arrow) surrounding a large cyst (c) containing anechoic fluid and a papillary projection (thin arrow).

gain is adjusted, whereas mucinous fluid has low-level echogenicity and appears hypoechoic, with tiny gray particles suspended within it (Fig. 5.3). 'Ground glass' echogenicity is seen within an endometrioma and represents fluid with a high density of solid particles within it (Fig. 5.4).

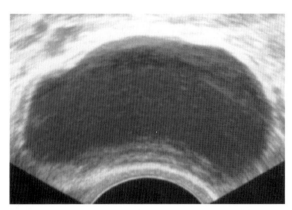

Figure 5.3   A benign mucinous cystadenoma with typical low-level echogenic fluid.

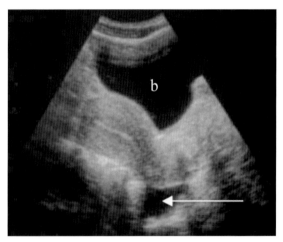

Figure 5.5   A transabdominal scan with a normal anteverted uterus. The full urinary bladder (b) is seen anteriorly and a small amount of fluid in pouch of Douglas posteriorly (arrow).

Transmitted movement of the transducer causes flow within the cyst and movement of particles can be seen with both low level and ground glass contents.

The presence of intra-abdominal fluid should be determined by examination of the woman in the Trendelenburg position. A small amount of anechoic fluid in the pouch of Douglas is a physiological finding and might be due to recent follicular rupture (Fig. 5.5). Ascites is diagnosed when anechoic fluid is present in the utero-vesicular fold.

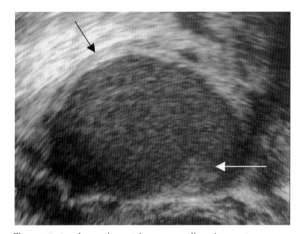

Figure 5.4   An endometrioma: a unilocular cyst containing echogenic fluid of 'ground glass' appearance with a condensation of material inferiorly (broken arrow). The cyst is located centrally and is surrounded by healthy ovarian tissue (arrow).

DOPPLER EXAMINATION

The Doppler assessment of the vascularity of a structure relies on the principle that a particle approaching the transducer reflects the ultrasound beam at a higher frequency then a particle that is stationary or moving away from the probe. Color Doppler enables visualization of blood vessels within the region of interest. The main role of color Doppler is to direct the position of the pulsed Doppler gate. Blood-flow characteristics, such as blood velocity and impedance to flow, are then examined using flow velocity waveform analysis.

The use of Doppler in examination of the uterus enables the identification of the base of a polyp and demonstration of a vascular connection between the uterus and a pedunculated fibroid. It has limited value in the preoperative diagnosis of malignancy of the uterus but is helpful in the characterization of adnexal masses.

Ideally, Doppler interrogation of the ovary should be carried out in the first 5 days of the cycle in a premenopausal woman. This reduces the possibility of obtaining Doppler signals from the corpus luteum or developing follicle. To start, the pulse repetition frequency (PRF) should be set to its minimum and the structure surveyed. This gives an overall picture of the vascularity of the structure and allows identification of large areas of continuously shifting flow or tumor lakes. The PRF can then be increased in a stepwise manner to identify those vessels with the flow of highest velocity. A pulsed Doppler range gate is then positioned over the vessel displaying the highest velocity to obtain a flow velocity waveform. The Doppler angle should then be adjusted carefully to obtain the loudest audible signal. The signal with the highest peak systolic velocity (PSV) is usually taken as the representative waveform. The waveform can be analyzed electronically to give four indices: PSV, time-averaged maximum velocity (TAMXV), resistance index (RI) and pulsatility index (PI). Low resistance flow is associated with a higher fraction of arterioles, and thus with neovascularization in a tumor. There has been considerable debate about the best cut-off values for these indices in the diagnosis of ovarian malignancy. A TAMXV > 12 cm s^{-1} is usually considered to be fast flow if seen in an intratumoral vessel. An RI < 0.5 is generally considered low resistance flow. The use of color Doppler energy (or Power Doppler imaging) has been shown to have no advantage over color Doppler imaging in the diagnosis of malignancy.

NORMAL ULTRASOUND APPEARANCES

The uterus

The position and relationship of the female pelvic organs vary considerably with posture and as a result of interactions with the surrounding viscera. The central location and large size of the uterus in the pelvis allow it to be used as a landmark for orientation. However, the position and flexion of the uterus itself can vary. In transvaginal sonography, with the image oriented so that the probe is positioned at the lowest point on the screen, an anteverted uterus projects from the anterior vaginal fornix to the right of the screen towards the bladder and anterior abdominal wall (Fig. 5.6A). Conversely, a retroverted uterus projects from the posterior vaginal fornix and extends to the left of the screen away from the bladder (Fig. 5.6B). The position of the body of the uterus in relation to the cervix, which is anchored in the midline, can also

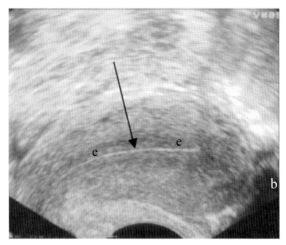

Figure 5.6A An anteverted uterus in the early proliferative phase. The midline echo is clearly visible as an echogenic line (arrow) surrounded by a thin layer of hypoechoic endometrium (e). The bladder is visible to the right of the uterine fundus, on the extreme right of the image.

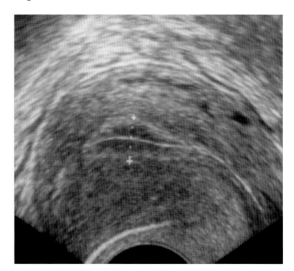

Figure 5.6B Measurement of the endometrium in a retroverted uterus in the late proliferative phase. The endometrium should be measured from the superior to the inferior endometrial/myometrial border encompassing both leaves of the endometrium, as indicated (+ − − − +). The midline echo should be at 90° to the sound beam to enable accurate measurement.

vary and a uterus might be anteflexed (angled forward) or retroflexed (angled backward) in relation to the cervix. A uterus that is axial lies in the same axis as the vagina and cervix; the ultrasound beam in this case is no longer perpendicular to the endometrium and consequently image quality might be less satisfactory.

The uterus is a pear-shaped, muscular, hollow organ situated in the true pelvis. It is found in the midline of the pelvis, anterior to the rectum and posterior to the urinary bladder. The appearance of the uterus varies depending on the age of the woman and the stage of the menstrual cycle at which she is scanned. The uterus is divided into four anatomic parts – fundus, corpus, isthmus and cervix. The fundus is the dome-shaped uppermost aspect of the uterus, the lateral-most part of the fundus extends into the interstitial part of each fallopian tube. The corpus extends from the fundus down to the cervix, the junction of the corpus and cervix is the isthmus, which is the site of development of the lower uterine segment in pregnancy.

The wall of the uterus is composed of three layers: parametrium, myometrium and endometrium. The parametrium is a thin layer of peritoneum that is highly echogenic on ultrasound and gives the uterus a bright outline. The myometrium is the muscular layer of the uterus, which is normally homogenous and echodense. The endometrium, the inner most layer of the uterus, varies greatly in response to the prevailing hormonal influence and timing within the menstrual cycle.

The size and shape of the uterus vary greatly in relation to parity and age. The bulk of the uterus consists of myometrium, which is the smooth muscle substance of the uterus and is continuous with the cervix. As the organ is predominantly made of one tissue type, its appearance is homogenous with a fine echodense texture. The thickness of the uterine walls is variable with age, parity and the presence of pathology. The area of myometrium closest to the endometrium is known as the junctional zone, and this might be less echogenic and is not always visible. The outer layers of the myometrium can be punctuated by small cystic spaces, which represent the arcuate vessels in cross-section, the flow within these vessels is classically slow and, with age, they might sclerose and calcify giving a hyperechoic appearance.

Various uterine developmental anomalies can be recognized on ultrasound, the most common being the subseptate uterus and the bicornuate uterus. The subseptate uterus will have a uniform and smooth external uterine contour. The bicornuate uterus is distinguished by the presence of a deep fundal indentation that divides the uterus into two distinct bodies with one unified cervix and isthmus (Table 5.1).

Table 5.1   Distinguishing ultrasound features of uterine abnormalities

Uterine morphology	Fundal contour	External contour
Normal	Straight or convex	Uniformly convex or with indentation < 10 mm
Arcuate	Concave fundal indentation with central point of indentation at obtuse angle (> 90°)	Uniformly convex or with indentation < 10 mm
Subseptate	Presence of septum, which does not extend to cervix, with central point of septum at an acute angle (< 90°)	Uniformly convex or with indentation < 10 mm
Septate	Presence of uterine septum that completely divides cavity from fundus to cervix	Uniformly convex or with indentation < 10 mm
Bicornuate	Two well-formed uterine cornua	Fundal indentation > 10 mm dividing the two cornua
Unicornuate with or without rudimentary horn	Single well-formed uterine cavity with a single interstitial portion of fallopian tube and concave fundal contour	Fundal indentation > 10 mm dividing the two cornua if rudimentary horn present

The endometrium

The endometrium is a specialized form of mucous membrane that is responsive to circulating hormones and a variety of drugs. The appearance of the endometrium is therefore highly variable, depending on the timing of the menstrual cycle and the effect of any drugs.

Measurement of the thickness of the endometrium conventionally includes both layers. This is because it is generally easier to visualize the junctional zone between endometrium and myometrium than it is to visualize the interface between the anterior and posterior layers of endometrium. In the absence of significant endometrial pathology, such as a polyp, the entire thickness of the endometrium appears uniform. The thickness and appearance vary with the timing of the cycle; a range of 5–14 mm is considered to be normal in women of reproductive age.

In the proliferative phase of the menstrual cycle, the functional layer becomes responsive to the increasing levels of estrogen. This causes the proliferation, lengthening and increase in tortuosity of the endometrial glands. The thickness of the endometrium is in direct relation to follicular development and rising estrogen levels. As the proliferative phase progresses, the endometrium not only thickens but also becomes less echogenic; however, the myometrial–endometrial interface and the interface between the opposing two layers of endometrium becomes more echogenic and the classic three-stripe endometrial echo is observed. Toward the end of the proliferative phase, with continued exposure to high levels of circulating estrogens, the entire endometrial complex becomes increasingly echogenic as a result of glycogen accumulation and edema.

After ovulation and the formation of the corpus luteum, increasing levels of progesterone cause a halt in endometrial proliferation. The endometrial glands, under the influence of progesterone, begin to secrete glycoproteins. The distinctive proliferative endometrium appears uniformly echogenic on ultrasound examination. If there is no pregnancy, the endometrium will not continue to grow, although it remains secretory. With the falling levels of estrogens and progesterone toward the end of the cycle, the functional layers begin to disintegrate and menstruation ensues. The endometrial appearance at this time is variable but it remains echogenic.

In postmenopausal women who are not on hormone replacement therapy (HRT), the normal endometrium appears homogenous and echo-poor compared with the adjacent myometrium. An endometrial thickness of 4 mm or less is considered normal.

The fallopian tubes

The fallopian tubes extend within the broad ligament from either cornu of the uterus to their fimbrial ends, which are usually located superior to the ovaries. The tube is made up of four parts: the interstitial portion, the isthmus, the ampulla and the infundibulum. The interstitial portion is located within the body of the uterus and can be clearly seen as a hyperechoic line extending from the lateral uterine angle to the origin of the broad ligament (Fig. 5.7); the isthmus and ampulla are rarely seen without the use of contrast media. The infundibulum can be seen if it is floating in peritoneal fluid (Fig. 5.8). Visualization of the tube is possible after distention either with contrast media or fluid in cases of hydro- or sactosalpinx.

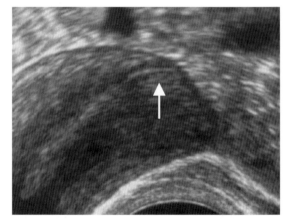

Figure 5.7 A view of the interstitial tube (arrow) appearing as a hyperechoic line extending from the cavity to the origin of the broad ligament.

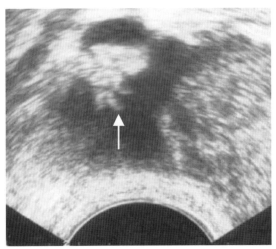

Figure 5.8 A view of the fimbrial end (infundibulum) of the tube (arrow) surrounded by free fluid in the pouch of Douglas.

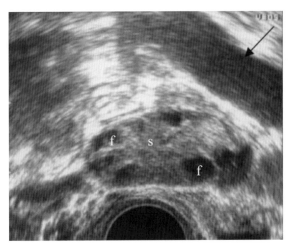

Figure 5.9A The left ovary seen medial to the left iliac vessels (arrow) using the transvaginal approach. A few small follicles (f) are seen in the cortex. The ovarian stroma (s), which occupies the central section of the ovary, appears moderately echogenic.

The ovaries

The ovaries are usually located in the ovarian fossa, inferior to the pelvic vessels on the lateral pelvic wall. However, they are mobile structures and can be found in the pouch of Douglas or above the uterine fundus; they can be located by following the broad ligament laterally. They appear as ellipsoid structures, which are slightly hypoechoic in comparison with the myometrium (Fig. 5.9).

Ovarian follicles are simple, anechoic cysts with clear and well-defined walls. They grow at an average rate of 2 mm/day until they reach 20–25 mm in diameter, just before ovulation. Strictly speaking, the diagnosis of an ovarian follicle can only be made on a follow-up scan that demonstrates normal follicular growth or signs of ovulation. However, in practical terms every simple ovarian cyst measuring less than 25 mm in size in a premenopausal woman can be classified as a follicle. Doppler examination of the follicles reveals only limited vascularity.

Corpora lutea can be solid, cystic or hemorrhagic. Solid corpora lutea are sometimes difficult to differentiate from the surrounding ovarian tissue and can be identified only by their high vascularity. Cystic corpora lutea can contain either anechoic fluid or low level echoes (Fig. 5.10). In comparison to follicles, their walls are thicker and often irregular. A hemorrhagic corpus luteum is

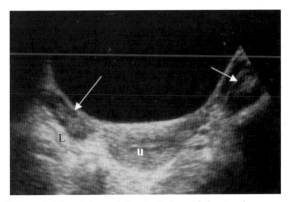

Figure 5.9B A transabdominal view of the ovaries (arrows) and uterus (u) in a transverse section. Note the hyperechoic endometrium and hypoechoic follicles within the left ovary (L).

recognized by the typical honeycomb appearance of its contents. The characteristic blood flow of a corpus luteum is halo-like and of high velocity and low resistance.

UTERINE ABNORMALITIES

Uterine fibroids

These are the most common gynecological tumor, being present in 50% of women over 40 years of

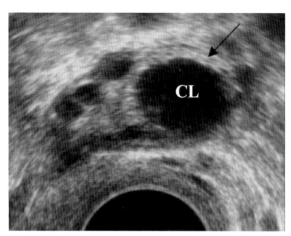

Figure 5.10 A cystic corpus luteum (CL) containing anechoic fluid. Note the thick echogenic cyst wall (arrow). See also Fig. 6.13.

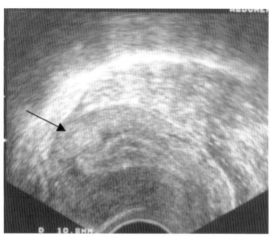

Figure 5.11 A small submucous fibroid indenting the uterine cavity in a retroverted uterus. The endometrium (+ – – +) is in the late proliferative phase with a clear midline echo, which is distorted by the fibroid (arrow). See also Fig. 6.5.

age. The vast majority are situated in the uterine body, although they can rarely be seen in the cervix and broad ligament. Women can present with a variety of symptoms ranging from menorrhagia to urinary frequency. The variable nature of clinical presentation is related to the size and position of the fibroid. Fibroids that lie within the myometrium without distorting the serosal surface or endometrial cavity are termed *intramural*. Those fibroids that distort the uterine cavity are *submucous* (Fig. 5.11) and a fibroid that distorts the serosal surface is called *subserous*. A large proportion of fibroids can be in more than one of these positions. Fibroids can also be *pedunculated* and submucosal, these fibroids will distort the endometrial cavity and might, if on a long stalk, prolapse though the cervix. Occasionally, a fibroid might be pedunculated and subserosal; these fibroids are often mistaken for an adnexal mass on clinical examination. Submucous fibroids should be classified according to the extent to which they extend into the uterine cavity. Hysteroscopic assessment of submucous fibroids classifies them into three types, a similar approach is possible with transvaginal ultrasound.

Fibroids are composed of smooth muscle fibers and fibrous connective tissue, which is arranged in concentric rings. In pregnancy, with the high levels of circulating estrogen, fibroids usually increase in size. The increase in size can outgrow the blood supply, leading to necrosis and degeneration, with resultant pain. In relation to pregnancy, submucous fibroids, which account for only 5% of all fibroids, are associated with infertility and miscarriage. They are also thought to increase the incidence of obstetric complications, such as antepartum hemorrhage, malpresentation and morbid adherence of the placenta. If large, cervical fibroids can cause obstruction of labor.

On ultrasound, fibroids might be single or multiple, and cause focal or generalized enlargement of the uterus. The outer contour of the uterus might be irregular because of the presence of focal subserous fibroids and the endometrial cavity might be distorted by the presence of submucous fibroids (Fig. 5.12). The myometrium is highly variable in echodensity depending on the size and position of the fibroid; the appearance of the myometrium is also affected by reflection and reduced transmission of ultrasound through a fibroid. This produces characteristic acoustic shadowing. There might also be areas of calcification, cystic degeneration and fluid levels within the fibroid. In pregnancy, a circumferentially calcified fibroid might be mistaken for a fetal head.

There might be areas of high velocity blood flow within the fibroid, especially if the fibroid is large. Those fibroids that have undergone central

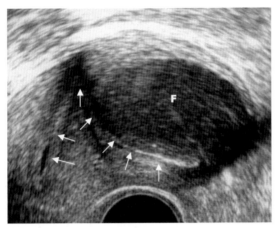

Figure 5.12 A large submucous fibroid (F) significantly distorting the uterine cavity (arrows). The fibroid is hypoechoic in relation to the surrounding myometrium. See also Fig. 6.5.

necrosis might demonstrate flow only in the peripherae. The use of Doppler in the evaluation of fibroids is limited because there is a wide range of flow and impedance values associated with fibroids. However, Doppler examination can be helpful in demonstrating the pedicle of a pedunculated fibroid, and thus helping to distinguish it from an ovarian fibroma.

Pedunculated subserous fibroids can be mistaken for ovarian tumors in the postmenopausal woman. Central cystic degeneration can mimic the appearance of an ovarian malignancy. If the ipsilateral ovary is not visible then careful Doppler interrogation can reveal a blood supply arising from the uterus and increased flow in the ipsilateral uterine artery.

Endometrial polyps

Endometrial polyps are a common finding in women of 35 to 50 years with abnormal vaginal bleeding, being present in up to 10% of cases. Women most commonly present with intermenstrual bleeding, and possibly dysmenorrhoea or infertility – it is postulated that the polyp prevents implantation of the blastocyst. Histologically, the polyp arises from the basal layer of the endometrium and is usually vascularized by a single vessel that passes through its stalk; this might be demonstrable on Doppler examination. Unlike

the endometrium from which they arise, endometrial polyps tend to be unresponsive to steroid hormones. Their appearance therefore remains similar throughout the menstrual cycle.

On ultrasound, endometrial polyps appear as distinct hyperechoic areas within the endometrium (Fig. 5.13). They are optimally visualized in the proliferative phase of the menstrual cycle when the hyperechoic polyp contrasts against the less echogenic endometrium. They are often found as isolated pathology, or they might be present within areas of endometrial hyperplasia or with endometrial carcinoma. The incidence of endometrial carcinoma arising within a polyp is less than 1%.

It can be more difficult to diagnose endometrial polyps in the secretory phase of the cycle because the echogenicity of the polyp and the endometrium is similar. The presence of fluid within the cavity will delineate the polyp from the endometrium. Thus, instillation of a small amount of fluid into the endometrial cavity, under aseptic technique, will aid in the identification of the polyp (Fig. 5.14).

Adenomyosis

This is a relatively common condition that affects women of reproductive age and is considered to be a variant of endometriosis. The histologic diagnosis of adenomyosis is made when endometrial

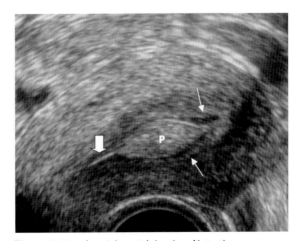

Figure 5.13 An endometrial polyp. Note the hyperechoic polyp (P) disrupting the midline echo (thick arrow) and the endometrium (thin arrows) around the polyp. See also Fig. 6.6.

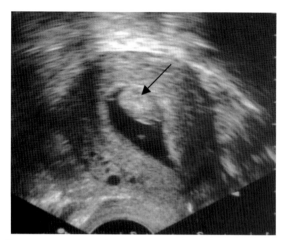

Figure 5.14 An endometrial polyp (arrow) protruding into the endometrial cavity that is distended with fluid during hydrosonography. See also Fig. 6.6.

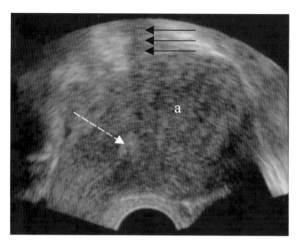

Figure 5.15 A large adenomyoma (a) seen at the fundus of the uterus casting an acoustic shadow (arrows). It is slightly distorting the endometrial cavity (broken arrow).

glands and stroma are seen within the myometrium. It is found to coexist with endometriosis in up to 20% of women. Adenomyosis typically presents in women who are in the latter part of their reproductive years and multiparous. The classic presenting symptoms are dysmenorrhea and menorrhagia. The disease is more common in women who have had previous uterine surgery, most commonly dilatation and curettage and cesarean section. On clinical examination, the uterus might be enlarged, especially on the posterior uterine wall, where adenomyosis is usually more extensive.

The ultrasound diagnosis of adenomyosis is problematic because there are no characteristic features. In most cases, the uterus appears normal or enlarged, and the posterior uterine wall might appear thickened. The myometrium can appear heterogenous with areas of both hyperechogenicity and hypoechogenicity representing areas of small myometrial cysts. These cysts contain the remnants of menstrual flow from the ectopic endometrium.

An adenomyoma is a focal, localized area of endometriosis and might be distinguishable as a focal echo-poor mass (Fig. 5.15). However, the appearances can be very similar to a uterine fibroid, which might be a coexistent pathology.

Management of adenomyosis is based on suppressing the cycling of the ectopic endometrial tissue and thus relieving symptoms. Principally, GnRH agonists and danazol are used for this. In a woman who has completed her family and in whom fertility is not an issue, hysterectomy might be considered.

Endometrial hyperplasia

The most common presenting symptom with endometrial disease is abnormal and/or irregular vaginal bleeding. The ultrasound findings are dependent on the age of the woman. A finding that is normal during reproductive years might be highly suspicious of pathology after the menopause. It is important, therefore, to obtain a complete history before the ultrasound examination.

Endometrial hyperplasia results from the prolonged action of estrogens that are unopposed by progesterone. Thus, it is more common to find this condition in women who have high circulating levels of estrogen, such as in women with polycystic ovaries, obesity, estrogen-producing tumors (e.g. granulosa cell tumor of the ovary) and women who are taking exogenous estrogens (e.g. hormone replacement therapy (HRT) and tamoxifen therapy; Fig. 5.16). The significance of endometrial hyperplasia lies not only in the symptomology but also because it is considered to a precursor of endometrial carcinoma.

The ultrasound appearance of endometrial hyperplasia is characteristic. The endometrium is usually thickened (> 10 mm) and demonstrates

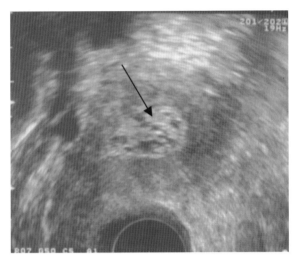

Figure 5.16   A large cystic, hyperechoic endometrial polyp (arrow) secondary to tamoxifen therapy.

increased echogenicity with occasional small cystic areas (Fig. 5.17). Small hyperechoic areas representing endometrial polyps might also be present. The three distinct forms of endometrial hyperplasia (cystic, adenomatous and atypical) are indistinguishable on ultrasound.

The final diagnosis of endometrial hyperplasia is made histologically. Therefore, in the presence of a history that is suggestive, together with suspicious ultrasound findings, endometrial sampling must be carried out.

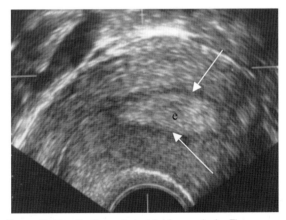

Figure 5.17   Cystic endometrial hyperplasia. The endometrium (e) is thick and hyperechoic in relation to the surrounding endometrium. It is irregular and cystic in appearance but a clear hypoechoic line demarcates the myometrial border (arrows).

The management of hyperplasia is dependent on its type and the patient's wishes regarding fertility. In all cases, any further investigations should be directed towards identifying and removing the source of the estrogen (i.e. discontinuation of HRT).

Cystic and adenomatous hyperplasia are unlikely to progress to endometrial carcinoma. Therefore expectant management is appropriate and any further investigations and treatment should be instigated only if there is recurrent bleeding. The presence of atypical hyperplasia indicates a high risk of coexistent, or progression to, carcinoma. Therefore, hysterectomy and bilateral salpingo-oophorectomy should be advised. In the younger patient who desires to maintain fertility, medical treatment with a prolonged course of progestogens (20 mg medroxyprogesterone/day for 8–12 weeks) and repeated currettage can be employed. In either case, long-term follow-up and early intervention in the presence of symptoms is paramount.

Drugs and the endometrium

Oral contraceptives

The most common oral contraceptive pill currently in use is the combined pill containing estrogen and progesterone. The estrogen and progesterone are usually taken for the first 21 days of the cycle, followed by a pill-free interval of 7 days to allow shedding of the endometrium. The endometrial appearances are uniform through the cycle. After prolonged use of the contraceptive pill the endometrium typically is thin, echogenic and regular in appearance. In the first few cycles of contraceptive pill use, however, a degree of stromal edema might be present. In such cases the endometrium appears thick and echogenic.

Clomiphene citrate

Clomiphene citrate is widely used in the treatment of anovulatory infertility. It acts by upregulating the production of pituitary gonadotrophins and hence causes the maturation of ovarian follicles. The endometrium continues to progress through its normal cyclical changes with clomiphene use.

RU 486 – mifepristone

The antiprogestogenic action of this synthetic steroid causes shedding of the endometrium. The ultrasound appearances are of highly disorganized endometrium, as would be expected during menses. It is now widely used in the medical termination of pregnancy.

Danazol

This synthetic derivative of ethisterone, with mild androgenic properties, is widely used in the treatment of endometriosis. It has minimal estrogenic and progestrogenic properties and causes the endometrium to become thin and atrophic with use.

Cyproterone acetate

This is an antiandrogen with progestogenic properties. It is used in the treatment of hirsutism in women and is often prescribed in combination with the combined oral contraceptive pill (Dianette). The use of cyproterone and its preparations can cause the endometrium to become thick and echogenic.

Tamoxifen

Tamoxifen is one of many steroid hormones with antiestrogenic properties. Its actions, however, are varied. It is used as an antiestrogen in the treatment and prevention of breast cancer. On the uterus, however, it has estrogenic properties, causing the proliferation of endometrium. These paradoxical effects are thought to result from the heterogeneity of the estrogen receptor – with response related to predominant subtype. The proliferation of the endometrium results in hyperplasia, metaplasia and can lead to carcinoma. Indeed, 50% of women taking tamoxifen will develop some type of endometrial pathology. Patients on long-term tamoxifen therapy have a six-fold increase in the risk of developing endometrial carcinoma, regardless of age.

On ultrasound, the endometrium is usually thickened (> 10 mm), echogenic and might have an irregular outline, with endometrial cysts often being present. Large endometrial polyps are char-

acteristic of tamoxifen therapy. These polyps can fill the entire uterine cavity and might be difficult to distinguish from the endometrium unless there is intracavity fluid present.

The presence of abnormal uterine bleeding together with thickened endometrium in women on tamoxifen therapy should warrant further investigation. Outpatient endometrial biopsy is not sufficient because tamoxifen causes subendometrial hyperplasia of the endometrial glandular epithelium. Therefore, the investigation of choice in this situation is formal endometrial curettage.

Hormone replacement therapy (HRT)

The use of cyclical estrogen and progesterone in women who are peri- and postmenopausal is common. The appearance of the endometrium is dependent on whether the woman is taking continuous combined estrogen with progesterone or cyclical estrogen and progesterone.

With continuous combined therapy, the endometrium should be uniformly thin (< 4 mm) and similar in appearance to that of a postmenopausal woman who is not taking HRT.

Cyclical HRT will cause changes in the endometrial appearance depending on when in a cycle the woman is examined. In such cases, ultrasound should be performed 7 days after the last progesterone tablet. At this time, the criteria for assessment of the endometrium are similar to all other premenopausal women.

Increased endometrial thickness (> 4 mm) in the presence of bleeding warrants further investigation with endometrial biopsy.

ABNORMALITIES OF THE FALLOPIAN TUBE

Hydrosalpinx describes the accumulation of serous fluid within one or both fallopian tubes. Hydrosalpinges can be mistaken for ovarian cysts, particularly in postmenopausal women in whom the ovaries might be atrophic and difficult to visualize. A hydrosalpinx is usually avascular and can appear either anechoic or echogenic on ultrasound. The distended fallopian tube can be confused with a ovarian cyst if the incomplete septations within the tube mimic the loculations of a multilocular cyst (Fig. 5.18). The terms 'beads on a string' or a

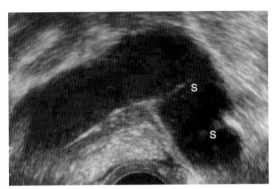

Figure 5.18 A hydrosalpinx containing anechoic fluid and incomplete septations (s). See also Fig. 6.18.

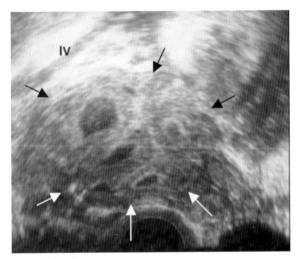

Figure 5.19 A tubo-ovarian abscess demonstrating thick irregular septations and echogenic fluid (arrows). The right external iliac vessels (IV) are visible laterally. This abscess was adherent to the lateral pelvic side wall.

'cogwheel appearance' also describe the appearances produced by the septations.

Tubo-ovarian abscess

A tubo-ovarian abscess typically appears as a multilocular mass with thick septations dividing areas of differing echogenicity. However, there is a wide variation in appearances (Fig. 5.19). Tubo-ovarian abscesses are usually well vascularized, bilateral and fixed in the pouch of Douglas. They can be difficult to characterize by ultrasound and clinical signs, which include fever, vaginal discharge and pelvic pain. Management is with broad-spectrum antibiotics until the pathogen is identified. As the cyst evolves, its septations break down and the locules become confluent. At this stage, vaginal drainage is possible under ultrasound guidance to avoid prominent blood vessels.

OVARIAN ABNORMALITIES

Polycystic ovaries

The polycystic ovarian syndrome was described by Stein and Leventhal in 1905 and is a triad of clinical symptoms, abnormal hormone profile and polycystic appearance of the ovaries on ultrasound. Universal agreement on the definition of polycystic ovarian syndrome is lacking but in the United Kingdom it is defined as polycystic ovaries together with either one or more clinical features (hirsutism, male-pattern baldness, obesity, amenorrhea, oligomenorrhea, acne) or raised serum concentrations of luteinizing hormone (LH) or testosterone.

A polycystic ovary is defined as an ovary that contains 10 or more cysts measuring 2–8 mm in diameter with an increase in ovarian stroma (Fig. 5.20). The increased stromal volume can be assessed by 3D ultrasound and is associated with raised serum androgen concentrations in women with polycystic ovaries. Polycystic ovaries also demonstrate an increase in stromal vascularity in comparison to that seen on Doppler interrogation of normal ovaries.

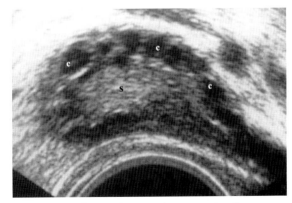

Figure 5.20 Polycystic ovary demonstrating the numerous small cysts (c) arranged peripherally and the typical increased volume of echogenic stroma (s). See also Fig. 6.10.

Polycystic ovaries are, however, commonly seen in up to 23% of asymptomatic women.

Multifollicular ovary

A multifollicular ovary is enlarged and contains six or more follicles of varying size arranged throughout the stroma of the ovary. This is in contrast to polycystic ovaries, in which the follicles are arranged centrapetally and are less than 9 mm in diameter. No increase in stromal volume is seen. The etiology of multifollicular ovaries is uncertain but might be due to a disordered hormonal environment, because they have been described in weight loss amenorrhea, puberty and the premenopause.

Luteinized unruptured follicle

If the ovulatory stimulus is inadequate to cause ovulation, or the follicle is too small to respond, then a luteinized unruptured follicle (LUF) can result. This appears as a simple anechoic cyst with a thick vascular wall, and might reach a diameter of 30 mm. Luteinized unruptured follicle syndrome has been linked to the use of non-steroidal anti-inflammatory drugs that inhibit the prostaglandin pathway essential for ovulation.

Functional cysts

Ultrasound examination can reveal the presence of follicular cysts in women with a history of irregular vaginal bleeding. These cysts appear similar to a follicle but are larger in size, and can occasionally reach more than 100 mm in diameter. They are usually poorly vascularized, thus differentiating them from luteal cysts, which have thicker and more irregular walls and, typically, a good blood supply.

The majority of functional ovarian cysts are detected incidentally in asymptomatic women. They are seen more often at the extremes of reproductive life when anovulatory cycles are commonplace.

The management of these cysts should be expectant as they usually regress spontaneously. A repeat examination after 6 weeks should be performed to confirm resolution. However, large functional cysts can cause pelvic pain, and occa-sionally ovarian torsion. In symptomatic women, intervention is sometimes necessary to alleviate symptoms.

True ovarian tumors that can be fully characterized using ultrasound

Histopathologic characteristics of ovarian tumors are highly variable and this is reflected in the wide spectrum of ultrasound findings. Certain types of benign ovarian tumor have pathognomonic features that enable a confident diagnosis using ultrasound alone.

Dermoid cysts

Dermoid cysts are present in about 2% of women and show a great variation in appearance (Figs 5.21, 5.22). These cysts can have cystic and solid areas and are usually poorly vascularized. They are characteristically located laterally in the ovary and are surrounded by a rim of normal ovarian tissue. They typically display mixed echogenicity and might include areas of calcification, due to bone or teeth, which cast acoustic shadows. Hair inside the cyst can be recognized by the presence of spicula-tions. *Struma ovarii* is a mature cystic teratoma made up predominantly of thyroid tissue. It has a multilocular appearance with thick septae and demonstrates increased vascularity.

Historically, management of dermoid cysts is an open ovarian cystectomy and routine bisection of

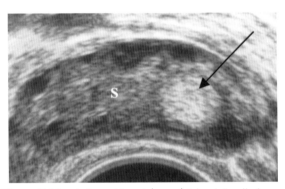

Figure 5.21 A dermoid cyst (arrow) lying laterally in the ovary surrounded by healthy ovarian tissue. The cyst appears hyperechoic in relation to the surrounding ovarian stroma (s). See also Fig. 6.15.

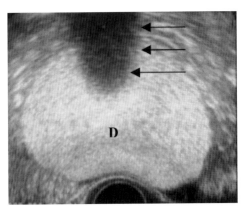

Figure 5.22 A large dermoid (D) casting an acoustic shadow, the 'iceberg' sign (arrows). The cyst appears hyperechoic in relation to the surrounding bowel but there is no ovarian tissue visible around the cyst. See also Fig. 6.15.

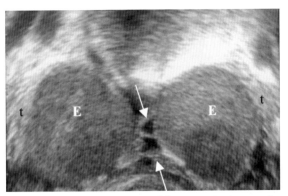

Figure 5.23 Endometriomata (E) 'kissing' in the pouch of Douglas. A rim of ovarian tissue (t) is visible around both cysts. Between the cysts there is an area of adhesions with typical anechoic fluid divided by thin septations (arrows). See also Fig. 6.14.

the contralateral ovary to exclude an occult tumor. However, if the contralateral ovary appears ultrasonically normal, this is unnecessary. Another option is to manage small, asymptomatic dermoids conservatively, with a repeat scan in 3–6 months to monitor growth. It is the authors' view that surgery in these cases leads to an excess of morbidity for a benign and often asymptomatic condition.

Endometrioma

Endometriomata are usually located centrally within the ovary and are surrounded by normal ovarian tissue (see Fig. 5.4). The ovaries might be 'kissing' in the pouch of Douglas (Fig. 5.23) or adherent to the uterus or pelvic sidewall. These masses are usually unilocular, have regular internal walls and contain echogenic fluid of a ground glass appearance. This fluid can be induced to move by gentle pressure on the cyst with the probe. Blood flow can be detected in approximately two-thirds of endometriomata.

The presence of endometriotic cysts might be associated with a hydrosalpinx. However, there is often no history of infertility or pelvic pain and detection is commonly made at the antenatal booking scan.

The management of these cysts should be aimed at controling pain and optimizing subsequent fertility. The use of the combined oral contraceptive pill, danazol and gonadotrophin-releasing hormone agonists are similarly effective, although symptom recurrence is common.

Ovarian masses that are difficult to classify using ultrasound

Many ovarian masses do not exhibit features that allow a specific ultrasound diagnosis to be made. In such situations we suggest that the role of the sonographer should be to provide as accurate a description of the mass as possible. This should include size, appearance, blood-flow characteristics and a differential diagnosis where appropriate.

REFERENCES AND FURTHER READING

Aslam N, Tailor A, Lawton F et al 2000 Prospective evaluation of three different models for the pre-operative diagnosis of ovarian cancer. British Journal of Obstetrics and Gynaecology 107: 1347–1353

Balen A H, Conway A S, Kaltsas G et al 1995 Polycystic ovary syndrome: the spectrum of the disorder in 1741 patients. Human Reproduction 10:2107–2111

Jurkovic D, Aslam N 1998 Three-dimensional ultrasound for diagnosis of congenital uterine anomalies. In: Merz E (ed) 3-D ultrasound in obstetrics and gynaecology. Lippincott Williams & Wilkins, Philadelphia, p 27–29

Tan S L, Zaidi J, Campbell S et al 1996 Blood flow changes in the ovarian and uterine arteries during the normal menstrual cycle. American Journal of Obstetrics and Gynecology 175:625–631

Valentin L 1999 Grayscale imaging and Doppler in pelvic masses. Ultrasound in Obstetrics and Gynecology 14:338–347

Chapter **6**

Ultrasound and infertility

Since the birth of the first IVF baby in 1978, a whole industry has developed to treat couples with problems associated with conception. 'Absolute infertility' was a diagnosis that once condemned couples to a life of childlessness, but this has now become relatively rare. With the advent of sophisticated assisted reproductive techniques, most health professionals prefer to use the term 'subfertility', implying a relative rather than absolute problem with conception.

Ultrasound has played a key role in the development of many of these techniques. It plays a vital role in the assessment and treatment of couples suffering from subfertility. Standard grayscale ultrasound imaging plays a primary role and is supported by the newer Doppler and 3D ultrasound techniques. A summary of the application of ultrasound technology to the management of subfertility is outlined below.

THE ROLE OF ULTRASOUND IN THE INVESTIGATION OF SUBFERTILITY

It is important to have some understanding not only of the leading causes of subfertility but also of the investigative processes used to determine a diagnosis. It is generally common practice to refer couples for assessment if they have not achieved conception following 1 year of unprotected intercourse, although this timescale can be tempered by a variety of factors, especially female age. The impact that age has on female fertility (and indeed success rates from fertility treatments) should not be underestimated and prompt referral, assessment and treatment should be instituted, particularly in women over 38 years of age.

The leading causes of subfertility are:

- ovarian/ovulatory dysfunction
- tubal dysfunction
- male factor problems.

Less common but equally important causes include:

- sexual dysfunction
- dysfunctional uterine environment
- cervical mucus hostility.

At least 25% of couples will have 'unexplained' subfertility and up to 30% will have more than one factor.

The assessment of a subfertile couple begins with a detailed history from both partners, as well as a thorough clinical examination. Investigations in the female patient are designed not only to detect any pathology but also to assess the normal reproductive cycle. Ultrasound is particularly useful at assessing both normal and abnormal female reproduction.

A general schema for investigation of subfertile couples is as follows:

- ovarian dysfunction
  - early menstrual serum level of follicle stimulating hormone (FSH)
  - midluteal progesterone level
  - pivotal transvaginal ultrasound (see below).
- tubal dysfunction. This can involve one of the following investigations:
  - X-ray hysterosalpingogram
  - laparoscopy with chromopertubation
  - hysterocontrast sonography (HyCoSy).
- male factor problems:
  - semen analysis.

Secondary investigations might be required but the above investigations will elucidate most major causes of subfertility.

Transvaginal ultrasound (TVS) is the method of choice for assessing the female reproductive organs.

It is helpful at this stage to introduce the concept of a 'pivotal' ultrasound scan (Table 6.1). Essentially, this involves performing a baseline transvaginal scan at an optimal time to ensure that

Table 6.1 The pivotal ultrasound (performed between days 8 to 12 of the menstrual cycle)

Area of the body	Information acquired
Uterus and uterine cavity	dimensions
	anomalies/tumors
Endometrium	thickness
	appearance
	hydrosonography (if indicated)
Uterine artery blood flow parameters	PSV (peak systolic velocity)
	PI (pulsatility index)
Ovarian morphology	normal/polycystic/multicystic
	position/mobility
	volume/antral follicle count
Follicular size	
Ovarian stromal and perifollicular blood flow parameters	PSV
	PI
Tubal patency	hysterosalpingo contrast sonography (HyCoSy)
Pelvis	presence or absence of free fluid/masses within pelvis

a maximal amount of information can be gained. If possible, this is best performed during the preovulatory phase of the menstrual cycle (usually days 8–12 of the cycle). At this stage in the cycle, information can be acquired about the uterine body, endometrium, fallopian tubes, ovaries and follicular development. The components of this pivotal scan can be altered depending on the level of technology available.

The female reproductive cycle also lends itself extremely well to assessment with Doppler ultrasound technology. One of the key events occurring within the ovary and endometrium is the formation of new blood vessels, or angiogenesis. This process can be directly assessed via Doppler, often giving valuable information that can be used to help predict treatment results.

Color Doppler imaging (CDI) uses the Doppler effect to display a color map of vessels within an organ. From this, measurements of velocity and resistance to flow can be taken. Color power angiography (CPA) is a newer modality that uses the amplitude of Doppler signals. Essentially, it represents the density of red blood cells within the vessels of the organ being studied. It is a more sensitive measure of overall blood flow within a particular organ.

The development of 3D ultrasound technology has extended the use of ultrasound in subfertility evaluation. This technology allows a volume of echoes to be captured rather than the more conventional 2D slices. This is done with the use of a specialized transducer, which moves in two planes. Once the volume of a particular organ is obtained it is generally analyzed by surface rendering software.

Uterine assessment

An understanding of the normal morphology and general dimensions of the uterus is important. The dimensions and appearance of the uterus should be recorded in both the longitudinal or sagittal plane (Fig. 6.1) and at 90° rotation in the coronal plane.

Transvaginal sonography is an excellent method of demonstrating uterine pathology. Leiomyomata (fibroids) are a common finding in women during the reproductive years. They can be subserosal, intra-

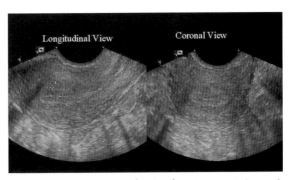

Figure 6.1 Longitudinal (sagittal) and coronal views of a normal uterus. 1, Longitudinal diameter; 2, transverse diameter; 3, endometrial thickness; + − − − + transverse diameter.

mural, submucosal or pedunculated (see Chapter 5). The presence of submucosal fibroids in particular is thought to interfere with embryo implantation. In addition, there is also an association with fibroids elsewhere in the myometrium and reduced fertility. The exact mechanism is unknown but might be related to an overall poor intrauterine environment impairing implantation.

Adenomyosis is a condition characterized by the presence of ectopic endometrium within the myometrium itself. Once a diagnosis only made at hysterectomy, adenomyosis is now increasingly being recognized with high resolution scanning. Ultrasound features of adenomyosis can be subtle and are often best appreciated with real-time scanning rather than hard-copy images (see Chapter 5). Recognized features include uterine enlargement without the presence of fibroids, often with an asymmetrical thickening of the anterior and posterior myometrium. The myometrium itself might have a heterogeneous appearance because of the presence of multiple small areas of ectopic endometrial tissue. More specific features might include myometrial nodules or cysts, possibly with discrete hemorrhagic foci. Although somewhat controversial, it does appear to be more prevalent in women with subfertility.

In addition to assessing uterine morphology, transvaginal ultrasound also allows an assessment of uterine mobility (fixity), the presence of free pelvic fluid (collecting in the pouch of Douglas) and the presence of lesions within neighboring organs, such as the bladder or rectum.

The advent of 3D ultrasound technology has also proved extremely useful in assessing uterine morphology and in particular helping to define uterine congenital abnormalities (Fig. 6.2).

Endometrial assessment

There are definitive changes of the endometrium throughout the menstrual cycle. Early in the menstrual cycle the endometrium is thin and is hypoechoic compared with the surrounding myometrium. As the follicular phase progresses, the endometrium thickens and takes on a characteristic trilaminar appearance (Fig. 6.3). Following ovulation the endometrium becomes more heterogeneous with a hyperechoic appearance compared to the surrounding myometrium (Fig. 6.4).

Lesions within the endometrium itself can also interfere with implantation. As well as the abovementioned submucous fibroids (Fig. 6.5), endometrial polyps (Fig. 6.6) can also be responsible for failure of implantation. These polyps can be identified with careful transvaginal scanning as effectively as more invasive procedures such as hysteroscopy. Saline contrast hysterosonography

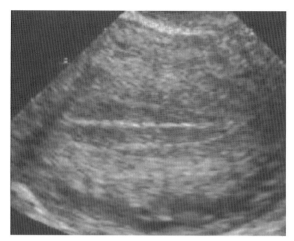

Figure 6.3 Longitudinal view of uterus demonstrating typical trilaminar appearance of proliferative phase endometrium.

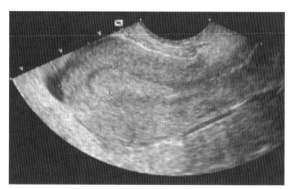

Figure 6.4 Longitudinal view of the uterus demonstrating typical hyperechoic appearance of secretory phase endometrium. 1, Longitudinal diameter; 2, transverse diameter; 3, endometrial thickness.

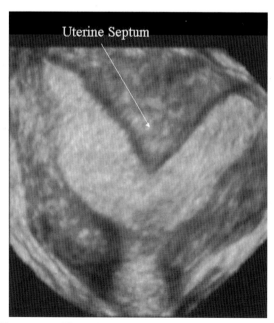

Figure 6.2 Three-dimensional image of a bicornuate uterus.

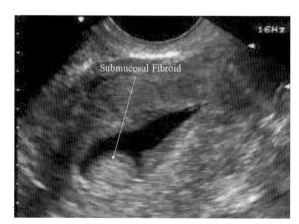

Figure 6.5 Submucous fibroid projecting into the uterine cavity. See also Figs 5.11 and 5.12.

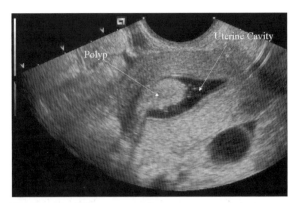

Figure 6.6 Saline contrast hysterosonography demonstrating the presence of an endometrial polyp. See also Figs 5.13 and 5.14.

(SCHS) can aid the diagnosis by further delineating the polyp.

Endometrial receptivity is a qualitative term used to describe a favorable situation with respect to implantation potential. This can be assessed during the pivotal scan by a combination of appearance and thickness, as well as estimating the uterine artery blood flow with Doppler ultrasound (Fig. 6.7). Typically, at the time of the pivotal scan during the late proliferative phase of the menstrual cycle, the following factors are regarded as markers of endometrial receptivity:

- minimum thickness of 7 mm
- trilaminar appearance
- uterine artery pulsatility index values (PI) < 3.0.

Assessing endometrial receptivity during investigation of subfertility can identify a group of patients who might otherwise have been classed as having 'unexplained' infertility. In addition, identifying these patients prior to treatment could afford the opportunity to institute therapy that can improve uterine or endometrial blood flow, and hence receptivity.

There is ongoing debate about the role of Doppler ultrasound assessment of uterine or endometrial blood flow in predicting likelihood of implantation.

There have been a number of studies that have shown differences in the uterine PI between women who have conceived and those who did not following IVF treatment. When the mean PI value within the uterine arteries is > 3.0 there is a

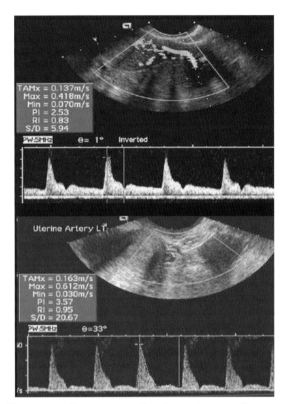

Figure 6.7 Uterine artery Doppler assessment. The upper panel shows a waveform typical of normal vessel resistance. The lower panel demonstrates a waveform from a vessel with elevated resistance.

reduced chance of successful implantation. More recently, interest has focused on subendometrial blood flow (Fig. 6.8). Using more conventional color Doppler it is possible to assess the degree of penetration of blood vessels into the endometrium. Absence of subendometrial vascularity correlates with a likelihood of failure of implantation.

Ovarian assessment

Transvaginal ultrasound is an excellent method of assessing the ovaries. In general, one should assess the following parameters with respect to the ovaries:

- appearance
- dimensions [length (l), width (w), depth (d)]
- volume (l × w × d × 0.5233)
- location/mobility/accessibility

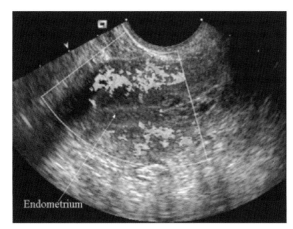

Figure 6.8 Color Doppler interrogation of the uterus demonstrating subendometrial blood flow.

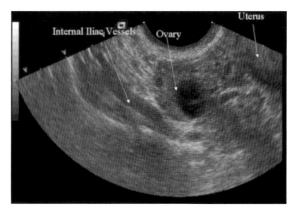

Figure 6.9 Transvaginal scan demonstrating a normal ovary and its anatomical relationships with the uterus and internal iliac vessels.

- dominant follicle
- stromal/follicular Doppler blood-flow parameters.

Using the transvaginal probe to view the uterus in a sagittal or longitudinal plane, the probe is then panned laterally to detect the ovaries. In this plane, measurements of length and width of the ovary can be obtained. By rotating the probe through 90° it will then be possible to measure the ovarian depth. In some situations, detecting the ovaries can prove troublesome. If there has been a previous hysterectomy then locating the ovaries can be difficult because the uterus can no longer be used as a reference point. Indeed, any surgery or pathological process within the pelvis can potentially disrupt the normal anatomical relationships and hinder the detection of the ovaries. In the postmenopausal woman the ovaries are often smaller and more homogenous with the surrounding tissues.

One of the advantages of scanning in the late preovulatory phase of the cycle is that at least one ovary will have a dominant follicle, which is usually readily visible as a hypoechoic area on the ovary. This, of course, applies only to women with regular menstrual cycles. If it is proving difficult to locate the ovaries, it might help to locate the internal iliac vessels and scan along their plane; the ovaries generally lie anterior to the internal iliac artery (Fig. 6.9).

The appearance of the ovaries is generally classified as:

- normal
- polycystic
- multicystic.

Polycystic ovaries (Fig. 6.10) are defined according to the following criteria (Adam's criteria):

- 10 or more cysts of between 2 and 8 mm arranged peripherally
- ovarian volume of > 8 cm³ (implying increased ovarian stroma).

Multicystic ovaries are distinguished from polycystic ovaries in that the cysts are spread throughout the ovary rather than peripherally.

The ovarian volume can be calculated from the measurements of length, width and depth using the formula l × w × d × 0.5233. In women with regular reproductive cycles the volume will vary

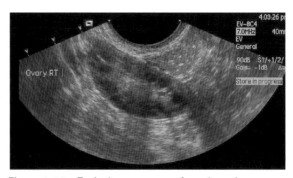

Figure 6.10 Typical appearance of a polycystic ovary demonstrating peripherally situated cysts and centrally increased ovarian stromal density. See also Fig. 5.20.

with the stage of the cycle and the presence or absence of a dominant follicle or corpus luteum. Postmenopausal women will normally have small volume ovaries that are approximately equivalent in size. Women with polycystic ovaries will often have an enlarged ovarian volume because of the associated increased stromal mass.

When the ovarian volume is less than 3 cm³ and there are fewer than five antral follicles, the 'ovarian reserve' is said to be reduced. This would imply that there is a significantly reduced chance of responding to ovarian stimulation during fertility treatment. It appears that this might be a more specific test than conventional early menstrual FSH estimation. Using 3D ultrasound technology it is possible to capture an image of the entire ovarian volume. Assessing the antral follicle count then becomes a relatively easy exercise (Fig. 6.11).

When scanning the ovaries in women who might require fertility treatment, it is important to assess not only their location but also their mobility and accessibility. This is particularly important for women who might undergo IVF treatment, in which access to the ovaries is imperative.

The presence of a dominant follicle (Fig. 6.12) can also be determined at the time of the pivotal ultrasound. This provides objective evidence of an ovulatory cycle. In addition, there is evidence to suggest that using Doppler to assess follicular blood flow can help identify those that contain better quality oocytes with greater fertilization

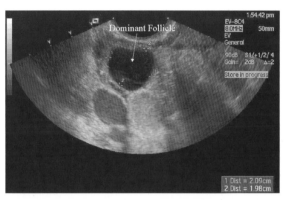

Figure 6.12 Normal ovary showing the presence of a preovulatory dominant follicle. Note the position of the two calipers, placed at 90° to each other, to obtain the mean follicular diameter of 20 mm in this plane.

potential and resultantly higher embryo implantation potential.

Apart from assessing intrinsic ovarian morphology and function, transvaginal ultrasound is also ideal for identifying ovarian pathology. Lesions such as functional or hemorrhagic cysts, endometriomata and dermoid cysts can generally be seen easily and, in most situations, a reasoned judgment can be made about the need for further treatment prior to embarking on fertility treatment. Simple or thin-walled cysts of less than 5 cm diameter are generally benign and usually resolve without any further treatment. Hemorrhagic cysts are commonly associated with bleeding into the corpus luteum (Fig. 6.13) and also generally resolve

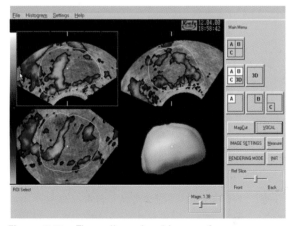

Figure 6.11 Three-dimensional image of an ovary obtained with surface rendering software.

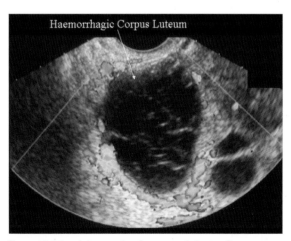

Figure 6.13 A hemorrhagic corpus luteum. Compare this with Fig. 5.10.

spontaneously. Fertility treatment should generally be deferred until resolution has occurred. Endometriomata (Fig. 6.14) are cysts that result from endometriosis occurring on the ovary. These cysts contain old blood and typically have a 'ground glass' appearance on ultrasound, with a uniform pattern of echoes. Dermoid cysts (Fig. 6.15) are benign tumours that result from totipotential cells found in the ovary. They can contain

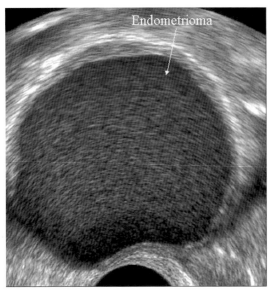

Figure 6.14 A large endometrioma demonstrating the typical 'ground glass' appearance. See also Fig. 5.23.

many different tissue types and have a variable appearance on ultrasound. They are often poorly defined and can easily be mistaken for bowel. Discrete echodense areas within the cyst resulting from a solid nodule of tissue, e.g. bone, characterize some dermoids.

It is well recognized that the presence of such ovarian lesions can negatively impact on ovarian stimulation, which is an integral part of many fertility treatments.

The presence of an adequate ovarian blood flow is essential to normal ovarian function. Although by no means conclusive, several studies have shown a relationship between ovarian stromal blood flow and the outcome of IVF treatment. Patients shown to have an ovarian stromal peak systolic velocity (PSV) of greater than 10 cm s^{-1} have higher clinical pregnancy rates than patients in whom the PSV is less than 10 cm s^{-1} (Fig. 6.16). Additionally, patients with polycystic ovaries tend to have stromal velocities that are significantly higher than normal ovaries. It is also known that they are at higher risk of ovarian hyperstimulation syndrome, particularly following IVF treatment. The detection of increased stromal flow in these patients can help to predict those most at risk.

The use of 3D CPA to assess ovarian vasculature has not been studied specifically in patients with subfertility. However it could become the assessment of choice because it is thought to be more sensitive than conventional 2D indices.

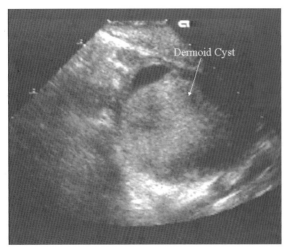

Figure 6.15 A dermoid cyst with characteristic poorly defined ultrasonographic features. See also Figs 5.21 and 5.22.

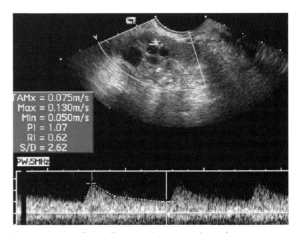

Figure 6.16 Color Doppler interrogation of an ovary demonstrating normal ovarian stromal blood flow.

Follicular assessment

Using color Doppler imaging, it is apparent that the PSV of blood flow surrounding the follicle is the best indicator of angiogenesis. A significant increase in PSV during the periovulatory period is also reported. It appears as though there is a relationship between follicular flow velocity and oocyte quality within a particular follicle. Presumably, follicles with good blood flow have a higher oxygen tension within the follicle, implying that the oocyte is less susceptible to hypoxia and damage (Fig. 6.17).

Certainly it has been shown that, in women undergoing IVF treatment, if the PSV of a particular oocyte is greater than 10 cm s^{-1} then there is an approximately 70% chance of the oocyte retrieved forming a grade I or II embryo after fertilization. This is compared with a less than 20% chance when there is low or no blood flow.

Fallopian assessment

Under normal circumstances, the fallopian tubes are not visible with ultrasound imaging unless there is fluid within the pouch of Douglas (rectovaginal space). However, when the tubes are damaged by infection they can become enlarged and form fluid-filled hydrosalpinges (Fig. 6.18). These

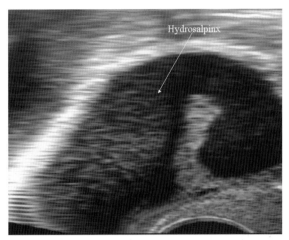

Figure 6.18 A hydrosalpinx. Note the presence of low level echoes within the distended fallopian tube, together with incomplete septations. See also Fig. 5.18.

are generally readily visible during scanning because the fluid within the tubal lumen provides a negative echo contrast. The presence of hydrosalpinges is an important prognostic feature. Where they are bilateral, it is believed that their presence could interfere with embryo implantation following IVF. The fluid contained within the tubal lumen appears to be embryotoxic. In this situation it is often advisable to consider removal of the hydrosalpinges, or at least proximal occlusion, prior to IVF treatment. The evidence where there is a unilateral hydrosalpinx is less clear.

An assessment of fallopian tube patency has a key role in the investigation of subfertility. Blocked fallopian tubes are a common cause of female subfertility. Conditions such as pelvic infection and endometriosis are relatively common and can be of an insidious nature. They can cause significant tubal damage without much in the way of symptoms to indicate this. In addition, any surgical procedure performed within the pelvis involves the risk of scarring and adhesions, which can impact on tubal function.

Determining tubal patency will help guide the clinician in the right choice of fertility treatment. Where the tubes are patent then the patient is more amenable to simpler fertility treatments, such as ovulation induction or intrauterine insemination, whereas in the situation of non-patent tubes, the patient will most likely require more sophisticated treatment, such as IVF.

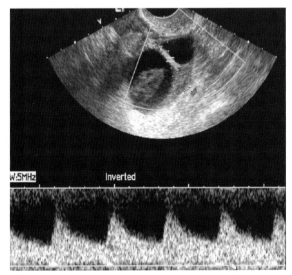

Figure 6.17 Color Doppler interrogation of an ovary demonstrating follicular blood flow.

Classically, the patency of the fallopian tubes has been assessed by:

- X-ray hysterosalpingogram (HSG): radio-contrast dye is infused into the uterine cavity via the cervix and a series of X-ray images captures the flow through the fallopian tubes.
- Laparoscopy with chromopertubation: a keyhole surgical procedure performed under general anesthetic. Methylene blue dye is infused in to the uterine cavity under direct vision.

Sonographic visualization of the fallopian tubes is also possible. Hysterosalpingo-contrast sonography (HyCoSy) involves the instillation of a positive contrast agent, such as Echovist® (Schering AG, Germany), into the uterine cavity during scanning. Flow of the contrast medium through the tubes and into the peritoneal cavity can be readily seen. This procedure can be performed as an adjunct to the pivotal scan. Using either pulsed or color Doppler, improved sensitivity for contrast flow can be obtained.

HyCoSy can provide similar information about tubal patency as the more traditional modes of investigation. When combined with saline contrast hysterosonography, the uterine cavity can equally be assessed. Three-dimensional CPA has also proved useful in assessing tubal morphology and patency. With conventional 2D HyCoSy it is often difficult to view the entire tubal length in a single scanning plane. By using power Doppler, which is sensitive to a slow flow of contrast medium, and by capturing the volume, it is possible to reconstruct a 3D image of the fallopian tube (Figs 6.19 and 6.20).

THE ROLE OF ULTRASOUND IN THE TREATMENT OF SUBFERTILITY

The development of transvaginal ultrasound has played a key role in the development of many fertility treatments. It is now widely used in the monitoring of fertility treatments and in a variety of invasive treatment procedures. A number of treatment procedures are available for couples experiencing subfertility. The choice of treatment depends not only on the etiology but also on the duration of subfertility and, in particular, the age of the female patient.

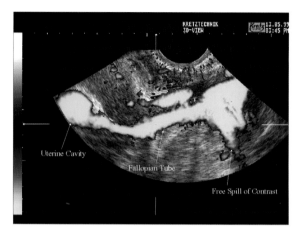

Figure 6.19 Three-dimensional color power Doppler HyCoSy demonstrating free peritoneal spill of contrast dye.

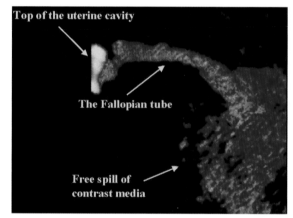

Figure 6.20 The same image as Fig. 6.19 following surface rendering of the three-dimensional image.

The treatment modalities available in which ultrasound plays a role are listed below.

Ovulation induction/intrauterine insemination

This procedure involves giving the patient medication to stimulate ovulation. Commonly used medications are clomifene citrate (an antiestrogen) or gonadotrophins. Ultrasound plays an essential role in monitoring these treatment cycles. Normally, patients are scanned around day 8 after starting ovarian stimulation, by which time it is possible to assess the size of the dominant follicle and the endometrial thickness and appearance. Not uncommonly, patients will produce multiple follicles. Scanning should be repeated until the leading follicle is between 16 and 18 mm in diameter. At this stage, a single injection of human chorionic gonadotrophin (hCG) is given to induce maturation of the oocyte and ovulation. This enables the couple to time intercourse or an insemination procedure with either the male partner's semen or donor semen.

When patients produce more than three follicles greater than 16 mm diameter, treatment should be abandoned because of the risk of a higher-order multiple pregnancy. Occasionally, ovarian hyperstimulation can occur, in which excessive numbers of follicles are produced.

In vitro fertilization (IVF)

This treatment procedure was originally developed for the treatment of tubal infertility but now has many indications. Transvaginal ultrasound plays a pivotal role at many stages of this treatment. Essentially, there are four key phases within a standard IVF cycle where ultrasound is invaluable:

1. Pituitary desensitization or 'downregulation' – the patient is given a gonadotrophin-releasing hormone agonist (GnRHa) to suppress the normal pituitary ovarian axis. In effect, this causes a 'temporary menopause'. This phase of treatment lasts around 2 weeks and improves the control of follicular development once superovulation is commenced. However, before commencing the next phase the patient is normally scanned to ensure downregulation has occurred. The typical features of downregulation are a thin endometrium (less than 4 mm) and quiescent ovaries containing only small follicles. Assessing ovarian stromal flow following downregulation can also be useful. Where the PSV is greater than 10 cm s^{-1} then a better ovarian response to superovulation and higher pregnancy rates can be expected.

2. Ovarian superovulation – once 'downregulation' is achieved, superovulation is commenced with daily injections of gonadotrophin (usually purified FSH or a combination of FSH and LH). The aim is to stimulate multiple follicular development with, on average, 10 or more follicles in both ovaries. Transvaginal ultrasonography is used to monitor follicular growth and the details are recorded on a folliculogram (Fig. 6.21). When the largest follicles (ideally more than three) are at least 18 mm in diameter and the endometrial thickness is at least 6 mm, then a single injection of hCG is given to induce maturation of the oocytes prior to collection (Fig. 6.22).

3. Oocyte collection – approximately 36 h after the hCG injection, the oocytes are retrieved from the ovary. The timing is important because oocyte maturation needs to have occurred but the oocytes must be retrieved before ovulation. The procedure itself is performed under transvaginal ultrasound guidance and, in most cases, with mild sedation only. A specialized needle guide is attached to the probe and each follicle is punctured and aspirated (Fig. 6.23). A two-way needle system can be used so individual follicles can be flushed with a medium to improve the collection of oocytes. Once the oocytes have been collected they are inseminated with sperm. In cases where there is a severe male factor problem, oocytes can be injected with individual sperm to achieve fertilization. This process is called intracytoplasmic sperm injection (ICSI).

4. Embryo transfer – this is normally performed 2–3 days after the oocyte collection. Usually one, two or three embryos are replaced into the uterine cavity by passing a fine silastic catheter through the cervical canal and into the cavity itself. This can be done under transabdominal ultrasound guidance to help guide positioning of the catheter within the uterine cavity (Fig. 6.24). At this stage, the endometrium should appear typically luteinized with a homogenous hyperechoic pattern. An assessment of uterine artery and endometrial blood flow prior to embryo transfer is sometimes useful. Where there is increased resistance to flow within the uterine arteries (PI > 3.0), then medication such as low-dose aspirin can be instituted in an attempt to improve the blood flow and increase the chance of successful implantation.

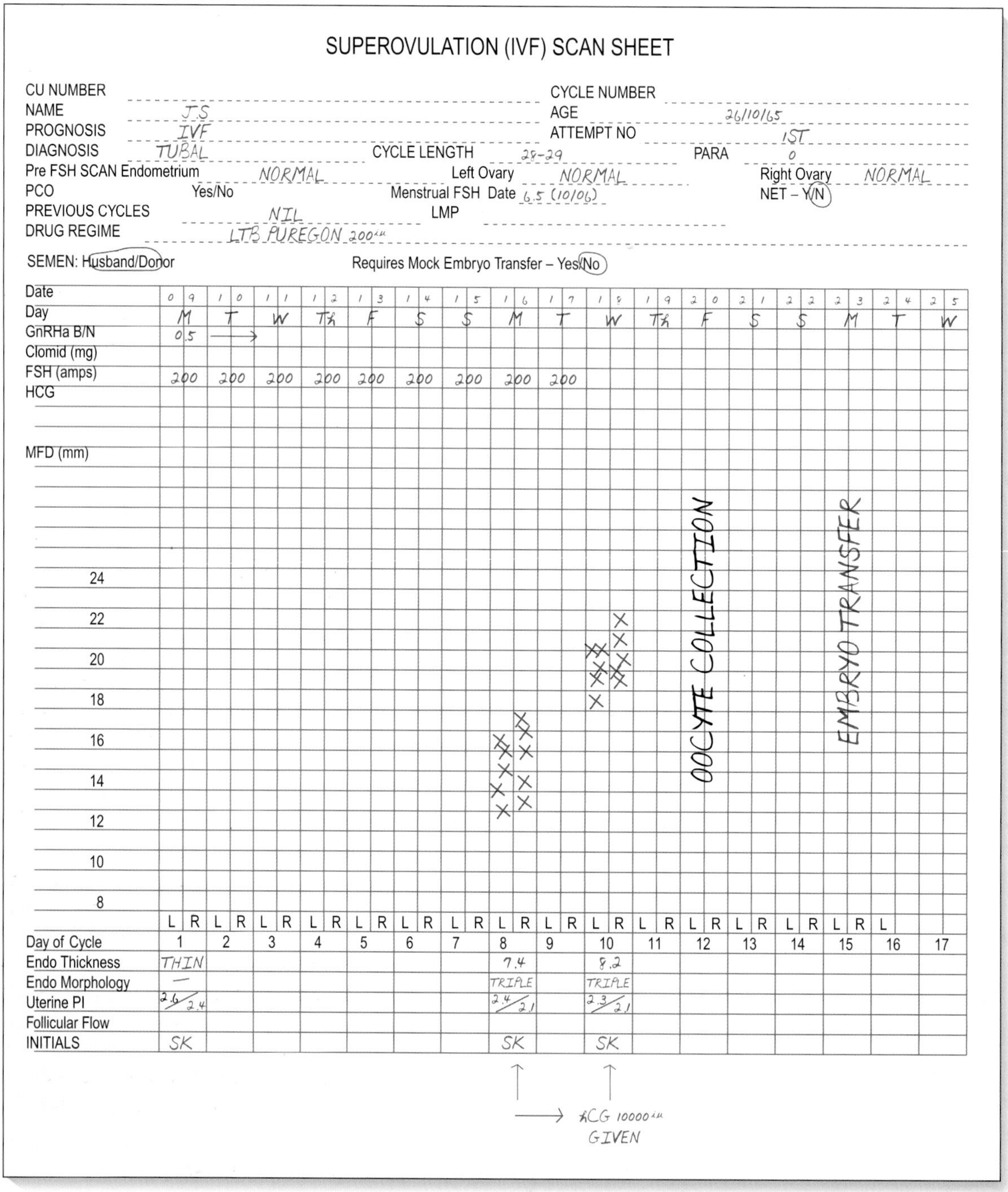

SUPEROVULATION (IVF) SCAN SHEET

CU NUMBER _____ CYCLE NUMBER _____
NAME _____ J.S. _____ AGE _____ 26/10/65 ____
PROGNOSIS _____ IVF _____ ATTEMPT NO _____ 1ST ____
DIAGNOSIS _ TUBAL _____ CYCLE LENGTH _ 28-29 _ PARA _ 0 _
Pre FSH SCAN Endometrium _ NORMAL _ Left Ovary _ NORMAL _ Right Ovary _ NORMAL _
PCO Yes/No Menstrual FSH Date 6.5 (10/06) NET – Y/(N)
PREVIOUS CYCLES _ NIL _ LMP _____
DRUG REGIME _ LTB PUREGON 200ıu _

SEMEN: Husband/Donor Requires Mock Embryo Transfer – Yes/(No)

Date	09	10	11	12	13	14	15	16	17	18	19	20	21	22	23	24	25
Day	M	T	W	TH	F	S	S	M	T	W	TH	F	S	S	M	T	W
GnRHa B/N	0.5	→															
Clomid (mg)																	
FSH (amps)	200	200	200	200	200	200	200	200	200								
HCG																	

MFD (mm)

OOCYTE COLLECTION

EMBRYO TRANSFER

	1	2	3	4	5	6	7	8	9	10	11	12	13	14	15	16	17
	L R	L R	L R	L R	L R	L R	L R	L R	L R	L R	L R	L R	L R	L R	L R	L R	L R
Day of Cycle	1	2	3	4	5	6	7	8	9	10	11	12	13	14	15	16	17
Endo Thickness	THIN							7.4		8.2							
Endo Morphology	—							TRIPLE		TRIPLE							
Uterine PI	2.6 2.4							2.4 2.1		2.3 2.1							
Follicular Flow																	
INITIALS	SK							SK		SK							

→ HCG 10000ıu GIVEN

Figure 6.21 Typical folliculogram demonstrating follicle monitoring during an IVF cycle.

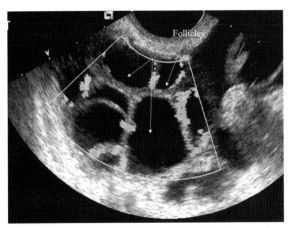

Figure 6.22 A stimulated ovary demonstrating multiple follicles with follicular blood flow during IVF treatment.

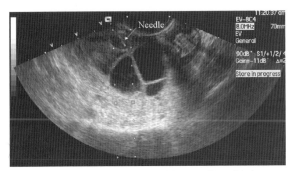

Figure 6.23 Oocyte collection. The needle, with its echogenic tip, can be visualized within one of the follicles, prior to aspiration of its follicular fluid and oocyte. The path of the needle guide is demonstrated (+ + +).

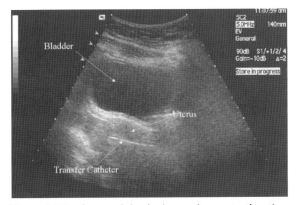

Figure 6.24 A transabdominal scan demonstrating the position of the catheter within the uterine cavity prior to embryo transfer. Note the appearance of the hyperechoic, luteinized endometrium.

Once the embryos have been replaced the patient is usually given progesterone supplementation to support corpora lutea function, because the GnRHa medication and the oocyte collection procedure may impair normal corpus luteum formation.

Oocyte donation

The use of donor oocytes has extended the boundaries of fertility treatment so that age is no longer a limiting factor. Essentially, the process involves the collection of oocytes from a known or anonymous donor. The donor ideally should be less than 35 years of age with proven fertility. She must undergo a cycle of IVF treatment as described above. The endometrium of the recipient must be prepared and be ready to receive the embryos at the correct phase of the donor's cycle.

Monitoring of the donor and recipient in tandem is crucial to the success of such a program. The donor is monitored as with a standard IVF cycle. For the recipient, a period of downregulation is often commenced in parallel with that of the donor. In the same way, downregulation is confirmed with the finding of a thin endometrium and quiescent ovaries at transvaginal ultrasound. When the donor begins superovulation, the recipient begins taking oral estrogen medication to stimulate endometrial proliferation. The recipient is scanned at similar intervals to the donor to ensure adequate endometrial growth. Ideally, by the time the donor is ready for oocyte collection the recipient's endometrium should be 7–8 mm thick with a typical triple layer appearance. The recipient is given progesterone to luteinize the endometrium at the same time that the donor is receiving the hCG injection prior to oocyte collection. At the time of embryo transfer the endometrium should be assessed to confirm that luteinization has occurred.

ULTRASOUND AND COMPLICATIONS OF FERTILITY TREATMENT

The development of sophisticated fertility treatments brings with it new complications. These can be complications arising as a result of the treatment procedures and also complications as a result of pregnancy.

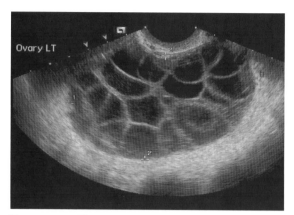

Figure 6.25   The appearance of an ovary demonstrating multiple follicular development characteristic of ovarian hyperstimulation syndrome.

Treatment-related complications

One of the most common and most feared complications is ovarian hyperstimulation syndrome (OHSS). This arises when the ovaries massively overrespond to stimulating medication, resulting in the development of multiple follicles (Fig. 6.25). It occurs in a mild or moderate form in around 5% of cycles and is severe in approximately 1–2% of cycles. The symptoms tend not to develop until the follicles have been luteinized (i.e. following oocyte collection) and are often aggravated if the patient conceives. Depending on the degree of severity, the patient can present with abdominal distention, nausea and vomiting and signs of dehydration.

In moderate to severe OHSS, ultrasonography will demonstrate enlarged ovaries, possibly with the presence of ascites. Patients might require hospitalization and the condition can be life threatening, with most of the recorded deaths being attributable to thromboembolic events secondary to dehydration.

In the majority of situations, OHSS is a self-limiting process that is prolonged if pregnancy occurs. Patients who are more likely to develop OHSS are those with polycystic ovaries, particularly if they have high ovarian stromal flow, or an elevated luteinizing hormone level prior to treatment. Those who have previously had OHSS are also at risk.

Transvaginal ultrasound can also play a useful role in draining ascitic fluid to provide symptom relief. Where there is significant ascites, this fluid will often collect in the pouch of Douglas. Using a needle guide attached to a transvaginal probe, drainage is a simple procedure.

Other complications related to treatment procedures are generally associated with the oocyte collection. These include vaginal or intra-abdominal bleeding and pelvic infection or abscess formation.

Pregnancy-related complications

Complications of early pregnancy are more common following fertility treatment. Both the risk of miscarriage and of ectopic pregnancy are higher in these patients and this should be considered when scanning in early pregnancy.

In patients who have undergone IVF treatment where more than one embryo has been replaced, it is important to consider the possibility of a coexistent intrauterine and ectopic pregnancy (heterotopic pregnancy). In nature the incidence of such an event is between 1 in 4000 and 1 in 30 000 pregnancies. Following IVF treatment the risk can be as high as 1 in 100 pregnancies.

ULTRASOUND AND MALE INFERTILITY

There is now a mounting body of evidence to suggest that a link exists between male subfertility and the development of testicular cancer. Although a thorough clinical examination is mandatory for all men with subfertility, many now advocate that routine scrotal ultrasound should be an integral component of the investigation process. Several studies have demonstrated an association with a variety of scrotal pathologies in subfertile men. Additionally, a number of testicular malignancies seen at ultrasound were not detected on clinical examination.

A description of testicular ultrasound features is beyond the scope of this chapter but its importance should not be underestimated.

REFERENCES AND FURTHER READING

Ayida G A, Balen F G, Balen A H 1996 The usefulness of ultrasound in infertility management. Contemporary Reviews in Obstetrics and Gynaecology 8:32–38

Dickey R P 1997 Doppler ultrasound investigation of uterine and ovarian blood flow in infertility and early pregnancy. Human Reproduction Update 3:467–503

Friedler S, Schenker J G, Herman A et al 1996 The role of ultrasonography in the evaluation of endometrial receptivity following assisted reproductive treatments: a critical review. Human Reproduction Update 2:323–335

Jacobsen R, Bostofte E, Engholm G et al 2000 Risk of testicular cancer in men with abnormal semen characteristics: cohort study. British Medical Journal 321:789–792

Pairletner H, Steiner H, Hasenoehrl G et al 1999 Three-dimensional power Doppler sonography: imaging and quantifying blood flow and vascularization. Ultrasound in Obstetrics and Gynecology 14:139–143

Sladkevicius P, Campbell S 2000 Advanced ultrasound examination in the management of subfertility. Current Opinion in Obstetrics and Gynaecology 12:221–225

Sladkevicius P, Ojha K, Campbell S et al 2000 Three-dimensional power Doppler imaging in the assessment of Fallopian tube patency. Ultrasound in Obstetrics and Gynecology 16:644–647

Chapter 7

Routine second trimester screening – assessing gestational age

All ultrasound examinations benefit from a methodical approach and this is especially true when measurements are required. However, a second trimester ultrasound examination should be more than a means of confirming gestational age because it provides an ideal opportunity for assessing fetal anatomy and therefore structural normality. In addition, assessment of placental morphology, amniotic fluid volume and the comparative interpretation of various measurements are all important pointers to potential problems. Such an examination is commonly referred to as a 'routine second trimester anomaly scan'.

The optimal time at which to offer the routine anomaly scan is the earliest gestation at which the necessary measurements and a full fetal anatomy survey can be performed and the latest gestation at which an acceptable range of options can be offered to the parents if an abnormality is detected. Although the measurements required to date the pregnancy accurately can be taken after 15 weeks of gestation, and most of the fetal anatomy can be evaluated at 18–20 weeks, it is frequently difficult to examine the fetal heart and the outflow tracts properly at this time. The optimal time to examine the heart is at 23–24 weeks, a gestation at which fetal viability must be considered. A compromise must therefore be made. We recommend that the routine anomaly scan is performed between 20 and 22 weeks because a full anatomical survey of the fetus, including assessment of the fetal heart, can be performed in the majority of cases at this gestation.

In the majority of normal pregnancies, measurement of the biparietal diameter (BPD) and femur length (FL) provide the most accurate assessment of gestational age in the second trimester. We recommend that measurements of the head circumference (HC), transcerebellar diameter (TCD) and abdominal circumference (AC) are also undertaken. They provide further confirmation of gestational age and aid in the exclusion of growth-related abnormalities and spina bifida. In addition, their inclusion encourages a systematic examination of the whole fetus.

As assessing gestational age, fetal anatomy, amniotic fluid volume and placental position are integral components of the same examination, we recommend the experienced sonographer adopts the following scanning sequence:

1. Determine the number of fetuses (see Chapter 3).
2. Determine the longitudinal lie of the fetus; confirm fetal situs is normal.
3. Check the fetal heart is beating.
4. Show the woman her baby's image on the screen.
5. Measure the BPD, HC and TCD, evaluate the intracranial anatomy and nuchal area on these two sections.
6. Return to a longitudinal section that demonstrates the full length of the fetal spine. Evaluate the spine including the sacrum and its skin covering. Note the position of the fetal stomach below the diaphragm.
7. Rotate the probe through 90° to obtain a transverse section of the fetal chest. Evaluate the four-chamber view of the fetal heart and both outflow tracts. Continue to evaluate the cross-sectional anatomy while sliding the probe down the fetal body to the AC section. Measure the AC.
8. Evaluate the cross-sectional anatomy of the lower fetal abdomen while sliding the probe down the fetal body to the sacrum. Find the femur and measure it.
9. Confirm the presence of three long bones in each limb. Confirm the presence of two hands and two feet and that the carrying angle of each is normal. Obtain a plantar view of each foot. Obtain a view of the fingers of each hand.
10. Evaluate the coronal section of the fetal face, the fetal lips, alveolar ridge and profile.
11. Observe the fetus for body and limb movements.
12. Evaluate amniotic fluid volume.
13. Localize the placenta relative to the internal os.
14. Confirm or assign gestational age.
15. Decide whether any further follow-up is necessary.
16. Discuss the findings with the woman.
17. Issue a written report accompanied by graphical representation of the biometric data.
18. Arrange further follow-up as appropriate.

We recommend the novice sonographer begins by learning how to accomplish the basic measurements of BPD, HC, TCD, AC and FL and uses the following scheme:

1. Determine the number of fetuses (see Chapter 3).
2. Determine the longitudinal lie of the fetus. Confirm fetal situs is normal.
3. Check that the fetal heart is beating.
4. Show the woman her baby's image on the screen.
5. Measure the BPD, HC and TCD. Evaluate the intracranial anatomy of these two sections.
6. Return to a longitudinal section, which demonstrates the full length of the fetal spine. Note the position of the fetal stomach below the diaphragm.

7. Rotate the probe through 90° to obtain a transverse section of the fetal chest. Slide the probe down the fetal body to the abdominal circumference section. Measure the AC.

8. Slide the probe down the fetal body to the sacrum. Find the femur and measure it.

9. Observe the fetus for body and limb movements.

10. Localize the placenta relative to the internal os.

11. Evaluate amniotic fluid volume

12. Confirm or recalculate gestational age.

13. Ask your teacher to confirm that the images you have taken are correct, that you have taken the measurements correctly and to finish the examination.

Having gained these skills we recommend you then progress to evaluating the fetal anatomy in full, as described previously.

FINDING THE LONGITUDINAL AXIS OF THE FETUS

Place the transducer on the maternal abdomen to obtain a midline longitudinal section of the uterus. Slide the transducer to each side of the abdomen until the fetal head is visualized. Repeat the process to identify the fetal heart within the fetal chest. Slowly rotate the transducer, keeping the heart in view, until a longitudinal section of the fetal body is obtained. By sliding or altering the angle of the transducer with respect to the maternal skin,

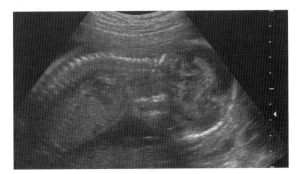

Figure 7.1 Longitudinal section of fetal head and upper spine. This is the section required to determine the fetal lie.

a longitudinal section of the fetal spine will be obtained. Rotate the transducer such that the fetal head and body are visualized on the screen together, as shown in Fig. 7.1.

Knowing the relationship of the longitudinal axis of the fetus to the maternal abdomen establishes fetal lie, is necessary to confirm normal fetal situs and is an important preliminary to obtaining accurate measurements of the fetal head and abdomen.

CONFIRMING NORMAL FETAL SITUS

Various severe cardiac diseases are associated with abnormal situs and identifying abnormal fetal situs is an important precursor to their diagnosis. Confirming normal fetal situs should therefore be one of the first objectives of the second trimester examination.

In the normal fetus, the stomach, cardiac apex and aortic arch lie on the left side of the body and the inferior vena cava lies on the right (situs solitus). Situs inversus is a mirror image of this arrangement. If some of the organs are correctly positioned but others are not this is termed situs ambiguous (or heterotaxy).

Determining which side of the fetus is its left side requires the correct understanding of, first, how the fetus is lying in the uterus and, second, how this position relates to the image orientation on the monitor. Let us consider the following example. The fetus is cephalic, lying with its spine uppermost, the left side of the fetus is therefore towards the maternal left. The maternal left appears on the right side of the image. The stomach and the cardiac apex should be visualized on the right side of the monitor (Fig. 7.2A). In Fig 7.2B the maternal left is to the right of the monitor. The fetus is breech, lying with its spine uppermost, the left side of the fetus is therefore towards the maternal right. The stomach and the cardiac apex should be visualized on the left side of the monitor. In Fig 7.2C the maternal left is to the right of the monitor. The fetus is cephalic, lying on its side with its spine to the maternal left. In transverse section the fetal spine will be visualized on the right of the monitor. The fetal stomach and the cardiac apex should be visualized posterior to the

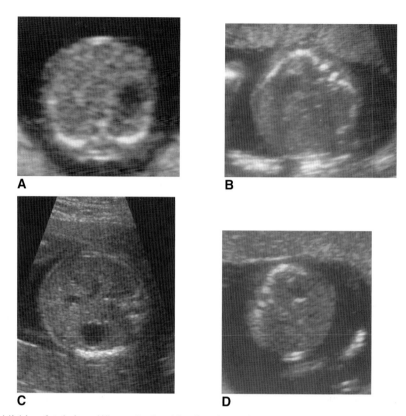

Figure 7.2 Establishing fetal situs. Where the fetal landmarks such as the stomach appear on the ultrasound monitor depends on the position of the fetus and orientation of the image. In all examples, the maternal left side is on the right side of the monitor. A. The fetus is cephalic, with its spine posterior. The fetal stomach should be visualized to the right side of the monitor if the situs is normal. B. The fetus is breech, with its spine uppermost. C. The fetus is cephalic, lying with its spine to the maternal left. The fetal spine should be visualized to the right side of the monitor and the stomach posteriorly if the situs is normal. D. The fetus is cephalic, lying with its spine to the maternal right. The fetal spine should be visualized to the left side of the monitor and the stomach anteriorly if the situs is normal.

spine, at the bottom of the image. In Fig 7.2D the maternal left is to the right of the monitor. The fetus is cephalic, lying on its side with its spine to the maternal right. In transverse fetal section the fetal spine will be visualized on the left side of the monitor. The fetal stomach and the cardiac apex should be visualized anterior to the spine, at the top of the image.

Variations of these themes are best worked out by mentally placing yourself in the uterus in the position occupied by the fetus and then working out where you expect the left side of the fetus to appear on the monitor.

MEASURING THE BIPARIETAL DIAMETER (BPD)

The BPD has traditionally been the most widely used ultrasound parameter in the estimation of gestational age. Although more recent data suggest that head circumference (HC) should be used in preference to BPD for dating purposes, the BPD is easy to obtain and, on a routine basis, is more accurate than the crown–rump length. A single optimal measurement of the BPD will predict the gestational age to within ± 5 days. It is more accurate at predicting the date of delivery than an optimal menstrual history. This last point has justified its use in all pregnancies.

The BPD is the maximum diameter of a transverse section of the fetal skull at the level of the parietal eminences. The BPD, occipitofrontal diameter (OFD) and head circumference can be measured from one of the following two sections:

- *Lateral ventricles view*: the correct section is demonstrated in Fig. 7.3, and should include the following features:
  - a rugby-football-shaped skull, rounded at the back (occiput) and more pointed at the front (synciput)
  - a long midline equidistant from the proximal and distal skull echoes
  - the cavum septum pellucidum bissecting the midline one-third of the distance from the synciput to the occiput
  - the two anterior horns of the lateral ventricles, symmetrically placed about the midline
  - all or part of the posterior horns of the lateral ventricles symmetrically placed about the midline. In earlier gestations (15–20 weeks),

the optimal view of the posterior horn is usually obtained in this section (see below). At later gestations (20–24 weeks), the optimal section for visualizing the posterior horn is slightly lower than the BPD section.

- *Thalami view*: the correct section is demonstrated in Fig. 7.4 and should include the following features:
  - a rugby-football-shaped skull, rounded at the back (occiput) and more pointed at the front (synciput)
  - a short midline equidistant from the proximal and distal skull echoes
  - the cavum septum pellucidum bisecting the midline one-third of the distance from the synciput to the occiput
  - the thalami
  - the basal cisterns.

There is no consensus as to which section is preferable. We recommend using the lateral ventricles view because this enables the anterior and posterior horns of the lateral ventricles to be examined and the head measurements to be taken from the same section. However, the thalami view is the section of choice in the American literature and in many departments in the United Kingdom. The BPD and HC measurements obtained from both sections are comparable.

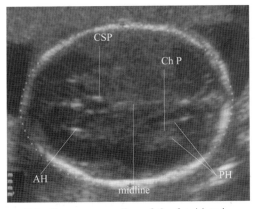

Figure 7.3 Transverse section of the fetal head demonstrating the landmarks required to measure the BPD using the lateral ventricles view. Note the rugby football shape, the centrally placed midline, the presence and position of the cavum septum pellucidum (CSP), and the appearance and position of the anterior horns (AH) of the lateral ventricles. Note the choroid plexus (ChP) within the distal posterior horn (PH) of the lateral ventricle and reverberation causing poor visualization of the proximal posterior horn.

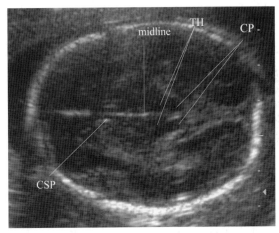

Figure 7.4 Transverse section of the fetal head demonstrating the landmarks required to measure the BPD using the thalami view. CP, cerebral peduncles; CSP, cavum septum pellucidum; TH, thalami.

Measuring the BPD from the lateral ventricles view

Obtain a longitudinal section of the fetus as described above. Small sliding movements of the transducer on each side of the fetal spine will give a longitudinal section of the fetal head that will demonstrate a strong midline echo (Fig. 7.5). By rotating the transducer through 90° a transverse section of the fetal head is obtained. If the midline is not in the exact middle of the section, alter the angle of the probe slightly on the maternal abdomen. This corrects for the angle of asynclitism. Once the midline is centrally placed do not alter the angle of the probe. Now assess the shape of the fetal skull. The required shape is that of a rugby football, with the more pointed end at the synciput. As the cavum lies one-third of the distance from the synciput to the occiput, identifying the cavum will allow you to determine which is the front and the back of the head. If the section is not the required ovoid shape, make minor rotational adjustments. If the landmark features listed above are not evident when the midline and shape are correctly imaged then the level of the section is wrong and should be corrected by small sliding movements of the probe up or down the fetal head.

The BPD is then measured on the frozen image. Place the intersection of the two arms of the first onscreen caliper on the outer aspect of the proximal skull surface. Place the intersection of the two arms of the second caliper on the outer aspect of the distal skull surface at right angles to the midline and at the widest diameter (Fig. 7.6). This BPD measurement includes the thickness of both parietal bones and is commonly described as an 'outer to outer' measurement.

Some centers include the thickness of only one (the upper) parietal bone when measuring the BPD. This measurement is commonly described as an 'outer to inner' measurement. The two techniques will produce BPD measurements that differ typically by 2–3 mm in the second trimester, approximately equivalent to 1 week of gestation. There is no consensus regarding which technique is more acceptable, although the 'outer to inner' method finds greater favor with the physicists. This is because the anterior edge of the parietal echo is less influenced by the equipment's controls than the posterior edge. The 'outer to inner' measurement is thus a more accurate representation of the true distance selected for measurement than the 'outer to outer'. What is critically important is that the technique used (including the section selected for measurement) corresponds to that employed when the reference data, that is the biometry

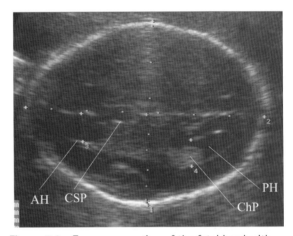

Figure 7.6 Transverse section of the fetal head with the callipers placed on the outer border of both the proximal and distal parietal bones (diameter 1). The measurement therefore produces an 'outer to outer' BPD measurement. The occipitofrontal diameter has also been measured in this image (diameter 2). Note the placement of the calipers to produce an 'outer to outer' OFD measurement. Measurements of the anterior and posterior horns of the distal lateral ventricle and distal hemisphere have also been taken (diameters 3, 4 and 1, respectively).

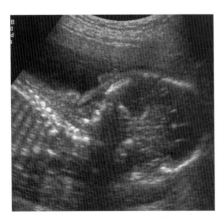

Figure 7.5 A longitudinal section of the fetal head and spine demonstrating the midline echo. Rotating the transducer through 90° should produce the sections demonstrated in Figs 7.3 and 7.4.

charts, were produced. We recommend using the 'outer to outer' technique because this measurement can be combined with the occipitofrontal diameter measurement to estimate the 'derived' HC measurement (see p. 102).

Problems

Incorrect angle.   If the angle of the probe on the maternal abdomen is incorrect, the midline echo does not lie centrally within the fetal skull (Fig. 7.7B and E). Similarly, the echoes from the lateral ventricles will not be visualized symmetrically about the midline. The angle of the probe to the maternal abdomen should be altered, without sliding or rotating the probe.

Incorrect rotation.   This is readily recognized because the visualized shape of the fetal skull is not that of a rugby football – it is usually too round – and/or not all the landmark features are seen. For example, visualizing the anterior horns together with the cerebellum indicates that the selected level at the back of the head is too low (Fig. 7.7F). This, in fact, is the suboccipitobregmatic view required for measurement of the TCD (see p. 103). Visualizing the orbits together with the posterior horns of the lateral ventricles indicates that the selected level at the front of the head is too low (Fig. 7.7D). A slightly higher level at the front of the head, between the orbits and the anterior horns, can produce the false impression of a lemon-shaped skull (see p. 101). Rotating the probe will correct the shape but you must be careful to maintain the correct angle.

Incorrect level.   Sliding movements of the probe will alter the level of section. A continuous midline indicates the selected level is too high (Fig. 7.7A). A section demonstrating the orbits and the cerebellum is too low. Be careful not to rotate or change the angle of the probe as you slide.

Midline not horizontal.   Having obtained the correct section displaying the required landmarks check that the midline is not lying at an angle to the horizontal (Fig. 7.7C). Dipping one end of the probe will orientate the head into the correct position.

BPD measurements in breech and transverse presentations.   In the second half of pregnancy, BPD measurements obtained from fetuses presenting transversely or by the breech can be unreliable. In these presentations the fetal head might be dolichocephalic (long and narrow) in shape. This produces a BPD measurement that is artifactually small for gestational age. The head circumference measurement, however, is unaltered by presentation and is therefore a reliable indicator of gestational age irrespective of fetal presentation.

OP/OA position.   Measurement of the BPD should only be taken when the fetal head is in the occipitotransverse (OT) position, because the landmarks are best recognized when the midline echo and the other landmarks are at 90° to the ultrasound beam. The BPD should therefore not be measured if the fetal head is directly occipitoposterior (OP), directly occipitoanterior (OA) or deep in the maternal pelvis. Tilting the woman into a 45° head-down position and/or partially filling the maternal bladder might displace and rotate the fetal head such that it can be measured. Alternatively, transvaginal imaging could be attempted. If these options are unsuccessful, estimation of gestational age could be made from measurement of femur length, but we recommend rescanning the woman at a later date to ensure that the intracranial anatomy is normal.

Evaluating the intracranial anatomy from the lateral ventricles view

It is important to observe the information presented in a section selected for measurement and thus to familiarize yourself with the range of normal appearances at a specific gestation. Once you have this experience you will immediately identify a finding that is not normal, even if you do not have the expertise to make the diagnosis. For example, make sure the cavum is normal in size and position. Similarly, make sure that the choroid plexus fills the posterior horn of the lateral ventricle and is of a homogeneous echogenicity. Evaluate the echo pattern in both halves of the brain to exclude any unusual echo-poor or echo-bright areas, ensuring that the echo pattern in both halves of the brain is similar and symmetrical about the midline. Are the intracranial contents of normal echogenicity or do they appear brighter than usual, such that you may have reduced the gain slightly? Abnormally echo-bright skull contents are

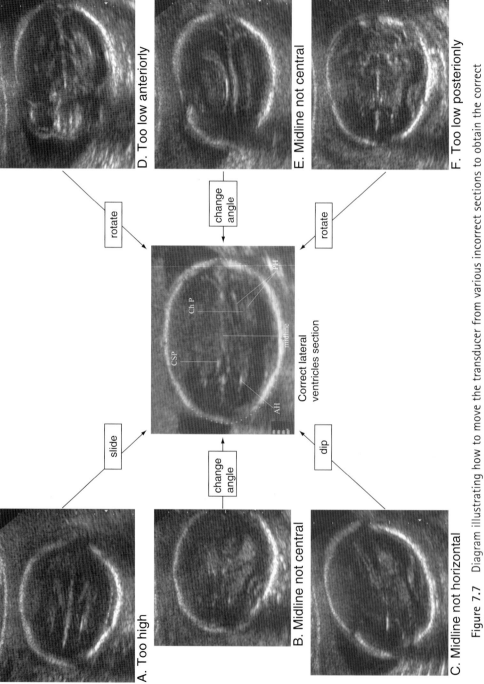

Figure 7.7 Diagram illustrating how to move the transducer from various incorrect sections to obtain the correct section on which to measure the BPD from the lateral ventricles view. CSP, cavum septum pelluctoum; ChP, choriod plexus; PH, posterior horn of lateral ventricle; AH, anterior horn.

unlikely to indicate a brain abnormality but rather skull hypomineralization, as seen in osteogenesis imperfecta type 11 or hypophosphatasia.

Skull shape

It is important to observe the normal shape of the fetal skull and appreciate how this varies, albeit subtly, with increasing gestation. As discussed above, the shape of the normal skull at 20–22 weeks is that of a rugby football. Abnormal scalloping of the frontal bones produces a more angular appearance to the front of the skull in this view. This is known as the 'lemon' sign and is associated with spina bifida. However, a similar appearance is demonstrated by the skull of the normal fetus early in the second trimester, before 16 weeks. It can also be obtained in a normal 20–22 week fetus from an incorrect BPD section, if the probe is rotated slightly too far toward the fetal orbits at the front of the skull. Conversely, fetuses with spina bifida rarely demonstrate a lemon-shaped skull after 24–26 weeks. These factors should be remembered if a lemon-shaped skull is suspected.

Measuring the BPD from the thalami view

Follow the same procedure as outlined above. From the anterior horns section, make a *very* slight rotation of the probe toward the fetal neck (i.e. the back of the head) to image the basal cisterns in preference to the posterior horns of the lateral ventricles. This is followed by a *very* slight sliding movement of the probe downward, toward the fetal body so that the lower border of the cavum is just visible together with the optimal view of the thalami.

The BPD is measured using the technique described above. The issue of ensuring the technique used (including the section selected for measurement) corresponds to that employed when the reference data were produced also applies. The range of problems described above are also relevant for this view.

Evaluating the intracranial anatomy from the thalami view

As discussed above, it is important to observe the information presented in a section selected for measurement and thus to familiarize yourself with the range of normal appearances at a specific gestation. Once you have this experience you will immediately identify a finding that is not normal, even if you do not have the expertise to make the diagnosis. For example, make sure that the thalami are of normal size, position and have a homogeneous echogenicity. Note that the normal third ventricle is a midline structure that lies between the two thalamic hemispheres and is usually too small to identify in the normal fetus. Exclude any unusual echo-poor or echo-bright areas and ensure that the echo pattern in both halves of the brain is similar and symmetrical about the midline. Are the intracranial contents of normal echogenicity or do they appear brighter than usual such that you may have reduced the gain slightly? Abnormally echo-bright skull contents are not indicative of a brain abnormality but rather of skull hypomineralization as seen in osteogenesis imperfecta type 11 and hypophosphatasia.

Skull shape

See the previous discussion of fetal skull shape.

Estimating gestational age from BPD measurements

We do not recommend relying upon estimates of gestational age produced by the ultrasound equipment software for the following reasons:

- estimation of gestational age should not be made from a single parameter
- manufacturers do not always state the origin of the charts provided, and these might not be appropriate for the equipment or the technique used
- monitoring growth and estimation of gestational age require different charts for statistical reasons.

Figure 7.8 illustrates a growth chart of the BPD (outer to outer). Note that gestational age (independent variable) is plotted on the *x*-axis and the BPD (dependent variable) is plotted on the *y*-axis. A growth chart should be used to determine if the parameter measured is within the normal range for the gestational age as calculated from a reliable menstrual history and/or a first trimester dating scan. In practical terms, you should measure the BPD and then you should plot it on a growth chart according to the gestational age. If the measurement

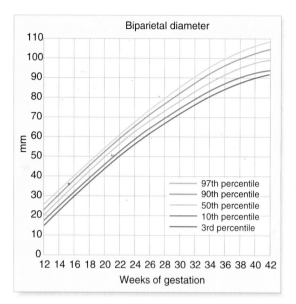

Figure 7.8 Growth of the BPD ('outer to outer') with increasing gestation showing 97th, 90th, 50th, 10th, and 3rd centiles (from Chitty et al 1994). This chart is reproduced in Appendix 8.

lies outside the normal range for the menstrual age then you must consider whether it is valid to ignore the menstrual dates and reassign an EDD based on the ultrasound measurements or whether the menstrual dates should be retained (see p. 110).

In cases where the gestational age is unknown or the menstrual history is unreliable, estimation of gestational age should be made from a dating chart, in which the BPD (independent variable) is plotted on the *x*-axis and the gestational age (dependent variable) is plotted on the *y*-axis, or from tables derived in the same manner (see Appendix 3). In practical terms, this means that, having measured the BPD, you should estimate the gestational age by use of the tables. The measurement can then be plotted on the growth chart according to the gestational age derived from the dating tables.

We recommend that dating charts are used in look-up table format and that all measurements are represented graphically on growth charts.

MEASURING THE HEAD CIRCUMFERENCE (HC)

This is measured from the same view as that used for the BPD. Figure 7.6 illustrates the section

required for measurement of the BPD using the lateral ventricles view. The HC is calculated by one of three basic methods:

1. *The two-diameter method.* The BPD and OFD are both measured using the outer to outer technique (Fig. 7.9 and see Fig. 7.6). The machine's software then calculates the HC using the formula πd derived from the formula for the circumference of a circle (2πr)

$$HC = 3.14 \, (BPD + OFD)/2$$

2. *The ellipse method.* The first onscreen cursor is placed on the outer table of the skull at the occiput. The second cursor is then placed on the outer table of the skull at the synciput. Using the appropriate control, a ready-formed ellipse of dots is moved out from between the two cursors until it matches the outline of the fetal skull (Fig. 7.10). On many machines, adjustment of the position of one or both the cursors can be made after the ellipse is formed to achieve a more exact match.

3. *The plot method.* The onscreen cursor marker is placed on the outer table of the skull. The correct position is then recorded in the machine's software by pressing the caliper 'enter' control. Sequential marks are plotted

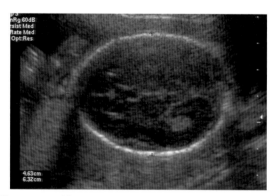

Figure 7.9 Measurement of the head circumference using the two diameter method (lateral ventricles view). The calipers are placed on the outer edge of both parietal bones to obtain the BPD and on the outer edge of the occipital and frontal bones to obtain the OFD. Both the BPD and OFD are therefore obtained using the 'outer to outer' technique.

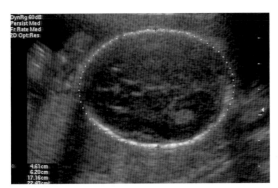

Figure 7.10 Measurement of head circumference using the ellipse method (lateral ventricles view).

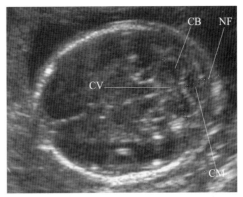

Figure 7.11 Measurement of the transcerebellar diameter. The calipers are positioned to obtain an 'outer to outer' measurement of the cerebellum. The cerebellar vermis (CV) can be seen as a slightly more echo-bright triangular-shaped structure lying between the two cerebellar hemispheres (CB). Note the normally sized cisterna magna (CM) lying between the cerebellum and the skull and the thickness of the normal nuchal skin fold (NF) overlying the skull at this point.

and recorded around the whole circumference. In some equipment, a continuous trace is produced rather than a series of dots. On many machines, adjustment of the last position(s) of the cursor can be made in case of error.

Growth of the HC is illustrated in Appendix 4. The literature now contains a number of datasets indicating the superiority of the HC over the BPD for pregnancy dating. For this reason, we include a chart for estimating gestational age using HC (two-diameter or 'derived' method) in Appendix 5.

MEASURING THE TRANSCEREBELLAR DIAMETER (TCD)

The cerebellum is dumb-bell-shaped and consists of two circular hemispheres separated centrally by the more hyperechoic triangular-shaped vermis. The section required to measure the TCD is the suboccipitobregmatic view, in which the anterior horns of the lateral ventricles and cavum are visualized at the front of the head together with the cerebellum at the back. Obtain the lateral ventricle view required for the BPD then rotate the probe slightly downward, toward the fetal neck. The posterior horns of the lateral ventricles will disappear from view to be replaced by the cerebellum. Ensure you do not rotate the probe too far toward the neck. Although this might not affect the TCD measurement, it will give a false impression of an enlarged cisterna magna and/or nuchal skinfold thickness. The TCD is measured at 90° to the long

axis of the cerebellum across its widest point, using the 'outer to outer' method (Fig. 7.11). In the second trimester, the TCD measurement (in millimetres) is numerically equivalent to the number of weeks of gestation of the pregnancy. It is therefore useful in the assessment of gestational age, especially when there is a discrepancy in gestational age equivalent between the BPD or HC and the femur.

MEASURING THE ABDOMINAL CIRCUMFERENCE (AC)

Figure 7.12 illustrates the section on which the AC is measured. The landmark features are:

- A circular section of the abdomen demonstrating an unbroken and short rib echo of equal size on each side.
- A cross-section of *one* vertebra visualized as a triangle of three white spots.
- A short length of umbilical vein. This should be imaged so that it is centrally placed between the lateral abdominal walls and is a third of the way along an imaginary line drawn from the anterior abdominal wall to the fetal spine.

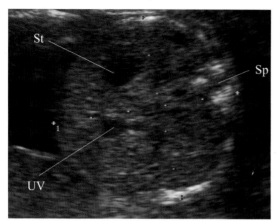

Figure 7.12 Transverse section of the fetal abdomen demonstrating the landmarks required to measure the abdominal circumference. Note the appearance of the normal single vertebra (Sp), the short length of umbilical vein (UV) and its position. Note also the appearance and position of the normally sized stomach (St).

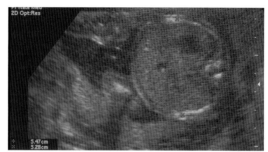

Figure 7.13 Measurement of the abdominal circumference using the two diameter method. The anteroposterior diameter (APAD) is obtained by placing one caliper on the outer border of the skin directly behind the spine and the second on the outer border of the anterior abdominal wall, following the direction of the umbilical vein. The transverse abdominal diameter (TAD) is obtained by placing the calipers on the outer borders of the widest part of the fetal abdomen, at 90° to the APAD.

- The stomach, usually visualized as a hypoechoic area in the left side of the abdomen.

Method

Obtain a longitudinal view of the fetus that demonstrates both the fetal heart and the fetal bladder. Slide the transducer laterally until the fetal spine is visualized. Rotate the transducer through 90° at the level of the fetal stomach to obtain a cross-section. The outline should be circular, if it is ovoid make a small adjustment of the rotation or the angle of the transducer. If the umbilical vein is not visualized as described above, make small sliding movements of the transducer to change the level of the section. Freeze the image.

The circumference of the abdomen is measured in the same way as the head circumference, using the two-diameter method. The anteroposterior diameter (APAD) is measured from the fetal spine to the anterior abdominal wall. The short section of umbilical vein should lie along this axis. The transverse abdominal diameter (TAD) is measured across the widest part of the abdominal circumference section at 90° to the APAD. Both diameters are measured using the 'outer to outer' technique (Figs 7.12 and 7.13). The machine's software then calculates the abdominal circumference (AC) using the formula πd derived from the formula for the circumference of a circle ($2\pi r$):

$$AC = 3.14 \ (TAD + APAD)/2$$

Growth of the AC is illustrated in Appendix 6.

Problems

Directly anterior fetal spine

The umbilical vein will not be seen in transverse section because it lies in the acoustic shadow produced from the fetal spine (Fig. 7.14A). In the second trimester it is nearly always possible to slide the transducer to a more lateral position on the maternal abdomen, or to dip one end of the transducer, to allow the umbilical vein to be imaged (Fig. 7.14B). Alternatively, you can complete the remainder of the examination, by which time the fetus might have moved into a more favorable position.

Non-circular outline

An oval outline indicates an oblique cross-section. This can be rectified by a slight change in rotation or angle – the choice depends on the position of the fetal body relative to the horizontal plane. If

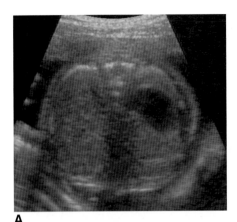

A

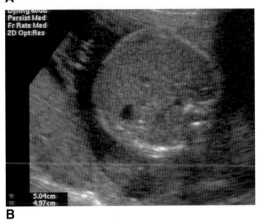

B

Figure 7.14 A. Transverse section of the fetal abdomen demonstrating how the acoustic shadow from an anterior fetal spine obscures the umbilical vein. B. The same fetus imaged from a lateral aspect on the maternal abdomen.

the longitudinal fetal spine is in the horizontal plane then rotation is required, if the longitudinal fetal spine is at an angle to the horizontal then angling is required.

Long length of umbilical vein

The umbilical vein travels up through the liver at approximately 45°. Thus, if the section on which you intend to measure the AC demonstrates a long length of umbilical vein, you know you have an oblique and incorrect section. If the longitudinal fetal spine is in the horizontal plane then angling is required, if the longitudinal fetal spine is at an angle to the horizontal then rotation is required.

MEASURING THE FEMUR LENGTH (FL)

This measurement is as accurate as the BPD in the prediction of gestational age. It is useful in confirming the gestational age estimated from BPD or HC measurements and can often be obtained when fetal position prevents measurement of the BPD or HC. As examination of intracranial anatomy is an important part of all ultrasound examinations, measurement of femur length should not replace that of the BPD or HC as the sole predictor of gestational age. The femur can be measured from 12 weeks to term.

Method

Measuring the femur is ideally undertaken after the AC has been measured. Slide the probe caudally from the AC section until the iliac bones are visualized. At this point, a cross-section of one or both femurs is usually seen. The upper femur should be selected for measurement. The lower femur is frequently difficult to image clearly because of acoustic shadowing from fetal structures anterior to it. Keeping the echo from the anterior femur in view, rotate the probe slowly until the full length of the femur is obtained. You might need to make a *small* sliding movement after each rotational movement to bring the probe back onto the femur. To ensure that you have the full length of the femur and that your section is not oblique, soft tissue should be visible beyond both ends of the femur and the bone should not appear to merge with the skin of the thigh at any point (Fig. 7.15). The end-points of the femur are often difficult to define when the femur is imaged lying horizontally but are much easier to define when the bone lies at a slight angle (5–15° to the horizontal). The angle of the bone relative to the horizontal can be manipulated by dipping one end of the probe gently into the maternal abdomen.

The measurement of the femur is made from the center of the 'U' shape at each end of the bone. This represents the length of the metaphysis. It is good practice to obtain measurements from three separate images of the same femur. These should be within 1 mm of each other.

Growth of the femur is illustrated in Fig. 7.16 and Appendix 9.

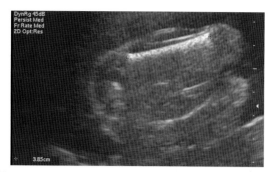

Figure 7.15 Measurement of the fetal femur. Note that soft tissue is visible beyond both ends of the bone. The femur length is the distance between the caliper markers.

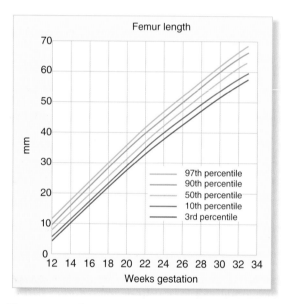

Figure 7.16 Growth of the femur with increasing gestational showing 97th, 90th, 50th, 10th and 3rd centiles (from Chitty et al 1994a) This chart is illustrated in Appendix 9.

As with the BPD, a growth chart should be used to determine if the FL measurement is within the normal range for the gestational age as calculated from a reliable menstrual history and/or a first trimester dating scan. In practical terms, you should measure the FL and then you should plot it on a growth chart according the gestational age. If the measurement lies outside the normal range for the menstrual age then you must consider whether it is valid to ignore the menstrual dates and reas-

sign an EDD based on the ultrasound measurements or whether the menstrual dates should be retained (see p. 108).

In cases where the gestational age is unknown or the menstrual history is unreliable, estimation of gestational age should be made from a dating chart, in which the FL (independent variable) is plotted on the x-axis and the gestational age (dependent variable) is plotted on the y-axis, or from tables derived in the same manner (see Appendix 7). In practical terms, this means that, having measured the FL, you should estimate the gestational age by use of the tables. The measurement can then be plotted on the growth chart according to the gestational age derived from the dating tables.

We recommend that dating charts are used in look-up table format and that all measurements are represented graphically on growth charts.

Problems

Fetal movements

Most problems arising with measuring the FL are due to a combination of fetal movements and slow use of the freeze button. The cine loop might be useful in such situations. If the end-points of the femur cannot be adequately visualized, unfreeze the image and seek another, better image. It is very easy to under- or overestimate the FL by 3–5 mm if a suboptimal image is measured.

One or both end-points are difficult to define

Dip one end of the probe gently in to the maternal abdomen, as described above.

The upper femur appears straight but the lower femur appears bowed

The slight bowing seen in the lower limb is a normal artifact of the imaging process. Unilateral femoral abnormalities are very rare but should always be considered as a possible, if unlikely, explanation for significant dissimilarity in the appearance of the two femurs. An experienced second opinion should be sought if necessary.

Gestational age equivalents of the BPD or HC and femur disagree

The estimation of gestational age obtained from measurements of femur length should agree with that obtained from the measurement of the BPD, HC and/or the TCD. If the femur length is small (below the 5th centile) compared to the BPD or HC (on the 50th centile) and TCD then all the long bones and the plantar view of the feet should be carefully measured to exclude skeletal dysplasia (see Chapter 8). A short femur is also a minor marker for chromosomal abnormalities, including trisomy 21.

BODY AND LIMB MOVEMENTS

In the majority of situations, movements of the fetal body and limbs will be only too apparent while attempting to obtain the required measurements. If the fetus appears to have remained uncharacteristically quiet during the examination, observe it and ensure that flexion and extension of the limbs and some body movements have occurred. Conditions such as arthrogryposis and severe anemia are associated with such loss of tone and movement.

PLACENTAL LOCALIZATION

The placenta is best identified by scanning the uterus longitudinally and is easily recognized by its more echogenic pattern compared with that of the underlying myometrium. Careful inspection will demonstrate the chorionic plate as a bright linear echo between the homogeneous echoes of the body of the placenta and the amniotic fluid (Fig. 7.17). The actual internal os might be difficult to identify transabdominally but its position can be assumed by visualizing the slight dimple at the upper end of the cervical canal. The cervical canal is best imaged by placing the probe in the midline, with its lower end just above the symphysis, slight dextrorotation may be necessary. The cervical canal lies directly posterior to the bladder, typically at about 45° to the horizontal.

The placenta can be fundal, anterior, posterior or lateral, in which case it will be visualized on both the anterior and posterior walls of the uterus. It might lie completely within the upper part of

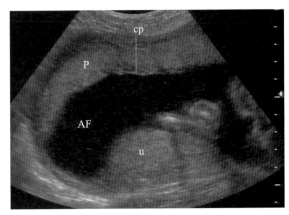

Figure 7.17   Localizing the placenta from a longitudinal, midline section of the uterus. Note the homogeneous echo pattern of the anterior wall placenta (P) and the bright echoes produced from the chorionic plate (cp) that demarcates the interface between the placenta and the amniotic fluid (AF). Posterior uterine wall (u).

the uterus, with its lower edge >5 cm from the internal os – such a position is usually described as 'upper' or 'not low'.

If the leading edge of the placenta lies within 5 cm of the internal os and/or appears to cover the internal os then its position should be described as 'low' and/or 'covering the os'. The term 'placenta praevia' should only be used after 28 weeks (see Chapter 9).

It is unnecessary to ask women to attend with a full bladder at the time of the 20–22 week scan as the majority will have an obviously fundal placenta. It is frequently possible to visualize the lower placental edge and the internal os, thus making the diagnosis of a low-lying placenta possible even with a partially filled bladder. If such views are suboptimal and a low-lying placenta is suspected, then a transvaginal examination should be performed or the woman should be scanned with a full bladder.

Problems

Braxton Hicks contractions

Figure 7.18 demonstrates how a Braxton Hicks contraction can be a trap for the unwary. These contractions cause a 'bunching-up' of the myometrium, particularly on the low posterior wall

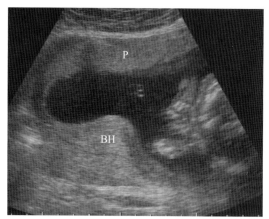

Figure 7.18   Longitudinal section of the uterus with an anterior placenta (P). A mass can be seen on the posterior uterine wall due to a Braxton Hicks (BH) contraction.

of the uterus, and are easily mistaken for a low posterior placenta (or a fibroid). Examination of the entire uterus will prevent this mistake because the placenta can be recognized elsewhere. Also, the lower edge of the placenta should always be sought by keeping the strong linear echo from the chorionic plate in view. Braxton Hicks contractions do not produce this echo. Finally, if there is still real doubt, the woman should be rescanned after 20 min, during which time the Braxton Hicks contraction will have disappeared.

Overdistention of the bladder

An overfull bladder compresses the uterus, causing the low anterior and low posterior walls to meet and simulating a low-lying placenta. This is best avoided by using the empty bladder technique in the first instance.

Abnormalities of the placenta are discussed in Chapter 9.

EVALUATING AMNIOTIC FLUID VOLUME

From early in the second trimester most of the amniotic fluid is fetal urine. Amniotic fluid is therefore produced by the fetal kidneys and removed by fetal swallowing and subsequent absorption by the fetal bowel. Disruption of this pathway will cause an abnormal reduction (oligohydramnios) or increase (polyhydramnios) in amniotic fluid

volume. Abnormal amniotic fluid volume is therefore an important indicator of a range of varying fetal abnormalities, and one that can be readily assessed during every examination.

Measuring amniotic fluid volume

Three methods of assessing amniotic fluid volume can be used:

1. visual assessment
2. measurement of the maximum vertical depth (MVD)
3. measurement of the amniotic fluid index (AFI).

Evaluation of amniotic fluid is described in detail in Chapter 9.

CONFIRMING OR ASSIGNING GESTATIONAL AGE

Interpretation of the measurements taken at the time of the routine 20–22 week ultrasound examination will depend on whether measurements have been taken at an earlier examination. If reliable measurements were taken at an earlier examination, then the EDD should have already been assigned, or confirmed, at that time. The second trimester measurements are thus used to assess fetal growth.

If the second trimester examination is the first of the pregnancy then the measurements are used: (i) to confirm the gestational age and the EDD based on the menstrual history; or (ii) to assign the gestational age and the EDD when the menstrual history is unknown or unreliable (see also Chapter 3). We recommend that the minimum measurements that should be taken for gestational age assessment are those of the BPD or HC and the FL.

Confirming gestational age in the second trimester

Confirmation of gestational age at the second trimester examination is based either on a reliable menstrual history or/and on measurements obtained from an earlier and reliable ultrasound examination. In both instances the gestational age of the second examination is known. Four outcomes are possible:

1. The measurements of the BPD or HC and the FL fall within the normal range for the gestational age when plotted on appropriate charts. This confirms the previously assigned EDD based either on the LMP or the early scan.

2. Measurements of the BPD or HC and the FL fall outside the normal range for menstrual age. In this case you should consider carefully the reliability of the menstrual history/early scan:
   - If there is uncertainty concerning the reliability of the previously assigned EDD then, in the majority of cases, it is considered acceptable practice to reassign the EDD based on the second trimester measurements. Estimate the gestational age from the BPD or HC using dating tables (see Appendices 3 and 5) and then replot the FL for the estimated gestation. If the FL is within normal range you should then assign the new EDD from the BPD-derived or HC-derived gestational age. Your AC measurement should further confirm the ultrasound date you have assigned.
   - If there is no reason to doubt either the optimal menstrual history (for example if the date of conception is indisputable) or the measurements from the earlier scan then the previously assigned EDD should be kept. The second trimester measurements in this case therefore indicate poor fetal growth. As early onset growth restriction is associated with chromosomal anomalies and/or poor outcome, karyotyping should be considered and the pregnancy should be monitored carefully.

3. The BPD or HC falls within normal range for the known gestational age but the FL is below the normal range. In this case you should repeat the measurements of the BPD or HC and FL and measure the TCD and AC. If all the measurements but that of the FL agree with the known gestational age, you should suspect a skeletal dysplasia or trisomy 21 (see Chapter 8).

4. The FL falls within the normal range for known gestational age but the BPD is below the normal range. Again, you should repeat the measurements of the BPD or HC and FL and

also measure the TCD and AC. If the HC and BPD are both below the normal range you should look for spina bifida or microcephaly, remembering that the majority of fetuses with spina bifida will have an abnormally shaped or absent cerebellum (see Chapter 10). If all the measurements are appropriate, with the exception of the BPD, look at the shape of the head – the most usual cause for a small BPD is dolichocephaly (narrow head) due to a breech or transverse presentation. Such circumstances emphasize why it is more appropriate to use the HC instead of the BPD with the FL to confirm the known gestational age. Some authors recommend the use of the cephalic index:

$$\text{Cephalic index} = \text{BPD/OFD} = 80 \pm 5$$

An index of less than 75 is seen in cases of dolichocephaly and makes the BPD measurement unreliable for estimating gestational age. An index of more than 85 is seen in brachycephalic heads (wide and short) and also makes use of the BPD for estimating gestational age unreliable. The cephalic index is constant throughout pregnancy.

Assigning gestational age for the first time in the second trimester

The gestational age is calculated for both the BPD or HC and FL using dating tables. Two outcomes are possible:

1. The gestational ages calculated from both the BPD or HC and FL dating tables agree to within 7 days. The ultrasound EDD is therefore derived from the gestational age (or the average if they agree to within 7 days of each other) as calculated from the dating tables.

2. The gestational ages calculated from the BPD or HC and the FL dating tables differ by more than 7 days. In this case you should repeat the measurements of the BPD or HC and FL and measure the TCD and AC. If a dating table is available for the TCD then this should be used. If a dating table is unavailable then the gestational age should be calculated from the relevant growth chart:

– If the gestational age equivalents of the TCD and AC agree with the BPD and HC then the pregnancy should be dated from the gestational age (or the average) as calculated from the BPD and HC dating tables. Having now established the gestational age, further management will depend on the severity of the FL shortening. As skeletal dysplasia and trisomy 21 are associated with FL outside the normal range, both these conditions should be considered. Less severe cases should be followed up in 2–4 weeks to confirm normal growth velocity of the FL.

– If the gestational age equivalents of the TCD and AC agree with the FL then the pregnancy should be dated from the gestational age (or the average) as calculated from the FL and TCD dating tables. If all the gestational age equivalents agree, with the exception of the BPD, look at the shape of the head – the most usual cause for a small BPD is dolichocephaly (narrow head) due to a breech or transverse presentation. In such circumstances it is appropriate to use the HC instead of the BPD together with the FL to assign the gestational age. If the BPD *and* HC are both below the normal range you should look for spina bifida or microcephaly, remembering that the majority of fetuses with spina bifida will have an abnormally shaped or absent cerebellum (see Chapter 10).

Determining gestational age in multiple pregnancy

If the fetuses are of different sizes then measurements from the larger fetus should be used to determine the gestational age.

WHAT TO DO WITH 'LATE BOOKERS'

Prediction of gestational age by ultrasound is most accurate when performed before 24 weeks of gestation. Gestational age cannot be predicted accurately after 28 weeks' gestation. Women who attend after 24 weeks fall into four categories:

1. Those in whom all measurements correspond with the menstrual age. These women do not need further ultrasound examinations unless clinically indicated.

2. Those who have an unreliable menstrual history or in whom fetal size is less than that predicted by menstrual dates. In these women an accurate EDD cannot be predicted. They should have serial ultrasound examinations to monitor fetal growth. Providing growth continues normally it is usually unnecessary to interfere with the pregnancy because of fetal concern.

3. Those in whom fetal size is greater than that predicted from the menstrual history. These women should be rescanned 3–4 weeks later to observe velocity of growth. An accurate EDD cannot be assigned in these cases.

4. Women with maternal diabetes mellitus might have large fetuses and pose a special problem if they book late. An accurate EDD cannot be assigned in these cases.

REFERENCES AND FURTHER READING

Altman D G, Chitty L S 1993 Design and analysis of studies to derive charts of fetal size. Ultrasound in Obstetrics and Gynecology 3:378–384

Altman D G, Chitty L S 1997 New charts for ultrasound dating of pregnancy. Ultrasound in Obstetrics and Gynecology 10:174–191

British Medical Ultrasound Society Fetal Measurements Working Party 1990 Clinical applications of ultrasonic fetal measurements. British Institute of Radiology, London

Royal College of Obstetricians and Gynaecologists 2000 Routine ultrasound screening in pregnancy: protocol, standards and training. Report of the RCOG Working Party July 2000. RCOG, London

United Kingdom Association of Sonographers 2001 Guidelines for professional working standards – ultrasound practice. United Kingdom Association of Sonographers, London

Chapter **8**

Routine second trimester screening – assessing fetal anatomy

An ultrasound examination is in the unique position of being both a screening test and a diagnostic test for fetal anomalies. Its clinical value is directly dependent on the skills of the sonographer, first, in obtaining the correct images for evaluation and measurement and, second, in the correct interpretation in each specific and unique clinical situation. Such examinations must only be performed by individuals who have undergone a supervised period of training that enables them to identify and distinguish between the range of normal findings, findings of uncertain significance and abnormalities at varying stages of gestation.

Although it is possible to describe the techniques for demonstrating the various organs, by far the best way of learning the anatomy is to spend as much time as possible studying normal fetuses and across the gestational age range. The majority of second trimester scans are now performed at 20–22 weeks, although a more limited assessment of fetal anatomy can be made, using the transabdominal probe, from 15 weeks.

A mental checklist, based on the scanning sequence described in Chapter 7 (see p. 94) is necessary to ensure that the study is complete.

Although it is necessary to examine the entire fetus and other uterine contents in detail, it is not always feasible to do this in the order suggested. If a fetal organ presents itself it might be better to examine it there and then, while it is in an optimal position. Later on, the fetus might have moved into a less favorable position for assessment of that particular part of its anatomy. We suggest that the measurements are always carried out early in the examination so that they are not forgotten.

In our opinion, it is not reasonable to expect all structural fetal abnormalities amenable to ultrasound detection to be diagnosed at a routine second trimester anomaly scan. If the approach in Chapter 7 is followed then no major structural abnormality should be missed. For example, anencephaly should not be missed in any ultrasound examination performed after 12 weeks of gestation. At the 20–22 week examination it is unreasonable to overlook large protruding masses such as encephalocele, cystic hygroma and abdominal wall defects. If the intracranial anatomy is evaluated routinely then all cases of spina bifida in which the 'lemon' and/or 'banana' signs are present, and/or hydrocephalus, should be detected at this stage. Abnormal fetal situs should be recognized. Similarly, severe limb reduction defects should be detected. Abnormal fluid collections such as ascites and pleural effusion should not be overlooked and severe oligohydramnios or polyhydramnios should also be recognized.

Severe examples of growth-related abnormalities, such as microcephaly and achondroplasia, might be detectable at this stage of gestation but such conditions are typically diagnosed later in pregnancy. Other conditions, such as duodenal atresia, congenital diaphragmatic hernia and progressive renal pelvic dilatation are typically detectable in the third trimester and are not apparent in the second trimester.

It is our opinion that no blame should be attached to a sonographer who fails to detect conditions, such as microcephaly, that can only be diagnosed by serial measurements. If, however, there is a discrepancy between the head measurements and the femur length, a competent sonographer should identify this fact and refer the woman for further examination so that microcephaly or skeletal dysplasia can be excluded.

THE INTRACRANIAL ANATOMY

As discussed in Chapter 7, examination of the intracranial anatomy should follow on naturally after taking the measurements of the biparietal diameter (BPD), head circumference (HC) and transcerebellar diameter (TCD). Demonstration of normal cerebral ventricles will exclude the most common cranial abnormalities, namely ventriculomegaly.

The cerebral ventricles

Figure 8.1 is a schematic diagram that illustrates the ventricular system. Cerebrospinal fluid (CSF) is produced by the choroid plexus and circulates through the ventricular system, around the brain and around the spine. It is absorbed by specific areas of the arachnoid. Excess production or failure of absorption leads to communicating hydrocephalus, whereas a block in any part of the ventricular system leads to obstructive hydrocephalus. Hydrocephalus describes the pathological increase in size of the cerebral ventricles and the head circumference. Ventriculomegaly describes the appearance of the lateral ventricles when their diameter is above the normal range for gestation. Thus not all fetuses with ventriculomegaly will develop hydrocephalus. It should be remembered that there is a difference in meaning between these two terms and it is therefore incorrect to use them interchangeably.

The easiest parts of the ventricular system to visualize with ultrasound are the lateral ventricles (Fig. 8.2). These are bilateral and have anterior, posterior and inferior horns. They contain the choroid plexus, which is normally apparent with ultrasound only in the posterior horn. The inferior horn is rarely seen in normal fetuses because it is lost in the echoes from the base of the skull. Figure 8.3 illustrates a pathological specimen of a fetal head at approximately the same level as Fig. 8.2 and demonstrates that ultrasound produces a very good representation of the anatomy. The remainder of the ventricular system is not readily visualized in the normal fetus.

The anterior horn

The anterior horns of the lateral ventricles are visualized in the same section as that required for the

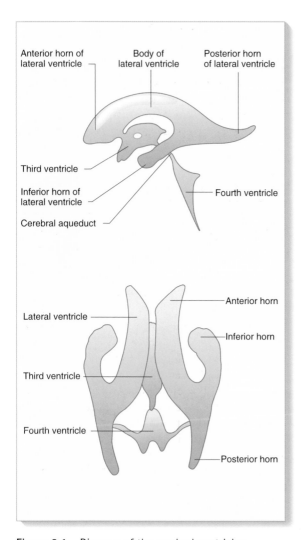

Figure 8.1   Diagram of the cerebral ventricles.

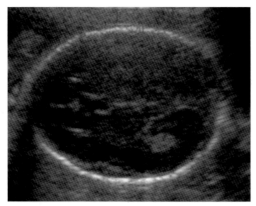

Figure 8.2   Transverse section of the fetal head demonstrating the ventricular system.

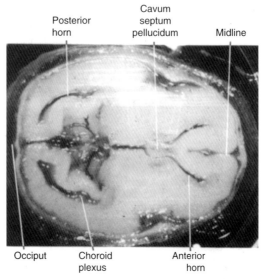

Figure 8.3   Pathological section of the fetal head. Note how well the ultrasound reflects the anatomy.

BPD (lateral ventricles view; see Fig. 8.2). Because of reverberation artifacts in the upper hemisphere of the brain, ventricular measurements are usually made only from the lower hemisphere. As can be seen in Fig. 8.3, the medial and lateral borders of the anterior horn lie in very close proximity at this level. With older imaging equipment it was rarely possible to differentiate between the linear echoes produced by these two interfaces. Thus the anterior horn 'measurement' in the normal fetus actually represents the distance of the anterior horn from the midline, rather than the actual size, i.e. depth of the anterior horn.

With modern equipment it is generally possible to observe the medial and lateral borders as separate echoes. It is important that the anterior horns of both hemispheres are observed and that they are equidistant from the midline. If they are not, the measurement taken will be incorrect. The 'measurement' of the anterior horn is made anterior to the cavum septum pellucidum, from the midline to the medial border of the ventricle. The intersection of the two arms of the caliper is placed on the distal border of the midline and the inner border of the ventricle (effectively, inner to inner). Make sure the measurement is taken at 90° to the midline echo, i.e. parallel to the BPD measurement (Fig. 8.4). It is important to distinguish between

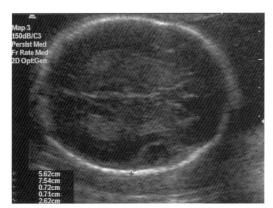

Figure 8.4 Measurement of the anterior horn of the lateral ventricle. This measurement is taken from the same section as that required for the BPD (lateral ventricles view). Note the placement of the calipers produces an 'inner to inner' measurement of the distance of the anterior horn complex from the midline and of the hemisphere. The AV/H ratio in this example is 7/26. The posterior horn measurement (7.1 mm) is also demonstrated.

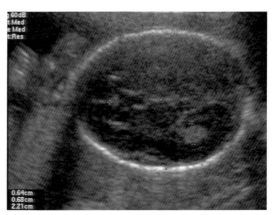

Figure 8.5 Measurement of the posterior horn of the lateral ventricle. Note that the choroid plexus almost fills the posterior horn at this level. Note how the placement of the calipers – across the maximum depth of the ventricle – produces an 'outer to outer' measurement of the posterior horn. The hemisphere measurement is obtained using the 'inner to inner' method. The PV/H ratio in this example is 6.8/22.1 or 7/22. The anterior horn measurement (6.4 mm) is also demonstrated.

the insula, which can be very prominent, and the lateral border of the anterior horn.

The posterior horn or atrium

The posterior horn, or atrium, contains choroid that is readily identified as a rounded, hyperechoic structure. The choroid plexus provides a very useful landmark with which to identify the position and extent of the posterior horn. The ultrasound appearance of the posterior horn differs from the anterior horn in that it has obvious depth. Assessment and measurement require visualization of both the medial and lateral borders and of the choroid. The section that demonstrates the optimal view of the posterior horn changes with gestation. Before about 20 weeks it is usually the BPD (lateral ventricles) view. With increasing gestation, a lower section of the head, obtained by sliding caudally from the BPD section, is frequently required. The measurement of the posterior horn is taken from the more medial edge of the medial border to the outer edge of the lateral border (outer to outer). Make sure the measurement is taken at 90° to the midline echo, i.e. parallel to the BPD measurement (Fig. 8.5). Occasionally, the

lateral border might not be visualized clearly and the lateral aspect of the choroid plexus is taken as the outer limit of the posterior horn.

The V/H ratio

The size of the anterior or posterior horn can be compared to the size of the cerebral hemisphere on the same (lower) side of the brain. The hemisphere is measured from the distal edge of the midline to the inner border of the skull at the level of the BPD (inner to inner). In practice, the anterior (AVHR) or posterior (PVHR) horn:hemisphere ratio (or V/H ratio) is, rather confusingly, expressed as a fraction (e.g. 7/25) rather than a ratio (e.g. 0.28). The normal ranges are illustrated in Fig. 8.6. As can be seen from Fig. 8.6, the AVHR should be less than 0.5 after 18 weeks of gestation. Measurements that falsely use the insula will give high AVHRs, implying an incorrect diagnosis of ventriculomegaly.

Choroid plexus cysts

As described above, the normal choroid is readily identified as a rounded, hyperechoic structure lying within the posterior horn. Cystic areas can be iden-

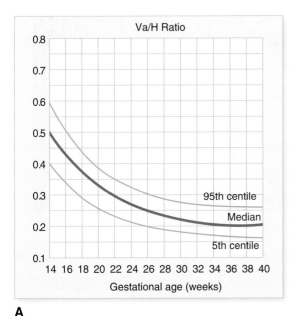

A

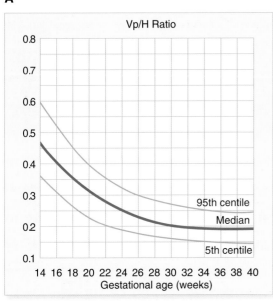

B

Figure 8.6 Size charts of the ventricular:hemisphere ratio with gestational age. A. Anterior horn (Va/H ratio) B. Posterior horn (Vp/H ratio) (with permission of Pilu and Nicolaides).

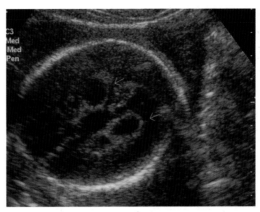

Figure 8.7 Transverse section of the fetal head at the level of the posterior horn demonstrating a choroid plexus cyst of 4.4 mm diameter in the lower choroid. Note poor visualization of the upper hemisphere although a second CPC of 4.9mm diameter can be identified.

tified within the second trimester choroid, and these are described as choroid plexus cysts (CPCs). Such CPCs are typically small (< 10 mm in diameter) and single (Fig. 8.7) and can be a unilateral or a bilateral finding. They are a common finding in the second trimester, with a reported prevalence of 0.5–2%. Most CPCs will resolve by 26 weeks and are usually of no pathologic significance to the developing fetus or infant. They constitute a 'minor marker' for chromosomal abnormalities because they are associated with an increased risk for trisomy 18. In the absence of other markers for trisomy 18, the maternal age-related risk is not significantly increased.

The circular and cystic appearance of CPCs often means they are readily noticed by the parents during the examination. It is therefore important that you can discuss the implications appropriately, and according to departmental guidelines, with the parents. Although CPCs are an innocuous finding in the majority of cases, their finding generates significant anxiety for parents. As with the detection of most 'not normal' findings, parental fears can be allayed by a sensitive and honest approach to the discussion. Such fears will almost certainly be fueled by a dismissive and/or uninformed approach.

Ventriculomegaly

Some authors advocate a numerical cut-off, typically 10 mm, rather than a ratio, to define ventriculomegaly in the second trimester. The value chosen refers to the posterior horn, or atrium, because its dilatation generally precedes that of the anterior horn. Other authors advocate posterior ventricle diameter growth charts and use a cut-off value that corresponds to the upper limit of the normal range (±2 standard deviations (SDs)) for the gestational age (Fig. 8.8). In ventriculomegaly, the choroid plexus, which normally fills the posterior horn, is surrounded by fluid (Fig. 8.9A). In severe cases it will be gravity dependent, hanging close to the medial border of the upper posterior horn and to the lateral border of the lower posterior horn (Fig. 8.9B).

The classic association of ventriculomegaly is with spina bifida. Mild ventriculomegaly (10–15mm) is also associated with chromosomal abnormalities, especially trisomy 21. Isolated ventriculomegaly can also be associated with fetal infection and other rare disorders such as lissencephaly and periventricular leukomalacia.

The thalami and third ventricle

The BPD (thalami view) section demonstrates two hypoechoic areas positioned symmetrically about the midline, posterior to the cavum; these are the two thalami (Fig. 8.10). The normal third ventricle is a tiny slit-like structure that lies on the midline between these two structures. It is usually visualized only when dilated. The basal cistern separates the lateral border of the thalamus from the brighter echoes of the hippocampus. Slight rotation of the

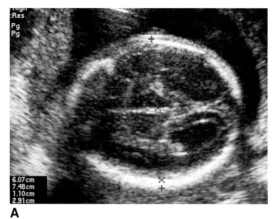

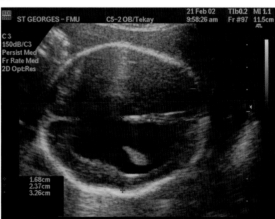

B

Figure 8.9 A. Mild ventriculomegaly at 22 weeks' gestation. The posterior horn measures 11 mm, above the upper range of normal for the gestational age of 22+ weeks. Note the amount of CSF relative to the size of the choroids and compare this with B. B. Severe ventriculomegaly at 24+ weeks' gestation. The posterior horn measures 23.7 mm, above the upper range of normal for the gestational age of 24+ weeks. Note the choroid in the posterior hemisphere is surrounded by CSF.

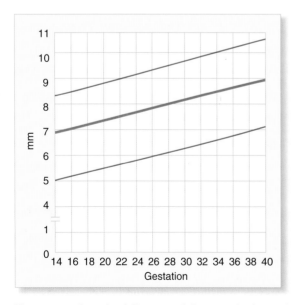

Figure 8.8 Growth of diameter of the posterior horn of the lateral ventricle with gestation (with 5th and 95th centiles) (with permission of Pilu and Nicolaides).

probe toward the fetal neck will demonstrate the cerebral peduncles that lie directly posterior to the thalami. The anterior part of the fourth ventricle can be seen directly posterior to the cerebellar peduncles and anterior to the cerebellar vermis (Fig. 8.11).

The cerebellum

The cerebellum lies within the posterior fossa and is best visualized using the suboccipitobregmatic

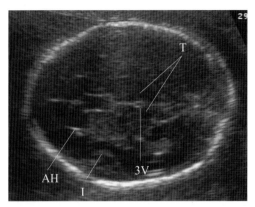

Figure 8.10 Transverse section of the fetal head demonstrating the two thalami (T) and the position of the third ventricle (3V) between them. The third ventricle is normally visualized clearly only when dilated. Note also the insula (I) and how easily this can be mistaken for the anterior horn (AH) of the lateral cerebral ventricle.

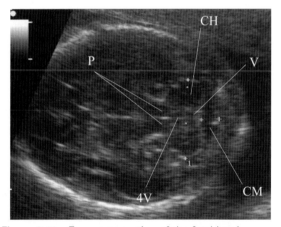

Figure 8.11 Transverse section of the fetal head demonstrating the cerebral peduncles (P), fourth ventricle (4V), cerebellar hemispheres (CH), cerebellar vermis (V) and cisterna magna (CM). This section is obtained by slight rotation of the probe towards the neck, from the BPD (lateral ventricles) section. Diameter 1 demonstrates measurement of the transcerebellar diameter (TCD).

view (see Figs 7.11 and 8.12A). Measurement of the transcerebellar diameter is described in Chapter 7. The cerebellum is dumb-bell-shaped, has two lateral lobes and a central, triangular-shaped, hyperechoic connection known as the vermis. Complete or partial absence or anterior displacement of the vermis is associated with the spectrum of Dandy–Walker malformations and other conditions, such

as Joubert's syndrome. A small, abnormally (banana) shaped or absent cerebellum is associated with spina bifida (see Chapter 10).

The cisterna magna

The cerebellum and cisterna magna lie within the posterior fossa and are best visualized using the suboccipitobregmatic view. The space between the cerebellum and the vault of the skull is the cisterna magna. This is a reservoir for cerebrospinal fluid. The diameter of the cisterna magna is taken as the horizontal distance between the outer border of the cerebellar vermis and the inner border of the skull (inner to inner) (Fig. 8.12A). Normal ranges for the cisterna magna have been published with the 95th centile ranging from 5 mm at 14 weeks to 9 mm at 27 weeks. Enlargement of the cisterna magna is associated with the Dandy–Walker spectrum and aneuploidy (trisomy 13, 18 and 21).

THE NUCHAL AREA

Nuchal fold

Edema of the skin at the occiput is associated with chromosomal defects, particularly trisomy 21, and other conditions including genetic syndromes. Thickening in this area identified in the second or third trimester fetus is called increased nuchal fold (NF) or increased nuchal skinfold thickness (NST) to distinguish it from the related, but different, increased nuchal translucency (NT) described in the first trimester fetus. Measurement of NF can be made from the suboccipitobregmatic view used for evaluation of the posterior fossa. The measurement is taken from the outer border of the occiput to the outer border of the skin echo (Fig. 8.12B). Care must be taken when making this measurement because the range of sections demonstrating the ideal view is very small. It is very easy to obtain a falsely increased nuchal fold if the skin over the upper neck is imaged rather than that over the base of the skull. Correct the section by rotating the probe cephalad, away from the fetal neck. Second trimester nuchal fold measurements of 6 mm or greater are considered to be increased.

Isolated increased NF is considered a strong marker for chromosomal abnormalities because of

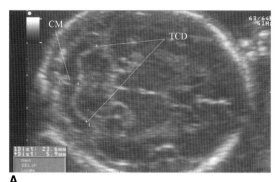

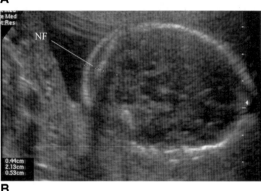

Figure 8.12 Suboccipito-bregmatic view of the head demonstrating the posterior fossa. A. The cisterna magna (CM) measures 5.9 mm, and transcerebellar diameter (TCD) measures 23.6 mm. Note the normal appearance and size of the cerebellar hemispheres and vermis. Note the positioning of the calipers from the outer border of the cerebellar vermis to the inner border of the skull to obtain an 'inner to inner' measurement of the CM. B. The nuchal fold (NF). Note the positioning of the calipers from the outer border of the skull to the outer border of the skin to obtain an NF measurement of 4.4 mm. Measurement of the TCD (21.3 mm) and CM (5.3 mm) are also shown

its association with trisomy 21. Karyotyping should therefore be discussed in such cases.

Cystic hygroma

The second major defect associated with the fetal neck is cystic hygroma. This condition arises during early embryonic development from a failure in the connection between the lymphatic and venous systems. Excess fluid thus collects in the cervical region and can be readily recognized on ultrasound as cystic areas under the skin. These can be limited to the posterior aspect of the fetal neck or might extend anteriorly, effectively encompassing the whole neck. Cystic hygromata have a characteristic appearance due to the presence of septa that typically radiate from the cervical spine to the skin (Fig. 8.13). This feature is useful in distinguishing between a cystic hygroma and an occipital encephalocele. The latter condition is also associated with a defect in the skull, whereas cystic hygroma is associated with an intact skull (see Chapter 10).

Cystic hygromata are frequently associated with chromosomal abnormalities, principally Turner's syndrome (45XO). Karyotyping should therefore be discussed in such cases. Because of its strong association with aneuploidy, other abnormalities (particularly fetal hydrops) are often present with cystic hygroma. The prognosis is dependent on the accompanying abnormalities but is poor in the presence of hydrops.

THE FETAL SPINE

The normal fetal spine is easily visualized because the ossification centers within the vertebrae produce high-level echoes. Obtain a transverse section of the fetal body at any level. Now, dip the probe or slide the probe around the maternal abdomen so that the fetal spine lies at the top of the image.

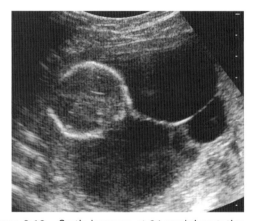

Figure 8.13 Cystic hygroma at 24 weeks' gestation. Transverse section of the head at the level of the thalami demonstrating a cystic mass containing septae. These septae produce the characteristic 'cart wheel' appearance of a cystic hygroma. Careful examination of the skull should reveal no defect in a case of cystic hygroma.

If the maternal abdomen is still flat, angling of the probe rather than sliding will be required to obtain this view. Rotating the probe through 90° will now demonstrate the spine in longitudinal section together with the overlying skin covering. Particularly note the upsweep of the sacrum (Fig. 8.14). Note the small distance between the spine and the fetal skin. This distance should be consistent along the length of the spine, if it is not then a slightly oblique view of the spine and skin covering is being imaged. Rotate the probe very slightly to achieve the correct view. The spine appears as two parallel lines of small echoes that come together at the sacrum. These echoes are thought to represent the ossification center of one lamina of the vertebral arch (posteriorly, i.e. immediately under the skin surface) and the ossification center of the same vertebral body anteriorly.

To obtain a coronal view of the spine, return to the longitudinal view of the fetal body. The ease with which this view can be obtained varies with fetal position. If the fetal spine is lateral, the coronal view of the spine is easily obtained by sliding the probe towards the relevant uterine side wall (Fig. 8.15). In this view, the three echoes from each vertebra derive from the ossification center of the vertebral body centrally and that of each lamina on either side. If the fetus is lying with its spine directly anterior or posterior then the coronal view is much more difficult to obtain. Begin with the longitudinal section of the fetal spine and then angle the probe through 90°. The angle of the probe to the maternal abdomen must be such that it produces a section that is virtually parallel to the scanning couch if a coronal spine view is to be obtained. As the spine is curved, it is rarely possible to view the whole spine in one coronal section (Fig. 8.15). Small sliding movements in this plane are needed to visualize all the vertebrae adequately in this view.

Rotating the probe through 90° from either the coronal or sagittal view will demonstrate the spine in transverse section (Fig. 8.16). In this view, each vertebra appears as three echoes which form a triangular or 'U' shape. The arms of the 'U' represent the ossification centers of the two lamina (immediately under the skin surface) and the vertebral body lying anteriorly. Note the small

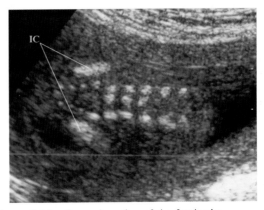

Figure 8.15 Coronal section of the fetal spine demonstrating the three echoes representing the ossification centers of each vertebra. The iliac crests (IC) can be seen on either side of the sacrum. Owing to the curvature of the normal spine note that the whole spine is not visualized in one image.

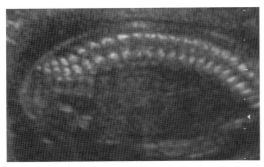

Figure 8.14 Longitudinal section of the fetal spine demonstrating the upsweep of the sacrum and the skin covering.

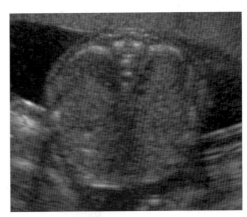

Figure 8.16 Transverse section of the fetal abdomen demonstrating the 'U' shape of a normal vertebra.

distance between the veretebra and the overlying skin.

The entire length of the spine, i.e. every vertebra, should be examined in all three sections. Care must be taken to keep the probe at right angles to the long axis of the spine when examining the spine transversely. This ensures that the triangular or 'U' appearance of each vertebra and the slight curve of the overlying skin are maintained – this is especially important when examining the sacrum.

THE FETAL CHEST AND DIAPHRAGM

The ribs are readily recognized in both longitudinal and transverse section. Abnormalities of the ribs are rare, although pathologic variations in size, shape and ossification are associated with skeletal dysplasias.

The most prominent structure in the chest is the fetal heart. The remainder of the chest is filled with the lungs, which produce homogeneous low level echoes (Fig. 8.17). With the obvious exception of the heart, single or multiple hypo- or hyperechoic areas within the chest are abnormal. Their differential diagnoses include diaphragmatic hernia, cystic adenomatoid malformation and tracheal occlusion (see Chapter 11).

The diaphragm can be identified in longitudinal and coronal section as a thin, echo-poor, cranially concave line that separates the lungs and heart in

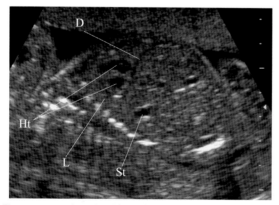

Figure 8.17   Longitudinal section of the fetal body illustrating the diaphragm (D), lungs (L) and heart (Ht). Note the concave shape of the diaphragm in this sagittal view and the normal position of the stomach (St) below the diaphragm.

the thorax from the stomach, liver and bowel in the abdomen (Fig. 8.17). It is important to appreciate the spatial relationships between these various organs in the normal fetus. Defects in the diaphragm are themselves rarely identified on ultrasound but can be assumed by the abnormal relative positions of one or more of these organs. A left-sided diaphragmatic hernia, for example, should be suspected if a cystic mass is seen in the left fetal chest with no stomach 'bubble' visible in the abdomen.

THE FETAL HEART

The fetal heart should occupy about one-third of the chest cavity with its apex pointing towards the left of the chest. Normal fetal situs should be confirmed before further examination of the heart is made (see Chapter 7). Three views of the heart should be sought routinely – the four-chamber view and the two outflow tract views.

The four-chamber view

First, obtain the abdominal circumference section and note the position of the fetal stomach. Slide the probe toward the fetal head until the heart is visualized. You might need to rotate the probe very slightly to obtain the four-chamber view. The two ventricles lie nearer to the chest wall than the two atria that lie nearer the fetal spine. The right ventricle lies nearer the anterior chest wall than the left ventricle and is characterized by the presence of the moderator band (Fig. 8.18). The left ventricle lies nearer the left fetal shoulder and is ipsilateral with the stomach in the normal fetus.

The moderator band and prominent papillary muscles are used to identify the morphologic right ventricle. The pulmonary veins are used to identify the morphologic left atrium. At least one of the four pulmonary veins can be readily visualized on the four-chamber view (Fig. 8.18).

The following should be observed in the four-chamber view:

- the two ventricles and ventricular walls should be of equal size
- the two atria and atrial walls should be of equal size

- the apex of the heart should point to the left of the fetal chest
- the moderator band should be seen in the right ventricle
- the foramen ovale should be seen moving in the left atrium
- at least one of the pulmonary veins should be seen entering the left atrium
- the motion of the mitral valve, between the left atrium and left ventricle, should be regular
- the motion of the tricuspid valve, between the right atrium and right ventricle, should be regular
- the atrioventricular valves should *not* insert into the interventricular septum at the same level. The insertion of the tricuspid valve is nearer the cardiac apex. This feature is known as the 'offset crux' of the heart
- the interventricular septum should be complete.

Echogenic foci

These circular hyperechoic structures, similar in shape and appearance to a small golf ball, are com-

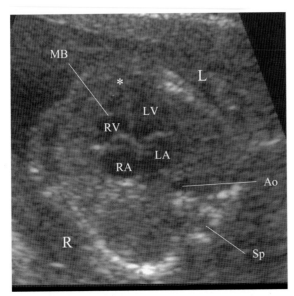

Figure 8.18 Four-chamber view of a normal fetal heart. Note the apex (*) of the heart points toward the left side. Note also the subtle difference in appearance of the right and left ventricles due to the presence of the moderator band in the right ventricle. Ao, aorta; L, left side of fetal chest; LA, left atrium; LV, left ventricle; MB, moderator band; R, right side of fetal chest; RA, right atrium; RV, right ventricle; Sp, spine.

monly seen in the second trimester fetus. They are thought to be due to mineralization within the papillary muscle. One echogenic focus identified in the left ventricle and attached to the mitral valve is the most common appearance (Fig. 8.19), although single right-sided and multiple foci have been reported. Most echogenic foci will resolve by the third trimester and are usually of no pathological significance to the developing fetus or infant. They constitute a 'minor marker' for chromosomal abnormalities because of their reported association by some authors with an increased risk for trisomy 21.

Owing to its bright appearance and regular movement, an echogenic focus is readily seen by both the operator and the parents. It is therefore important that you can discuss its finding appropriately, and according to departmental guidelines, with the parents.

Abnormalities detected on the four-chamber view

Identifying a normal four-chamber view should exclude abnormalities that result in a disparity of size between the two ventricles. Impaired function of the tricuspid or mitral valve will result in enlargement of the affected atrium with hypoplasia of the corresponding ventricle. For example, an enlarged right atrium will result from regurgitation of the tricuspid valve, whereas hypoplastic left heart syndrome should be suspected if the left ventricle is small. Coarctation should be suspected if

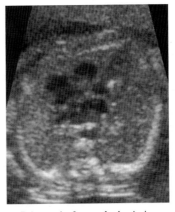

Figure 8.19 Echogenic focus. A single hyperechoic mass can be seen lying within the left ventricle. Careful observation will demonstrate that it is typically associated with the mitral valve.

there is disproportion between the two ventricles with enlargement of the right ventricle. Ebstein's anomaly is associated with enlargement of the right atrium at the expense of the right ventricle, due to the abnormal implantation of the tricuspid valve.

A normal interventricular septum should exclude significant ventricular septal defects (VSD), in particular, the submembraneous type. A normal offset crux should exclude atrioventricular septal defect (AVSD). Both VSDs and AVSDs are associated with choromosomal abnormalities, the latter being characteristic of trisomy 21.

The aortic outflow tract

Rotating the probe slightly toward the right fetal shoulder from the four-chamber view will demonstrate the long axis view of the aorta or aortic outflow tract view (Fig. 8.20). This view should demonstrate the left ventricle, continuity of the interventricular septum with the (anterior) wall of the aorta, the aortic valve and a short section of the ascending aorta directed toward the right fetal shoulder.

Most VSDs are perimembraneous or subaortic in position. The former are probably best imaged from the four-chamber view; imaging the aortic outflow tract provides the best method of detecting the latter. Inability to obtain a normal aortic outflow view is most commonly due to poor technique, especially in the novice. However, this view will be abnormal in cases of overriding aorta, aortic stenosis, double outlet right ventricle and Fallot's tetralogy.

The pulmonary artery outflow tract

Return to the four-chamber view and slide the probe towards the fetal head. Only a small movement is required to demonstrate the long axis view of the pulmonary artery or pulmonary artery outflow tract view (Fig. 8.21). This view should demonstrate the right ventricle, continuity of the right ventricular wall with the wall of the pulmonary artery, the pulmonary valve and the main pulmonary artery directed toward the fetal spine. The pulmonary artery branches into three (the main – which becomes the ductus arteriosus – the left and the right) a short distance after leaving the heart. This can be seen in this view. Inability to obtain a normal pulmonary artery outflow view is most commonly due to poor technique, especially in the novice. The pulmonary artery outflow view will be abnormal in cases of double outlet right ventricle and pulmonary stenosis.

The cross–over

It will be noted from the above that the direction of the two outflow tracts differs and that they cross over each other when leaving the heart.

The normal cross-over of the aorta and pulmonary artery excludes transposition of the great arteries. This is an important diagnosis to make

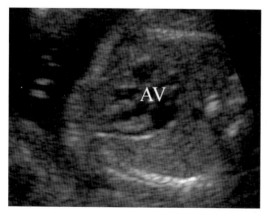

Figure 8.20   The aortic outflow tract. Note the normal continuity between the interventricular septum and the aortic root in this view. AV, aortic valve.

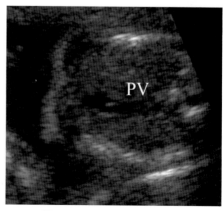

Figure 8.21   The pulmonary artery outflow tract. PV, pulmonary valve.

prenatally because it is one of the few cardiac conditions where prior knowledge before delivery enables immediate postnatal intervention.

Three further views complete the examination of the fetal heart – the short axis, ductal arch and aortic arch views. These views are important in assessing the relative size of the various vessels, the relationship of the great vessels to other structures and therefore in the recognition of associated abnormalities. How to obtain these views is described in Chapter 11.

Fetal heart rate

The fetal heart should have a regular beat and rate (110–150 bpm), although it is not uncommon for bradycardic episodes of several seconds to be observed during the second trimester examination. The fetal heart should be observed to confirm normal rhythm and symmetry of movement between the atria and ventricles and between the left and right sides of the heart.

THE FETAL ABDOMEN

Obtain a view of the fetal abdomen suitable to measure the abdominal circumference (see Chapter 7). A single, left-sided stomach 'bubble' will be seen in the majority of fetuses after 16 weeks' gestation. Confirming a normally situated single stomach bubble is important in the exclusion of gastrointestinal tract obstruction (see Chapter 11)

Cord insertion

Slide caudally to the site of insertion of the umbilical cord (Fig. 8.22A). Within the cord itself, the two umbilical arteries can be observed leaving the fetal abdomen just superior to the fetal bladder and immediately inferior to where the single umbilical vein enters. If any doubt remains, color Doppler can be used to confirm arterial flow in both umbilical arteries as they pass on either side of the fetal bladder. Vessel number can also be evaluated from a transverse section of the cord in the amniotic fluid (Fig. 8.22B) although this is frequently difficult before 22 weeks of gestation. Abnormalities of the umbilical cord are discussed in Chapter 9.

Confirming a normal cord insertion is important in the exclusion of abdominal wall defects, the

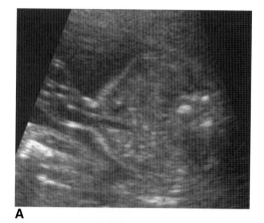

A

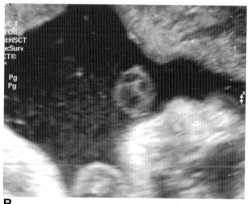

B

Figure 8.22   A. Insertion of the umbilical cord into the fetal abdomen. Note the direction of the two arteries within the fetal abdomen. B. Transverse section of the normal umbilical cord at 24 weeks demonstrating the presence of two arteries and one vein.

most common of which are omphalocele and gastroschisis (see Chapter 11).

Major blood vessels

Return now to a transverse section of the fetal abdomen and follow the umbilical vein into the liver. Note it runs through the liver at approximately 45° to the fetal spine. The umbilical vein, together with the extra hepatic portal vein, enters the portal sinus, which gives rise to the left portal vein, the right portal vein and the ductus venosus (Fig. 8.23). Most of the blood that is being returned to the fetus from the placenta passes through the ductus venosus to the right atrium.

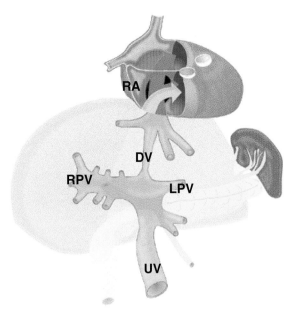

Figure 8.23   The relationship between the umbilical vein and the ductus venosus. DV, ductus venosus; LPV, left portal vein; RPV, right portal vein; UV, umbilical vein.

The fetal aorta is best located from a longitudinal, coronal section of the fetal abdomen. It can be followed down to the iliac bifurcation and into each leg as the femoral artery (Fig. 8.24). The inferior vena cava is visible alongside the aorta in the upper abdomen (Fig. 8.25). Note that this passes through the diaphragm and can be seen entering the right atrium. The aorta passes behind the diaphragm.

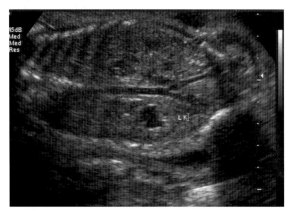

Figure 8.24   Longitudinal section of the fetal abdomen demonstrating the iliac bifurcation of the aorta.

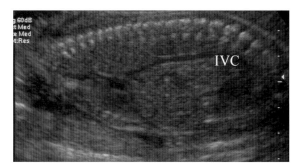

Figure 8.25   Longitudinal section of the fetal abdomen demonstrating the course of the inferior vena cava (IVC).

The gall bladder

The gall bladder can also be visualized on a cross-sectional view of the fetal abdomen, typically very slightly below that required for the AC (Fig. 8.26). The gall bladder can be distinguished from the stomach by its elongated shape and its more anterior position on the right side of the fetal abdomen.

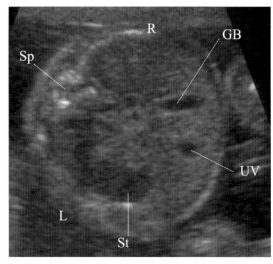

Figure 8.26   Transverse section of the fetal abdomen demonstrating the gall bladder. Note its elongated shape and anterior position on the right side of the abdomen compared to that of the stomach on the left. GB, gall bladder; L, left side of fetal abdomen; R, right side of fetal abdomen; Sp, spine; St, stomach; UV, umbilical vein.

The spleen

The fetal spleen is not normally visualized in the second trimester fetus, although it can be seen on the left of the abdominal cavity in the third trimester.

The bowel

The bowel, liver and spleen are usually indistinguishable in the normal second-trimester fetus. It is important to observe the fetal abdomen in both longitudinal and cross-section to exclude evidence of obstruction or areas of increased echogenicity (Fig. 8.27).

Echogenicity in the abdomen

Echogenic bowel

Localized areas of increased echogenicity in the small bowel (Fig. 8.27) are usually of no pathologic significance. The diagnosis of echogenic bowel is necessarily subjective, with echogenicity equal to that of fetal bone being the most commonly used criterion. Intra-amniotic bleeding is the most common cause of echogenic bowel but it has been described in association with cystic fibrosis (CF). This is a useful marker for CF where there is a family history, but is of no value in screening. Echogenic bowel is a minor marker for chromosomal abnormalities, in particular trisomy 21. It is also a marker for congenital infection when present in a small and/or growth-restricted fetus.

Echogenic foci in the liver

Localized areas of increased echogenicity in the liver are rare but are associated with infection, most commonly varicella or chicken pox.

THE URINARY TRACT

The fetal kidneys can be seen transabdominally from 14 weeks' gestation and are easily visible at 20–22 weeks. They are best located from a transverse section of the abdomen. By sliding caudally from the section required for measurement of the AC, look closely in the paraspinal gutters.

The first clue that you have found the kidney is the hypoechoic area – delineated by a hyperechoic bright border – that represents the renal pelvis (Fig. 8.28). If the fetal spine is directly anterior then both kidneys can be seen on the same section; if the spine is lateral then the lower kidney is usually hidden in the acoustic shadow from the spine. To see the lower kidney, the probe should be rotated around the maternal abdomen in an

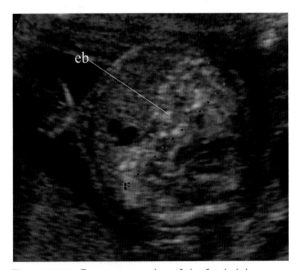

Figure 8.27 Transverse section of the fetal abdomen demonstrating echogenic bowel (eb). Note the area of increased echogenicity is confined to a small area of the abdomen, suggesting only part of the bowel is affected at this gestation.

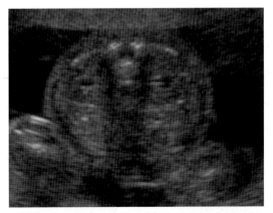

Figure 8.28 Transverse section of the fetal abdomen demonstrating both kidneys and renal pelves. Note the spine is anterior, enabling both kidneys to be imaged. In this plane the acoustic shadow of the spine hides the umbilical vein.

attempt to bring the spine to the top of the screen.

Having located the kidneys in the transverse plane, bring one kidney into the center of the screen by sliding the probe across the maternal abdomen. Rotate the probe through 90° keeping that kidney in view until a longitudinal, sagittal section of the kidney is obtained (Fig. 8.29). If the upper and lower limits of the kidney are difficult to see, make tiny lateral sliding movements of the probe. Fetal breathing movements aid in the identification of the renal end-points. Note the appearance of the renal pelvis in this view. The echogenicity of the renal cortex is very similar to that of the fetal lungs, i.e. low-level, homogeneous echoes.

Renal size is assessed from longitudinal, antero-posterior and transverse diameter measurements. The maximum longitudinal renal diameter should be measured from a longitudinal, sagittal section of the fetus, rather than a longitudinal, coronal section. Slight rotation of the probe from the long axis of the fetus might be necessary to obtain the maximum longitudinal axis of the kidney. Take care to ensure that the adrenal, lying immediately superior to the anterior pole of the kidney, is not included in the renal measurement. Rotate the probe through 90° to obtain a view of the kidney in transverse section. Make small sliding movements of the probe up and down the renal axis to obtain the optimal transverse section. The maximum transverse and AP diameters of one kidney should be taken from the same image (Fig. 8.30). All three renal diameters are measured using the same method – by placing the intersection of the two arms of the onscreen calipers on the outer aspects of the renal outline ('outer to outer'). Only rarely will both kidneys be visualized optimally in transverse section on the same image. The two kidneys should therefore be imaged and measured independently. Charts showing normal values for these parameters are available (see Appendix 10).

Renal pelvic size is typically reported using the AP pelvis diameter only. The AP pelvis diameter and maximum transverse and AP renal diameters are measured from the same section. The AP pelvis

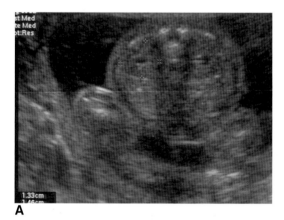

A

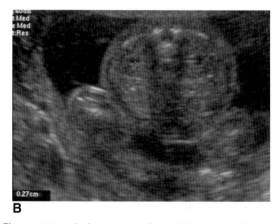

B

Figure 8.30   A. Anteroposterior and transverse diameter measurements of the left kidney shown in Fig. 8.28. Note the calipers are positioned to obtain an 'outer to outer' measurement of both diameters (13.3 mm and 14.6 mm respectively). B. Anteroposterior (AP) diameter measurement of the right renal pelvis shown in Fig. 8.28. Note the calipers are positioned to obtain an 'inner to inner' measurement of the AP pelvis (2.7 mm).

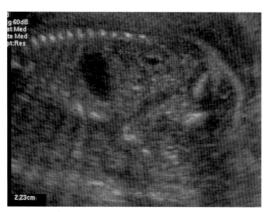

Figure 8.29   Sagittal section demonstrating the longitudinal diameter (22.3 mm) of the left kidney imaged in Fig. 8.28.

diameter is measured by placing the intersection of the two arms of the onscreen calipers on the inner aspects of the renal pelvis outline ('inner to inner').

Mild renal pelvic dilatation

The normal renal pelvis fluctuates in size, although this does not appear to correlate simply with fetal bladder volume. Controversy remains as to what constitutes normal renal pelvic size in the fetus. An AP diameter of 5 mm is commonly taken as the upper limit of normal renal pelvic size in the second trimester and 10 mm in the third trimester. The definition of mild renal pelvic dilatation (RPD) also varies between authors. Some use quantitative criteria to distinguish between mild, moderate and severe RPD, whereas others use qualitative criteria, such as calyceal dilatation.

Mild RPD can be a unilateral or a bilateral finding (Fig. 8.31). It is a common finding in the second trimester, with a reported prevalence ranging from 0.7 to 2.8%. It constitutes a 'minor marker' for a range of chromosomal abnormalities, including trisomy 21. In the absence of other markers for trisomy 21, the maternal age-related risk is not significantly increased.

In a small number of cases mild RPD is the first sign of progressing prenatal urinary tract dilatation that can result in postnatal uropathies, including pelviureteric junction obstruction (PUJO), duplex kidney and reflux. For this reason, we suggest that all cases of mild RPD should be rescanned between 32 and 36 weeks to exclude worsening dilatation.

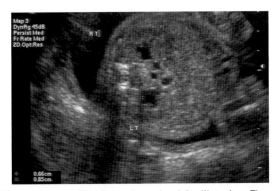

Figure 8.31   Mild bilateral renal pelvic dilatation. The right AP pelvis measures 6.6 mm and the left 8.5 mm. Compare the appearances to those of the normal renal pelves in Fig. 8.28.

Postnatal ultrasound investigations should be recommended in those fetuses demonstrating progressive dilatation (AP pelvis > 10 mm in the third trimester).

The fetal bladder is usually readily visible in both transverse and longitudinal sections of the fetal abdomen and pelvis transabdominally from 12 weeks of gestation. The fetus empties its bladder every 30–45 min. Demonstration of fetal bladder filling implies that renal function is present.

THE FETAL LIMBS

Chapter 7 describes how to obtain measurements of the fetal femur. This is often the only long bone measured, although a visual assessment of the other long bones should be made. Normal values for all the long bones are available.

To visualize the tibia and fibula, obtain the view required to measure the femur. Keeping the lower end of the femur (at the knee) in view, rotate the probe slowly until some part of the two bones of the lower leg is seen. Continue to rotate the probe until the AP view of the lower leg, demonstrating both tibia and fibula, is obtained (Fig. 8.32A). You might need to accompany each rotational movement with a small sliding movement of the probe to keep the bones of the lower leg in view. The tibia and fibula are very similar in length and appearance. Ensure that both bones are straight and not bowed, and are of similar echogenicity to the other long bones. Should measurements be required, images of the tibia and fibula should be sought separately (Fig. 8.32B). Attempting to measure both tibia and fibula from the same image will rarely provide optimal sections of both bones.

Two views of the lower leg are useful for evaluation of the foot. The first AP view, as described above, demonstrates both the tibia and fibula in longitudinal section. In this view only a cross-section of the talus should be seen and *not* the whole foot (Fig. 8.32A). If the plantar or footprint view of the foot is obtained in this section, talipes should be suspected (Fig. 8.33). The carrying angle of the foot can be assessed from the second, lateral view of the lower leg. This section demonstrates only one (usually the tibia) bone in longitudinal section. In this view, the foot should be seen in sagittal section. The normal carrying angle of the

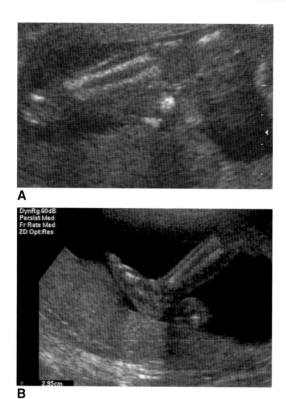

A

B

Figure 8.32 A. The tibia and fibula in longitudinal section. Note that only the talus of the foot can be seen in this plane in the normal fetus. B. Measurement of the tibia (29.5 mm).

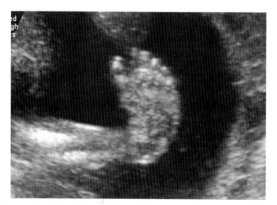

Figure 8.33 Abnormal carrying angle of the foot in talipes. Compare this appearance to the normal appearance shown in Fig. 8.32A.

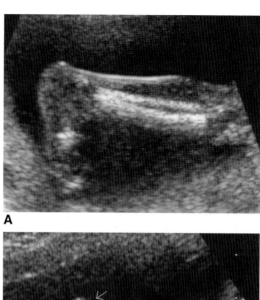

A

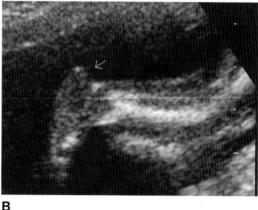

B

Figure 8.34 A. Lateral view of the lower leg demonstrating the normal carrying angle of the foot. Note the position of the foot, the shape of the normal heel and of the normal sole of the foot. Note also that only one of the two lower limb bones, the tibia, can be adequately seen in this view. B. Lateral view of the lower leg demonstrating a rocker-bottom foot. Note the protruding heel and convex shape of the sole of the foot compared to the normal appearances of A.

view of the foot can be obtained by rotating the probe through 90° from this view (Fig. 8.35A). It is difficult to count the toes but you should attempt to do so to exclude polydactyly or syndactyly. Also look at the position of the big toe relative to the second toe to exclude a sandal gap (Fig. 8.35B).

Talipes, rocker–bottom feet and sandal gap

Three minor markers of chromosomal abnormalities involve the foot. Talipes is a relatively common

foot to the lower leg can now be assessed (Figs 8.34A and 8.32B), together with the shape of the calcaneus or heel and the sole of the foot (to exclude rocker bottom foot; Fig. 8.34B). A plantar

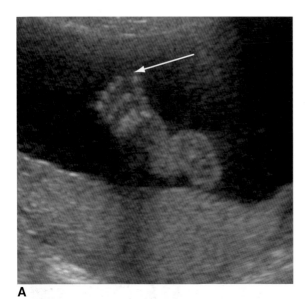

A

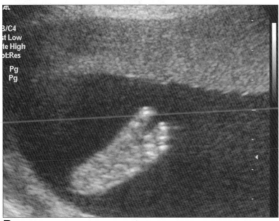

B

Figure 8.35   A. Plantar view of the normal foot. Note the appearance of the toes, especially the big toe (arrow) and second toe. B. Plantar view of a foot with a sandal gap. Note the appearance of the big toe and second toe.

finding in chromosomally normal fetuses, with a reported incidence is 1 in 1000 (see Fig. 8.33). It has a slightly higher association with trisomy 18, 13 and triploidy. Rocker-bottom feet are associated with trisomy 18 whereas sandal gap is associated with trisomy 21 and triploidy.

The humerus is located and measured in the same way as the femur. Return to the section demonstrating the four-chamber view of the heart and

slide the probe in a cranial direction until the clavicles are visualized. At this point a cross-section of the humerus is usually seen. Keeping this bright echo from the humerus in view, rotate the probe slowly until the full length of the humerus is obtained. You might need to make a *small* sliding movement after each rotational movement to bring the humerus back into view. To ensure that you have the full length of the humerus and that your section is not oblique, soft tissue should be visible beyond both ends of the humerus and the bone should not appear to merge with the skin of the upper arm at any point (Fig. 8.36).

To visualize the radius and ulna, keep the lower end of the humerus (at the elbow) in view and rotate the probe slowly until some part of the two bones of the lower arm is seen. Continue to rotate the probe until the AP view of the lower arm, demonstrating both radius and ulna, is obtained. You might need to accompany each rotational movement with a small sliding movement of the probe to keep the bones of the lower arm in view. As with the leg, ensure that you have obtained the maximum length of each bone before making your assessment and/or measurement. You should ensure that both bones are visualized. The radius and ulna differ in appearance and this should be noted (Fig. 8.37). The ulna is longer, thinner and extends further toward the elbow or humerus than the radius. Remember that the radius and the thumb are on the same side of the lower arm. Ensure that the radius and ulna are straight and not bowed and are of similar echogenicity to the other long bones.

The normal carrying angle of the hand to the lower arm can now be assessed (Fig. 8.37). Fixed

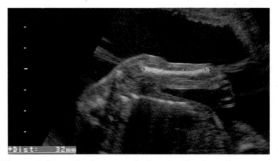

Figure 8.36   The humerus in longitudinal section, demonstrating its measurement (32 mm).

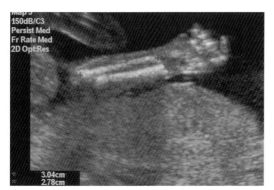

Figure 8.37 The radius and ulna in longitudinal section. In this image the radius is the more posterior bone and measures 27.8 mm. The ulna lies anterior to the radius in this image and measures 30.4 mm. Note the relative lengths and positions of the two bones. Note also the position and appearance of the normal (clenched) hand.

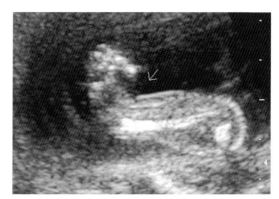

Figure 8.38 Fixed flexion deformity of the hand. Compare the position and appearance of this abnormal hand to the normal hand shown in Fig. 8.37.

flexion deformities are easily excluded using this view (Fig. 8.38). Patience is necessary to assess the hand properly. Counting fingers is difficult because the fetus often has a closed fist. Useful information can still be obtained, however, because it is often possible to exclude overlapping of the fingers using this view (Fig. 8.39A). The outstretched hand view is necessary to confirm the normal appearance of the four fingers and thumb and to exclude clinodactyly, polydactyly or syndactyly (Fig. 8.39B and C). Expecting to obtain this view with every fetus during routine screening examination might be unrealistic.

Fixed flexion deformity, overlapping fingers, clinodactyly, polydactyly, syndactyly

Fixed flexion of the wrists and overlapping fingers is associated with trisomy 18 whereas clinodactyly is associated with trisomy 21. Postaxial polydactyly is more typical of trisomy 13 and syndactyly of triploidy.

THE FETAL FACE

To demonstrate the soft tissues of the face, start with the BPD section. Slide the probe caudally until the orbits can be visualized. Increase the

angle of the probe by about 45° toward the front of the face then slide the probe toward the front of the face until the section shown in Fig. 8.40 is obtained. During this maneuver, the lens of the eye, eyelid and the mouth can be seen. Slide the probe a little further forward until just the fetal lips and nostrils are seen (Fig. 8.41). Sliding the probe very slightly back toward the face again will demonstrate the bright echoes of the alveolar ridge (Fig. 8.42). These two views are required to exclude a cleft of the upper lip and gum (or alveolus), respectively.

The normal palate is not routinely visualized with ultrasound. It should not be confused with the tongue, which is easily demonstrated from transverse sections of the head, at the level of the mandible (Fig. 8.43).

Cleft lip and palate

Facial clefting occurs in about 1 in 700 births. Approximately 35% of the total number of clefts are of the lip and palate whereas 25% involve the lip and alveolar ridge only (Fig. 8.44). Isolated cleft palate is the most common of the three conditions occurring in 40% of cases.

Over 80% of cases of cleft lip, with or without cleft palate, are isolated conditions. However, cleft lip is associated with chromosomal abnormalities (principally trisomy 13 and trisomy 18), exposure to teratogens including antiepileptic drugs and a large number of genetic syndromes.

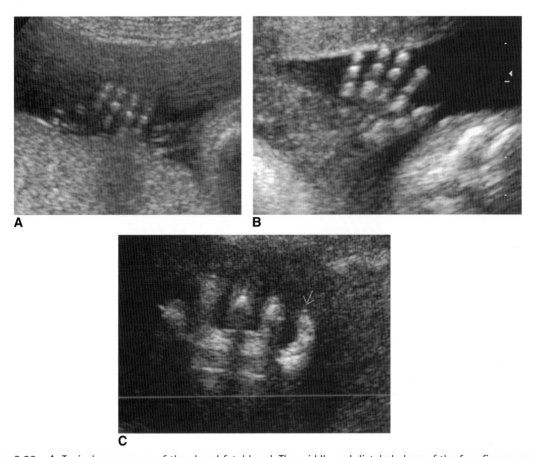

Figure 8.39 A. Typical appearance of the closed fetal hand. The middle and distal phalanx of the four fingers can be seen. Note the parallel position of the normal fingers. B. The outstretched hand. In this view all three phalanges of the four fingers and the two of the thumb can be visualized. Note the appearance of the normal little finger. C. Clinodactyly. The absence of the middle phalanx of the little finger produces incurving of the little finger. Compare this appearance to the normal appearances of Figs 8.39 A and B.

Median cleft lip is typically associated with holo-prosencephaly.

A profile of the fetal face requires a midline sagittal section, obtained by rotating the probe through 90° from the coronal view of the fetal face. The ease with which this view can be obtained varies with fetal position. If the fetus is lying in the OP position the profile is easily obtained (Fig. 8.45A). If the fetus is lying in the OT position then the angle of the probe to the maternal abdomen must be such that it produces a section that is virtually parallel to the scanning couch in order for the fetal profile to be obtained.

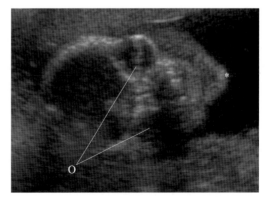

Figure 8.40 Coronal section of the fetal face demonstrating the orbits (O) and soft tissues. Note that this is *not* the correct view to exclude a cleft of the upper lip. *chin.

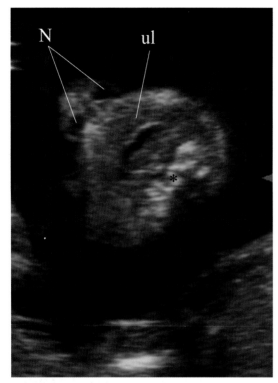

Figure 8.41 Coronal section of the fetal face demonstrating the lips and nostrils. The mouth is slightly open. Note that *this* is the view required to exclude a cleft in the fetal lip, and not that shown in Fig. 8.40. N, nostrils; ul, upper lip; *chin.

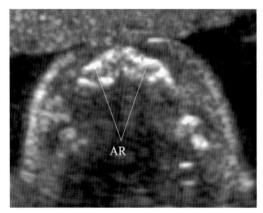

Figure 8.42 Transverse section of the head demonstrating the alveolar ridge (AR). Note that this is the view required to exclude a cleft of the alveolar ridge.

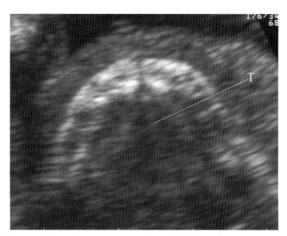

Figure 8.43 Transverse section of the head demonstrating the tongue (T). Note that this view does not demonstrate the palate, which is difficult to image when normal.

Micrognathia, cleft lip, frontal bossing, flattened face

A normal fetal profile can exclude various abnormalities, including minor markers of aneuploidy. Micrognathia, or receding chin (Fig. 8.45B), is associated with trisomy 18 and triploidy together with various genetic syndromes such as Robert syndrome. The prominent premaxilla that is frequently present with a bilateral complete cleft of the upper lip (Fig. 8.45C) is best identified from the fetal profile. Some skeletal dysplasias, including thanatophoric dysplasia and achondroplasia, are associated with a bulbous forehead or frontal bossing. By contrast a flattened face is associated with trisomy 21.

THE FETAL SEX

It is possible to determine the sex of the fetus transabdominally from 14 weeks but it is frequently difficult to make a definitive diagnosis until several weeks later. The diagnosis depends upon the fetus having its legs apart and on recognizing the echo patterns characteristic of the male and female respectively. The male scrotum and penis can be identified (Fig. 8.46). The testes can be visualized in the scrotum in the third trimester. The female labia are smaller in size than the male scrotum and have an appearance similar to two lips between the

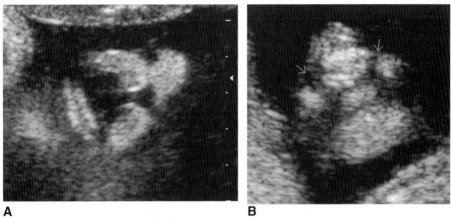

Figure 8.44   A. Transverse view of the head demonstrating left-sided unilateral cleft of the lip and alveolar ridge. Note the distortion of the nasal tissue on this side. Compare this appearance with that shown in Fig. 8.42. B. Bilateral cleft lip (arrows). Compare this appearance with the normal appearance shown in Fig. 8.41.

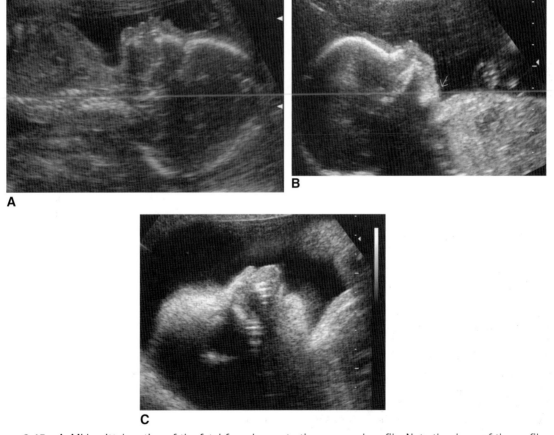

Figure 8.45   A. Midsagittal section of the fetal face demonstrating a normal profile. Note the shape of the profile, particularly the size and angle of the normal chin. B. Midsagittal section of the fetal face demonstrating micrognathia (arrow). Compare the shape of the profile with that shown in A and C. C. Midsagittal section of the fetal face demonstrating the prominent premaxilla associated with a bilateral complete cleft of the lip. Compare the shape of the profile with that shown in A and B.

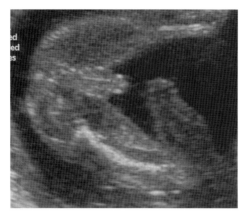

Figure 8.46 Male genitalia at 22 weeks' gestation.

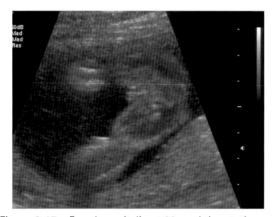

Figure 8.47 Female genitalia at 22 weeks' gestation.

fetal legs (Fig. 8.47). You should not make the diagnosis unless the views obtained are unequivocal and do not diagnose a female by an apparent lack of male parts. Identifying fetal gender is important in women who are carriers of sex-linked conditions such as heamophilia. In these conditions only the male fetus is affected.

Parents seem to be equally divided as to whether they wish to know the sex of their fetus. We suggest that you do not ask the parents if they wish to know the sex of their baby, but if they want to know you should try to tell them. Asking the parents seems to put them under pressure to make a decision one way or the other and many parents assume that if you have asked the question the fetus must be a male. Never guess; if you are unsure, say you do not know.

REFERENCES AND FURTHER READING

Chitty L S, Chudleigh P M, Wright E et al 1998 The significance of choroid plexus cysts in an unselected population: the results of a multicentre study. Ultrasound in Obstetrics and Gynaecology 12:1–7

Chudleigh P M, Chitty L S, Pembrey M, Campbell S 2001 The association of aneuploidy and mild fetal pyelectasis in an unselected population: the results of a multicenter study. Ultrasound in Obstetrics and Gynaecology 17:197–202

Cleft Lip and Palate – A Guide for Sonographers. CLAPA 2001

Grandjean H, Larroque D, Levi S 1999 The performance of routine ultrasonographic screening of pregnancies in the Eurofetus Study. American Journal of Obstetrics and Gynecology 181:446–454

Pilu G, Nicolaides K 1999 Diagnosis of fetal abnormalities: the 18–23-week scan. Parthenon Publishing, New York, p 134

Prefumo F, Presti F, Mavrides E et al 2001 Isolated echogenic foci in the fetal heart: do they increase the risk of trisomy 21 in a population previously screened by nuchal translucency? Ultrasound in Obstetrics and Gynecology 18:126–130

Snijders R J M, Nicolaides K H 1994 Fetal biometry at 14–40 weeks' gestation. Ultrasound in Obstetrics and Gynecology 4:34–48

The British Medical Ultrasound Society 2002 Prenatal diagnosis of congenital heart disease. BMUS Bulletin 10:1:4–34

The Royal College of Obstetricians and Gynaecologists 2000 Routine ultrasound screening in pregnancy: protocol, standards and training. Report of the RCOG Working Party, July 2000. RCOG, London

Thompson M O, Thilaganathan B 1998 Effect of routine screening for Down's syndrome on the significance of isolated fetal hydronephrosis. British Journal of Obstetrics and Gynaecology 105:860–864

United Kingdom Association of Sonographers 2001 Guidelines for professional working standards – ultrasound practice. United Kingdom Association of Sonographers, London

Chapter 9

The placenta and amniotic fluid

PLACENTAL LOCALIZATION

With the exception of women undergoing chorion villus sampling, accurate assessment of placental position is not necessary when examining the first trimester uterus. Because of positional changes of the body of the uterus in early pregnancy, the placental site can change relative to the internal os. We therefore do not recommend reporting placental position in normal cirumstances until the routine 20–22 week scan. Localizing and reporting placental position in the second trimester is described in Chapter 7.

'Placenta previa' is a term relating placental position to the lower segment. Before 28 weeks the uterus does not have a true lower segment. If the placenta overlaps or encroaches on the internal os before 28 weeks it is better to define it as low-lying and retain the term 'placenta previa' until after 28 weeks gestation.

Is localizing the placenta at 20–22 weeks worthwhile?

Yes. Approximately 95% of women will have an obviously fundal placenta at this gestation and, therefore, will not have placenta previa in later pregnancy. The remaining 5% will have a low-lying placenta at 20–22 weeks and should therefore be rescanned in the third trimester. One in five of these women will have a true placenta previa.

OBSTETRIC MANAGEMENT OF THE WOMAN WITH A LOW-LYING PLACENTA AT 20–22 WEEKS

If the woman has had no bleeding it is probably only necessary to request a rescan in the third trimester. If the woman has bled or if she has lost several previous pregnancies she might be admitted to hospital or advised to refrain from sexual intercourse.

PLACENTA PREVIA

Classification

Figure 9.1 illustrates the most commonly used classification of placenta previa. The typing of placenta previa from I to IV was developed before the introduction of ultrasound. Placenta previa was typed on vaginal examination under general anesthesia, usually in early labor. Hence, the existence of type III, in which the placenta partially covers an open internal cervical os. Since the widespread introduction of ultrasound, placenta previa is generally classified as 'major' and 'minor'. Minor previa is diagnosed when the placenta encroaches into the lower segment of the uterus, whereas major previa describes the leading edge of the placenta encroaching to, or covering the internal cervical os.

The clinical problem

If the placenta overlies the internal os, then vaginal delivery can occur only through the placenta. With the major degrees of placenta previa, life-threatening bleeding will occur when the uterus contracts and the placenta separates. In some cases this will not occur until the woman goes into labor, but it

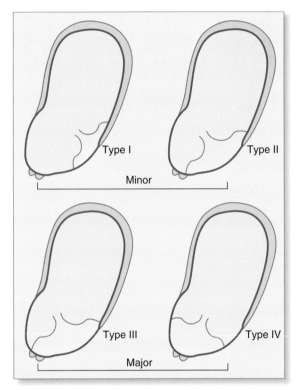

Figure 9.1 The typing of placenta previa.

could occur at any time during the pregnancy, either spontaneously or in response to premature contractions. Women known to have major degrees of placenta previa are usually kept in hospital (with cross-matched blood permanently available) and are delivered by elective cesarean section at about 39 weeks, or earlier if they have had a large hemorrhage.

Method of diagnosis

The lower uterine segment, which forms during the third trimester of pregnancy, is covered anteriorly by the bladder. The presence of fluid in the bladder will help identify the anterior lower segment. The posterior aspect of the lower segment can then be determined by projecting the upper edge of the bladder onto the posterior wall of the uterus (Fig. 9.2). Unless the placenta is quite clearly in the fundus, the internal os and the lower edge of the placenta should be demonstrated on the same scan.

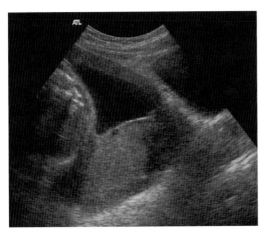

Figure 9.2 Identifying the lower segment in the third trimester. The area covered by the bladder is the lower segment. By projecting this backward the lower segment can be defined posteriorly. The placenta can be seen on the posterior wall. Note the bright echoes from the chorionic plate.

Problems

The most common problem is locating the lower edge of a posterior placenta. The presenting part of the fetus attenuates the ultrasound such that few echoes are obtained from the posterior myometrium. Scanning in laterally from the sides of the uterus can overcome this problem and allow the lower edge of the placenta to be seen. Alternatively, placing the woman in a head-down position might displace the presenting part so that the posterior myometrium above the internal os can be visualized.

Use of a transvaginal probe inserted a few centimetres into the vagina will easily overcome this problem. The higher resolution gained by using a 6–7.5 MHz transducer, together with the fact that the fetal presenting part is no longer lying within the path of the ultrasound beam, allows clear visualization of the posterior lower segment. We recommend transvaginal scanning only for women with a questionable low posterior placenta on abdominal scanning.

Reporting placenta previa

When reporting placenta previa, information other than just the classification is useful to the clinician.

It should be noted whether the placenta is anterior or posterior, because the surgeon could encounter and even cut through the placenta during cesarean section if it is positioned anteriorly.

In the case of a minor placenta previa, a clinical decision has to be made regarding suitability for a trial of vaginal delivery. In this instance, the distance of the leading placental edge from internal cervical os and the relative position of the fetal head in relation to the leading placental edge are important. These factors, together with gestational age and any previous episodes of antepartum hemorrhage, are considered when assessing the pregnancy for delivery.

Clinical management of the woman with placenta previa

If the woman has bled during pregnancy or has a major degree of placenta previa, the obstetrician will advise hospital admission. Two units of blood, correctly cross-matched, should be kept available. Serial scans to monitor fetal growth and placental position will be requested, although fetal growth is rarely affected in women with placenta previa. The woman with a major degree of placenta previa will be delivered by cesarean section at 39 weeks, or before if she has had a sizeable hemorrhage.

Controversy remains over the management of women with minor degrees of placenta previa. The problems are as follows:

What to do with women with asymptomatic placenta previa?

Whereas most obstetricians would advise admission for women with major degrees of placenta previa, it is probably unnecessary to admit those with minor degrees of placenta previa if they do not bleed. Bleeding in these women is very unlikely to be life threatening.

How reliable is the interpretation of the ultrasound examination?

In skilled hands, ultrasound placentography has a negligible false-positive rate. Many obstetricians who perform ultrasound have abandoned the typing of placenta previa and simply report the distance in centimeters of the lower edge of the placenta from

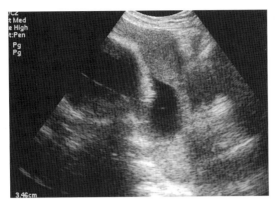

Figure 9.3 Longitudinal, midline section of the uterus demonstrating measurement of the distance (34.6 mm) from the lower edge of the posterior placenta to the internal os.

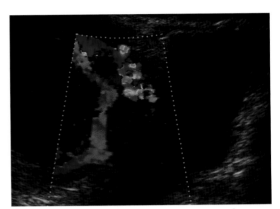

Figure 9.4 Longitudinal, midline section of the uterus demonstrating the vessels connecting the succenturate lobe with the body of the anterior placenta overlying the cervical os. The connecting vessels are better imaged using color Doppler.

the internal os (Fig. 9.3). In the case of minor previa, the woman is scanned finally at 37–38 weeks gestation in a slightly head-down position. If the biparietal diameter (BPD) is below the lower edge of the placenta, most clinicians would await the spontaneous onset of labor. If not, the woman is usually offered an elective cesarean section.

NORMAL VARIATIONS IN PLACENTAL MORPHOLOGY

Succenturate lobe

This is defined as one (or more) accessory lobes of the placenta that is attached to the bulk of the placenta by blood vessels. Making the diagnosis is important because it is possible to have a fundal placenta together with a succenturate lobe that is centrally placed over the internal os. These women have the same problems as those with placenta previa. Very rarely, the intervening vessels overlie the internal cervical os (vasa previa) and can rupture during labor (Fig. 9.4). This leads to massive fetal bleeding. Finally, the succenturate lobe might be retained after delivery and could be the source of postpartum hemorrhage or infection.

Placental lakes

These lie within the bulk of the placenta and are filled with slowly moving blood (Fig. 9.5). They probably represent the intervillous space in an area

lacking fetal villi. Although there is a relationship between the presence of placental lakes and uteroplacental insufficiency, it is so weak to be of little apparent significance.

Placental cysts

These are found immediately beneath the chorionic plate (Fig. 9.6). The smaller ones are blood vessels viewed in cross-section. The larger ones are distinct entities caused by the deposition of fibrin in the intervillous space. They have no apparent significance.

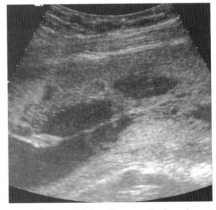

Figure 9.5 Placental lakes in an anterior placenta. Note the lakes lie within the bulk of the placenta.

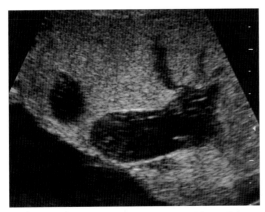

Figure 9.6   Placental cyst. Note the position of the mass, immediately beneath the chorionic plate.

Highly echogenic areas

Echogenic areas seen in the placenta in late pregnancy represent normal changes that occur with increasing gestation (see below).

PLACENTAL GRADING

This is a classification of the normal changes that occur in the placenta during the course of a pregnancy; it is often known as Grannum grading, after its author. It used to be thought that a Grannum grade III placenta was associated with mature fetal lungs and placental dysfunction. This concept has been largely rejected and placental grading is rarely used. It is included here for completeness and

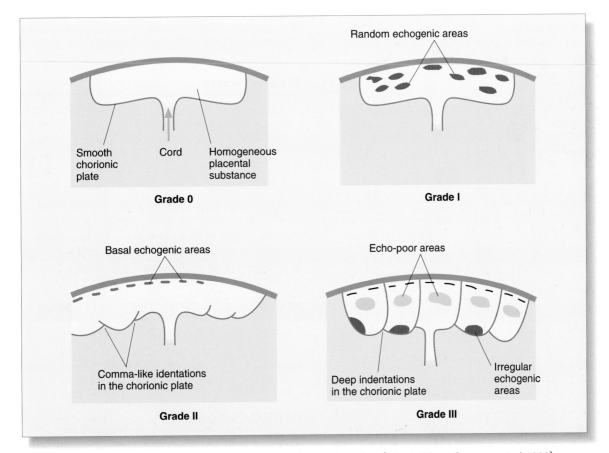

Figure 9.7   Diagram of the ultrasound appearances of placental grading (adapted from Grannum et al 1982).

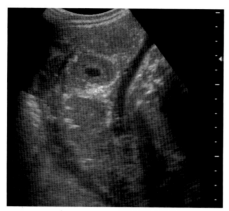

Figure 9.8   Grannum grade III anterior placenta at 38 weeks' gestation.

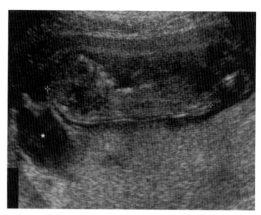

Figure 9.9   A posterior placenta in the first trimester demonstrating a retroplacental clot (*).

because it illustrates the varying appearances of the normal placenta.

Figure 9.7 illustrates the Grannum grading criteria and Figure 9.8 the ultrasound appearances associated with a Grannum grade III placenta.

PLACENTAL ABRUPTION

About 3% of the pregnant population will bleed after 28 weeks' gestation. Approximately one-third of these women will have suffered a placental abruption, in which all or some of the placenta separates from the underlying myometrium before the fetus has been delivered. If this is a major abruption, it is usually clinically apparent because of abdominal pain and a peculiar 'woody hardness' to the uterus. Ultrasound has no place in the diagnosis of major abruption, although it might be needed to determine whether the fetus is still alive.

Minor abruptions

These can produce few or no symptoms. The woman presents with slight abdominal pain and/or an antepartum hemorrhage. The diagnosis is difficult to make either clinically or by ultrasound. The main role of ultrasound in these cases is in excluding placenta previa, although occasionally a retroplacental clot can be seen as a hypoechoic area between the placenta and the myometrium (Fig. 9.9). It must be stressed, however, that ultrasound is very unreliable in refuting

or confirming the diagnosis of minor abruption and should not be part of the routine management of this clinical diagnosis. Recurrent antepartum hemorrhage and abruption can be associated with uteroplacental insufficiency, hence assessment of fetal wellbeing would be indicated in this situation.

PLACENTA CIRCUMVALLATA

In the normal placenta, the fetal membranes insert into the edge of the placenta. In placenta circumvallata they insert some distance along the fetal surface, leaving an area of placenta free of membranes. The site of insertion is usually marked by a depression in the surface of the placenta. The membrane-free area tends to separate and bleed, but rarely causes more than a little spotting. However, the condition has a high incidence of fetal growth restriction. It is probably responsible for a small proportion of all antepartum hemorrhage.

BLEEDING FROM THE MARGINAL SINUS

This is often a brisk, moderately heavy bleed that is often mistaken clinically for placenta previa. It is not commonly diagnosed on ultrasound but very occasionally the subsequent clot can be seen (Fig. 9.10).

CHORIOANGIOMA

This is a very rare vascular tumor of the placenta (Fig. 9.11). Such tumors vary both in appearance

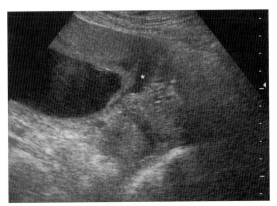

Figure 9.10 A placenta demonstrating a clot (∗) in the marginal sinus.

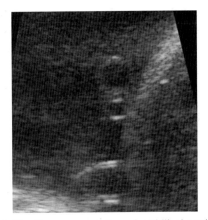

Figure 9.12 Transverse section of umbilical cord demonstrating the normal vein but only a single artery. Compare this appearance with that of the normal three-vessel cord shown in Fig. 8.22B.

and in size and occasionally appear to be separate from the placenta. They are usually benign and, if less than 5 cm in diameter, rarely cause a problem. Larger tumors are very vascular and can act as a fetal arteriovenous anastomosis. In this situation, a fetal hyperdynamic circulation can result in high-output cardiac failure with subsequent polyhydramnios and hydrops fetalis.

UMBILICAL CORD

Two–vessel cord

The absence of one umbilical artery is relatively common, with a reported incidence of approximately 1% (Fig. 9.12). Associated malformations are thought to be present in as many as 50% of cases, with the cardiac and renal systems being most commonly affected. The likelihood of the pregnancy being affected by intrauterine growth restriction is also thought to be increased, making follow-up growth scans part of the routine management.

Coiling of the umbilical cord

Reduced coiling of the umbilical cord is associated with uteroplacental insufficiency. Hypercoiling of the cord is also associated with poorer neonatal outcomes, because of associated abnormalities. There is no established, reproducible method of assessing umbilical vessel coiling reliably. Hence coiling is not used clinically to indicate the need for regular scans or detailed fetal assessment.

Nuchal cords

Nuchal cords, or wrapping of the umbilical cord round the fetal neck, is of dubious clinical value when discovered on ultrasound. In the majority of cases, a normal pregnancy outcome is expected. Occasionally, a nuchal cord will be noticeably short, often in association with a breech or malpresentation. This should be noted on the report because the clinician would be well advised not to attempt an external cephalic version.

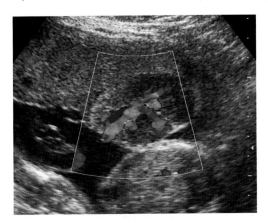

Figure 9.11 A chorioangioma – Colour Doppler flow.

Umbilical cord masses

These are primary in nature, originating from the remnants of the allantoic or vitelline duct. These embryologically derived cysts can coexist with an exomphalos. The use of color Doppler will help differentiate cord masses of vascular origin and their relationship to the umbilical vessels. More commonly, hypercoiling of the umbilical cord or excessive Wharton's jelly gives the false appearance of a cord cyst or tumor. These findings should be noted on the ultrasound report, because the pediatrician will assess the neonate clinically after delivery.

ASSESSMENT OF AMNIOTIC FLUID VOLUME

The amniotic fluid volume increases from approximately 250 mL at 16 weeks to 1000 mL at 34 weeks, declining thereafter to approximately 800 mL at term. The amniotic fluid volume reflects the status of both the mother and the fetus and is altered in many physiological and pathological conditions. Ultrasound has a potential role in the management of such conditions, by the assessment of amniotic fluid volume.

As outlined in Chapter 7 there are three methods for assessing amniotic fluid volume:

1. *Subjective assessment* – With experience, it is possible to classify amniotic fluid volume into the broad categories absent, low, normal, increased and excessive. Although reliable in the hands of an experienced operator, this method has proved impossible to standardize in clinical and research terms.

2. *Single deepest pool* – The size of the deepest, cord-free pool of amniotic fluid is assessed with the ultrasound probe perpendicular to the maternal abdomen (Fig. 9.13). The vertical depth of the largest pool is measured. When this method was first introduced, a 1-cm pool was considered acceptable in normal pregnancy, but subsequent studies have suggested that a minimum depth of 2–3 cm is a more appropriate threshold.

3. *Amniotic fluid index* – This is a semiquantitative technique for assessing amniotic fluid

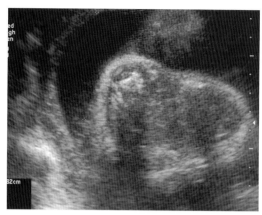

Figure 9.13 Assessment of amniotic fluid volume by measurement of the deepest pool of amniotic fluid (5.82 cm). The calipers are positioned to produce a vertical measurement from the outer edge of the chorionic place to the inner edge of the uterine wall.

volume. Using the maternal umbilicus as a reference point, the abdomen is divided into four quarters. With the ultrasound probe held in the longitudinal axis of the mother and perpendicular to the floor, the largest vertical pool depth in each quadrant is recorded (Fig. 9.14). The sum of these measurements represents the amniotic fluid index (AFI). Although the AFI is known to vary with gestational age, an AFI < 5 cm is classified as oligohydramnios and an AFI > 25 cm is classified as polyhydramnios. Even though this method is accepted as superior to the single deepest pool technique, considerable intra- and interobserver variation exists.

Although the importance of quantifying the amniotic fluid volume is unquestionable, a practical and reproducible technique for the accurate assessment of amniotic fluid volume has yet to be introduced into clinical practice.

OLIGOHYDRAMNIOS/ANHYDRAMNIOS

Oligohydramnios/anhydramnios is defined as reduced/absent amniotic fluid volume for a given gestational age (Fig. 9.15). The finding of anhydramnios in the first and second trimesters is usu-

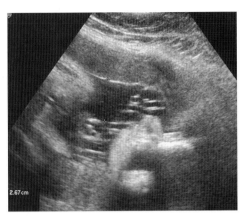

Figure 9.14   Assessment of the largest vertical pool in a single quadrant (2.67 cm) avoiding the umbilical cord. The amniotic fluid index is calculated from the sum of this measurement in all four quadrants.

ally associated with a poor prognosis because of the subsequent development of lethal fetal pulmonary hypoplasia. Prolonged oligohydramnios/anhydramnios is also associated with limb contractures, such as talipes.

Causes of oligohydramnios/anhydramnios

There are three main pathological reasons for the finding of reduced or absent amniotic fluid:

1. *Uteroplacental insufficiency* – Oligohydramnios is an early feature of uteroplacental insufficiency and is associated with decreased fetal biometry particularly the abdominal circum-ference. Other ultrasound features, such as echogenic bowel, mild cardiomegaly and abnormal uteroplacental/fetal Dopplers, aid in the confirmation of uteroplacental insufficiency as the cause for the reduced amniotic fluid volume.

2. *Amniotic membrane rupture* – The maternal history of persistent vaginal loss and dampness would suggest a diagnosis of prelabor membrane rupture. The latter is often associated with anhydramnios rather than oligohydramnios. The finding of normal amniotic fluid volume or oligohydramnios, however, does not exclude this diagnosis. Hence, ultrasound is of limited diagnostic value when this diagnosis is suspected.

3. *Abnormal fetal renal function* – Unilateral renal problems in the fetus are usually associated with normal amniotic fluid volume. Conversely, bilateral renal agenesis, polycystic kidney disease, multicystic dysplasia and bladder outflow obstruction characteristically present with anhydramnios on ultrasound (Fig. 9.16).

Pitfalls

Physiological changes in amniotic fluid volume

Amniotic fluid volume decreases markedly with advancing gestation, especially in the third

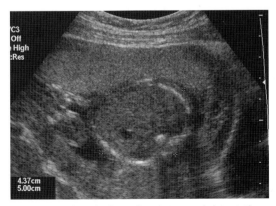

Figure 9.15   Oligohydramnios at 35 weeks' gestation. The largest vertical pool measures 1.8 cm and the AFI is 3.0 cm.

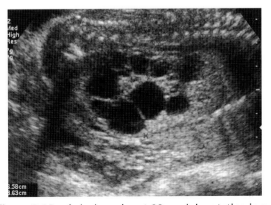

Figure 9.16   Anhydramnios at 28 weeks' gestation in a fetus with polycystic kidney disease. Note the grossly enlarged and echo-bright stroma of the cystic kidney.

trimester. Hence the significance of reduced amniotic fluid volume in late gestations is debatable.

Estimation of amniotic fluid volume

Measurement of the AFI or single deepest pool is at best a proxy for the amniotic fluid volume. As described above, these methods are far from reproducible.

Management

Anhydramnios as a consequence of renal pathology or early/midtrimester membrane rupture is frequently associated with a poor prognosis. If oligohydramnios is due to uteroplacental insufficiency, the management will depend on the severity of growth restriction and the gestation of the pregnancy.

Oligohydramnios of unknown etiology is of dubious clinical significance. Given the poor reproducibility of subjective and objective amniotic fluid estimations, one could question the value of reporting this when present as an isolated finding. The exception to this recommendation would appear to be prolonged or post-term pregnancy, where reduced amniotic fluid volume can be associated with poorer fetal and neonatal outcomes.

POLYHYDRAMNIOS

Polyhydramnios is defined as excess amniotic fluid volume for a given gestation of pregnancy. This is a physiological finding in approximately 1% of pregnancies in the third trimester. The prognosis in pregnancies with polyhydramnios is dependent on the cause of the condition. In idiopathic/physiologic cases, the prognosis is usually very good, with the only complication being premature delivery due to uterine overdistention.

Causes of polyhydramnios

Increased amniotic fluid/fetal urine production

Polyhydramnios can occur as a result of increased urine production. The most common reasons for this are maternal diabetes mellitus and constitutional fetal macrosomia. Infrequently, polyhydramnios can be due to conditions that predispose to a fetal hyperdynamic circulation, such as fetal anemia due to rhesus disease or parvovirus infection, or arteriovenous fistulae associated with chorioangioma or sacrococcygeal teratoma. The latter are the only causes of polyhydramnios before 25 weeks' gestation (Fig. 9.17).

Decreased fetal swallowing

Upper gastrointestinal tract obstruction of intrinsic origin (esophageal atresia or duodenal atresia) or extrinsic origin (thoracic tumor or diaphragmatic hernias) are the readily detectable causes of polyhydramnios (Fig. 9.18). A much rarer cause is fetal neurogenic disease, which is much more difficult to detect on ultrasound. The latter is often insidious, late in onset and is only detected if there are other features of neurogenic origin such as poor fetal tone and joint fixity.

Idiopathic polyhydramnios

When a definitive cause is not suspected antenatally, a label of idiopathic polyhydramnios is used. It might be more appropriate to label these cases as physiological rather than idiopathic polyhydramnios.

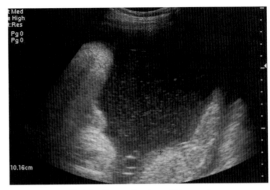

Figure 9.17 Polyhydramnios in a 24-week pregnancy in which the fetus is severely anemic due to Rhesus incompatability. The largest vertical pool measures 10.16 cm.

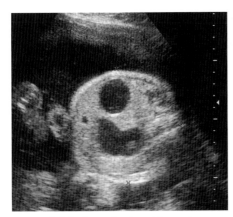

Figure 9.18 Polyhydramnios in a 32-week pregnancy in which duodenal atresia is suspected. The largest vertical pool measures 12.5 cm.

Pitfalls

These are similar to those seen with the diagnosis of oligohydramnios.

Management

The prognosis and management of polyhydramnios is dictated by the cause, e.g. improved diabetic control with fetal macrosomia or fetal karyotyping and amniodrainage with duodenal atresia. Up to 20% of cases of polyhydramnios are associated with fetal abnormality, hence this finding should be investigated thoroughly when it is detected.

Even cases of idiopathic polyhydramnios should be highlighted to the obstetric/pediatric team. Esophageal atresia is associated with a tracheo-esophageal fistula in 80% of cases, leading to the finding of a near-normal stomach bubble on antenatal ultrasound. Hence, neonates are usually checked for a patent esophagus before active feeding is encouraged, to avoid aspiration in affected cases.

REFERENCES AND FURTHER READING

Grannum P A T, Berkowitz R L, Hobbins J C 1982 The ultrasonic changes in the maturing placenta and their relation to fetal pulmonic maturity. American Journal of Obstetrics and Gynecology 133:915–922

National Institute of Child Health and Development 2001 Conference summary: amniotic fluid biology – basic and clinical aspects. Journal of Maternal and Fetal Medicine 10(1):2–19 Review

Oyelese Y 2001. Placenta previa and vasa previa: time to leave the Dark Ages. Ultrasound in Obstetrics and Gynecology 18:96–99

Sherer D M, Langer O 2001. Oligohydramnios: use and misuse in clinical management. Ultrasound in Obstetrics and Gynecology 18:411–419

Chapter 10

Craniospinal abnormalities

One in 50 babies born in the United Kingdom are born with a congenital abnormality, and in one in 100 this will be a major abnormality. Neural tube defects (NTD) account for half of the major anomalies and have an incidence that varies from 2 to 5 per 1000 births. The cause of NTDs is unknown but they are currently thought to be related to a relative deficiency in folic acid in the mother. The two most common forms of NTD are spina bifida and anencephaly, and they are equal in occurrence.

Anencephaly (absence of the cranial vault) is incompatible with life so prenatal diagnosis is desirable. Prenatal diagnosis is also desirable in cases of spina bifida because only about half of the infants with open spina bifida will survive 5 years and the vast majority of the survivors have major degrees of handicap. More than 90% of infants born with NTD are born to women who have not had a previously affected child. In the past, estimation of maternal serum alphafetoprotein (sAFP) was commonly used as a screening test for NTDs. Second trimester ultrasound examination is now considered to be the most sensitive screening method for detecting NTDs.

ALPHAFETOPROTEIN (AFP)

Alphafetoprotein is virtually undetectable in the adult but is easily detectable in embryonic and fetal life. It is a protein that the embryo produces from the yolk sac and the fetus produces from its liver. In the normal fetus, AFP is excreted into the amniotic fluid via fetal urine and crosses the placenta to enter the mother's blood.

The level of AFP in the fetal blood reaches a peak at 16–18 weeks and this is reflected in the levels of AFP in the amniotic fluid. In maternal blood, AFP continues to increase in concentration until 32 weeks, probably due to increasing placental permeability.

Most laboratories report the maternal serum AFP (MSAFP) levels in multiples of the median (MoM) rather than absolute concentration, as this corrects for the physiological change in AFP levels with gestation. It is also necessary to set the upper limit of normal to a level that will not include too many false positive cases of normal pregnant women; this level is generally taken as 2.5 MoM. About 2 per 100 women will have a MSAFP value above this level. In areas where the incidence of neural tube defects is 2–3 per 1000 births, the chance of a woman with a MSAFP > 2.5 MoM having a fetus with a neural tube defect is approximately 1 in 20 prior to the introduction of periconceptual folate therapy. However, having a normal MSAFP is not a guarantee that the fetus does not have a neural tube defect; a MSAFP > 2.5 MoM will only detect about 85% of cases of open spina bifida.

A woman who has had a child or fetus with a neural tube defect has a 1 in 20 chance of recurrence. If she has had two affected pregnancies the chance is increased to 1 in 10. Periconceptual folate therapy appears to reduce these recurrence risks by approximately one half. A normal MSAFP is not adequate reassurance in these cases and it is important that these women are offered an ultrasound examination after 12 weeks to exclude anencephaly, followed by a detailed ultrasound examination after 18 weeks to evaluate the spine and the intracranial anatomy.

WHAT TO DO WITH A WOMAN WITH A RAISED MSAFP

Ideally, no woman should be offered a MSAFP test before the gestational age of the pregnancy has been confirmed and multiple gestation and anencephaly excluded by ultrasound examination. Box 10.1 lists the causes of raised MSAFP. If a raised value is obtained, the test should be repeated to exclude laboratory error and a detailed ultrasound examination should be performed.

> **Box 10.1 Causes of raised maternal serum alphafetoprotein**
>
> Laboratory error
> Idiopathic
> *Should be detected by ultrasound after 7 weeks*:
>   incorrect gestational age
>   multiple pregnancy
>   hydatidiform mole
>   intrauterine death
> *Should be detected by ultrasound after 12 weeks*:
>   anencephaly
> *Should be detected by ultrasound at the 20–22 week routine anomaly scan*:
>   spina bifida
>   omphalocele/gastroschisis
> *Can be detected by ultrasound at or after the 20–22 week routine anomaly scan*:
>   obstructive uropathies
>   esophageal atresia
> *Diagnosable by fetal bladder puncture*:
>   Finnish-type congenital nephrosis (the urine AFP is very raised in these cases)

Traditionally, there have been two possible ways of managing the woman: amniocentesis or high-resolution ultrasound. In the past, amniocentesis was frequently performed to estimate the AFP level in the amniotic fluid. If this was raised (and if there is a second band of acetylcholinesterase on electrophoresis) the woman was usually offered a termination of pregnancy. This approach has two main disadvantages:

1. Amniocentesis carries a risk of causing a miscarriage of about 1 in 100. In about 19 of every 20 cases of raised MSAFP the fetus will be normal, so for every five cases of NTD detected by amniocentesis, one normal pregnancy will be lost.
2. There is a small false-positive rate associated with this method (about 1 in 400). In such cases a normal fetus might be aborted.

The current preferred method is to perform a detailed ultrasound examination. In skilled hands it should be possible to decide if the fetus is abnormal, to specify the type of anomaly and to say how extensive it appears. Although there will be a few cases in which a small abnormality will be missed, the false-positive rate should be the same or less than that of amniocentesis and studies of amniotic fluid AFP. The method that involves ultrasound does not carry the risk of the amniocentesis and has the added advantage of being able to visualize the abnormality such that a prognosis may be given.

Raised MSAFP is associated with intrauterine growth restriction. In cases of raised sAFP and where the ultrasound examination identifies a structurally normal fetus, serial growth scans should therefore be considered.

HOW TO LOOK FOR SPECIFIC ABNORMALITIES

Anencephaly

As ossification of the fetal skull is normally completed by 11 weeks, the diagnosis of absence of the cranium or anencephaly can be made reliably after this gestation. There appears to be a natural progression of this condition from initial acrania with associated exencephaly in the first trimester, to anencephaly. Toward the end of the first trimester, the absence of the cranial bones (acrania) can be observed. However, the fetal brain is present and

can therefore be identified (exencephaly), although it frequently appears abnormal in appearance (Fig. 10.1A). As gestation progresses, the exposed brain becomes eroded, producing the classic 'frog's eyes' appearance of anencephaly in the second trimester, in which the fetal skull ends just above the orbits (Fig. 10.1B).

The diagnosis of anencephaly can be missed in the first trimester because the brain can appear normal and the absence of the skull bones (i.e. acrania) is overlooked. The most common reason for missing the diagnosis in the second or third trimester is that the fetal head cannot be visualized and is assumed to be deep in the maternal pelvis. Such women should always be examined using transvaginal imaging. If this is refused then they should be re-examined with a full bladder and should be tipped head down. If the fetal position is still not favorable, the woman should be re-examined 1 week later; do not confirm gestational age by measurement of the femur and send her away.

It is unreasonable to expect every anomaly that is amenable to ultrasound detection to be identified by routine ultrasound screening but anencephaly is a diagnosis that should not be overlooked after 14 weeks of gestation. In the majority of cases, failure to identify an anencephalic fetus after 14 weeks would be considered negligent.

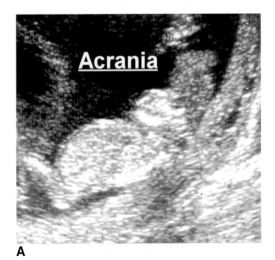

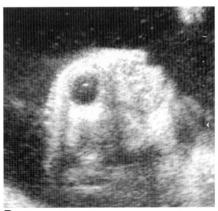

A **B**

Figure 10.1   The varying appearances of anencephaly. A. At 12 weeks, absence of the skull bones (acrania) can be identified. Note the appearance of the fetal brain (exencephaly). Compare this image with the normal appearances in Fig. 3.18. B. At 23 weeks the fetal brain tissue can no longer be visualized. Note the typical frog's eyes appearance.

Spina bifida

As discussed in Chapter 8, the spine and skin covering should be examined in sagittal, transverse and coronal views. Before a spine can be passed as normal every vertebra must be examined in transverse, longitudinal and coronal section.

Extreme care must be taken to ensure the correct sections are obtained for evaluation. It is easy to miss a small or subtle defect because the technique is less than rigorous. Figure 10.2A illustrates an apparently normal spine in longitudinal view but a slight sideways movement demonstrates a defect (Fig. 10.2B). The splaying of the abnormal verte-bral arch produces a 'V'- or 'U'-shaped appearance in transverse section (Fig. 10.3A), compared with the normal triangular shape (Fig. 10.3B). The abnormal vertebrae will cause a bowing of the two outer parallel lines seen in the coronal view of a normal spine (Fig. 10.4). The sagittal view will demonstrate the spinal defect only if the vertebral arch is absent or if kyphoscoliosis is present. However, the sagittal and transverse views are preferred for detecting the meningocele or meningomyelocele usually associated with open spina bifida.

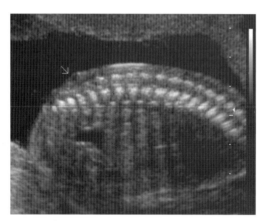

Figure 10.2A Longitudinal view of the lower spine and sacrum demonstrating an apparently normal spine and skin covering. Careful examination of the lower spine demonstrates a break in the line of echoes from the spine and a small meningocele (arrow).

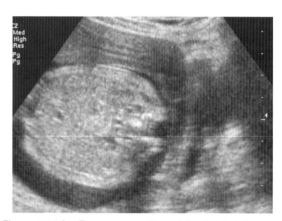

Figure 10.3A Transverse section of the fetal abdomen demonstrating splaying of the vertebra in spina bifida. The spinal defect is associated with a meningomyelocele. The sac contains obvious strands of nervous tissue. Compare the abnormal shape of this vertebra with that of the normal vertebra shown in Fig. 8.16.

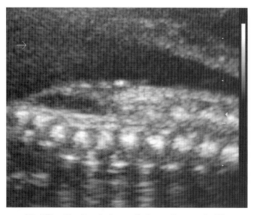

Figure 10.2B Sagittal view of the spine and skin covering demonstrating a meningocele overlying the lumbar spine. Note the appearance of the spinal defect that can be estimated to extend from L2 to S3.

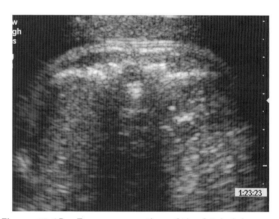

Figure 10.3B Transverse section of the fetal abdomen demonstrating the appearance of a normal vertebra. Note the triangular shape made by the three ossification centres, the flat skin covering anterior to them and compare to the abnormal appearances of Fig. 10.3A.

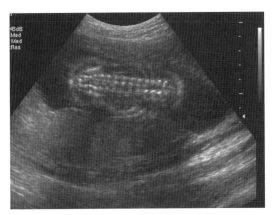

Figure 10.4 Coronal view of the fetal abdomen demonstrating the appearance of the normal spine. Note the parallel appearance of the three ossification centres in the upper spine and how these taper towards the base of the spine and the two iliac crests

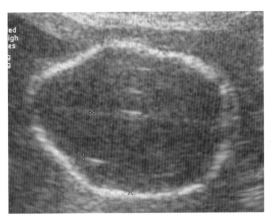

Figure 10.5 Transverse section of the head demonstrating scalloping of the frontal bones, described as the 'lemon' sign in a fetus with spina bifida. Compare this appearance to that of the skull shape of the normal fetus shown in Fig. 7.3.

In open spina bifida there is an absence of skin covering the defect. The normal skin outline is thus disrupted in both the transverse and sagittal views by the cystic mass of the meningocele that overlies the bony vertebral defect (see Figs 10.2A, 10.2B and 10.3A). Small, linear, high-level echoes within the mass, thought to represent nerve fibers, can enable the differentiation to be made between a meningomyelocele and a meningocele that contains CSF only.

It is not always possible to obtain an adequate longitudinal view of the fetal spine, especially if the fetus is lying on its back. In such cases, detailed study of the spine in transverse section can also be impossible. If you are unsure of the integrity of the spine and skin covering, always bring the woman back.

The lemon and banana signs

Open spina bifida is frequently associated with the 'lemon' and the 'banana' signs. The 'lemon sign' describes the abnormal scalloping of the frontal bones, which produces a more angular appearance to the front of the skull than is seen in the normal fetus (Fig. 10.5). However, this appearance should be used as a marker for spina bifida only between 16 and 24 weeks, because the normal fetal skull can give similar appearances before 16 weeks. As discussed in Chapter 7, this appearance can also be produced in a second trimester fetus from an

incorrect BPD section that is rotated slightly too far toward the fetal orbits. After 24–26 weeks fetuses with spina bifida rarely demonstrate a lemon-shaped skull so a normally shaped skull should not be used to exclude spina bifida after this gestation.

The 'banana sign' describes a crescent or banana-shaped cerebellum that consequently produces an abnormally small transcerebellar diameter (TCD) (Fig. 10.6). The cisterna magna is also frequently obliterated or reduced in size in such

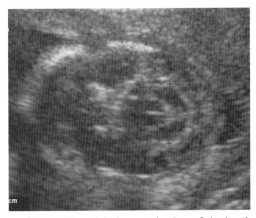

Figure 10.6 Suboccipitobregmatic view of the head demonstrating the small and abnormally shaped cerebellum described as the 'banana' sign. Compare this appearance with that of the normal cerebellum shown in Figs 7.11 and 8.12A.

cases. The banana sign will be present in some cases of open spina bifida, whereas in others the cerebellum cannot be identified within the posterior fossa because it has herniated into the foramen magnum. This is known as the Arnold–Chiari malformation type II.

The banana sign is the more sensitive of the two signs for the detection of spina bifida in the second trimester. Both these intracranial signs of spina bifida, and the Arnold–Chiari malformation, are thought to result from traction on the brainstem.

In women at high risk of carrying a fetus with spina bifida, nearly all cases of open spina bifida can be identified before 20 weeks using the lemon and banana signs. In low-risk women around 80% of cases will be detected.

Cases of closed spina bifida are rarely detected with ultrasound because the intracranial signs are absent and MSAFP levels, if performed, are normal.

Hydrocephalus

As discussed in Chapter 8, hydrocephalus describes the pathological increase in the size of the cerebral ventricles and head circumference. These features are commonly associated with spina bifida towards the end of gestation. Ventriculomegaly describes the appearance of the lateral ventricles when their diameter is above the normal range for gestation. Often the first clues to the presence of spina bifida are a lemon-shaped skull and ventriculomegaly (Fig. 10.5 and 10.7). Ventriculomegaly occurs in about 80% of fetuses with spina bifida. Its presence

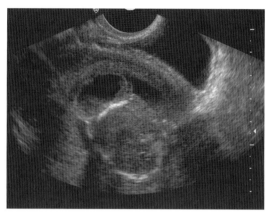

Figure 10.8 Transverse section of the head of a 22-week fetus, demonstrating a large encephalocele that contains most of the contents of the posterior fossa.

makes the prognosis much worse because mental retardation is more common if both conditions are present.

The method of measuring the ventricles is described in Chapter 8. The diagnosis of ventriculomegaly is made from assessment of ventricular size and not on the presence or absence of a large head. Although fetuses with ventriculomegaly can develop a large head in late pregnancy, biparietal diameter (BPD) and head circumference (HC) are commonly reduced in comparison with the femur and abdominal circumference (AC) in cases of spina bifida with ventriculomegaly in the second trimester. Indeed, if the BPD and HC are found to be small in comparison with the femur, this should prompt a careful search for spina bifida (or microcephaly).

Hydrocephalus can occur in the absence of spina bifida; a condition known as isolated hydrocephalus. This tends to be more severe than hydrocephalus associated with spina bifida. The recurrence risk for isolated hydrocephalus is about 1 in 30 unless it is due to the more rare type due to sex-linked aqueduct stenosis. Aqueduct stenosis carries a recurrence risk of 1 in 4. Thus sex-linked aqueduct stenosis should be suspected in a woman who has had a previous male infant with hydrocephalus; her subsequent male fetuses carry a 1 in 2 risk of the same condition. In such cases, parental testing for mutation of specific genes by chorion villus sampling can be offered.

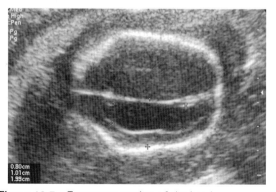

Figure 10.7 Transverse section of the head demonstrating ventriculomegaly in a 20-week fetus with spina bifida. Note the typical lemon shape of the skull.

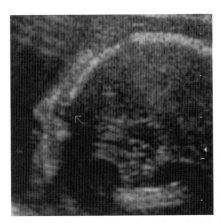

Figure 10.9 Occipital meningocele with a skull defect (arrow) measuring 7 mm in a fetus at 24 weeks' gestation.

Encephalocele

This rare form of NTD can be considered to be a high spina bifida. There is a bony defect in the cranial vault, usually in the occiput (although it can be in the frontal, nasal or parietal bones) through which a sac composed of dura mater protrudes. In most cases, the sac contains parts of the brain and prognosis is poor (Fig. 10.8). Very rarely, the sac contains only CSF, in which case it is referred to as an occipital meningocele and has a good prognosis (Fig 10.9).

Encephaloceles are usually isolated lesions but can occasionally be associated with multicystic kidneys (Potter's type III renal dysplasia) and polydactyly; a condition known as Meckel–Gruber syndrome. This is an autosomal recessive condition and so has a 1 in 4 chance of recurrence (see Chapter 12). The recurrence rate for isolated encephalocele is 1 in 20. When an encephalocele is detected it is therefore important to examine the remaining fetal anatomy carefully, especially the fetal kidneys, to ensure that the correct diagnosis is made and therefore that the appropriate information is discussed with the parents. Conversely, as bilateral renal dysplasia is frequently associated with oligohydramnios, a marked reduction in amniotic fluid volume should always initiate careful examination of the renal tract, the intracranial contents and the integrity of the skull.

Microcephaly

Microcephaly means a small brain enclosed within a small skull. It is not a neural tube defect. The time of onset of this condition and its progression are variable. Some cases are severe and are therefore amenable to prenatal detection. Others are mild and some only develop after birth. Many infants with the severe condition die soon after birth and those that survive are not only severely mentally retarded but are also dwarfed.

Microcephaly can be caused by viral infections (especially rubella), irradiation, maternal heroin addiction and some drugs (antiepileptics, alcohol and cocaine). A few cases are associated with an autosomal recessive mode of inheritance; in most cases the cause is never established.

Ultrasound diagnosis of microcephaly is not easy. Some cases undoubtedly develop late in pregnancy and will not, therefore, be detected at the 20–22 week routine anomaly examination. Furthermore, microcephaly is not a structural abnormality but a variable slowing of the growth rate of the fetal head. This calls for careful, serial measurements of all growth parameters, starting as early in the pregnancy as possible. Ideally, gestational age should be established by an early estimation of crown–rump length performed transvaginally. Serial measurements of the BPD, HC, AC and femur length should be performed. Calculation of the ratio of the head circumference (H) to the abdominal circumference (A) and plotting this ratio on the appropriate H/A ratio chart is also recommended. It is frequently easier to interpret the growth profile of the relevant organs when represented by one value, namely the H/A ratio, than by the comparison of two. Figure 10.10 illustrates a typical case; the poor head growth leads to a decline in the H/A ratio but the diagnosis in this case could not be made with certainty until 24 weeks.

The diagnosis of microcephaly is best made by serial measurements that demonstrate poor head growth despite normal growth of the fetal femur and abdominal girth. Diagnosis from a single measurement should be made only if the BPD and HC are more than three standard deviations below the mean but other fetal parameters are of normal size.

As the diagnosis is often not made until after 20 weeks, it is possible that the diagnosis will not become apparent until after the gestation at which the referring clinician is prepared to terminate the

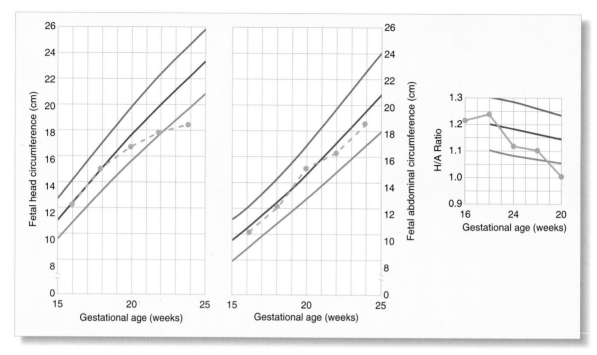

Figure 10.10 Charts of head circumference, abdominal circumference and head/abdomen (H/A) ratio (mean ± two standard deviations) demonstrating the growth pattern in a case of microcephaly.

pregnancy. Careful discussion is needed to decide at what gestation serial scans should cease.

OTHER ABNORMALITIES

Agenesis of the corpus callosum

The corpus callosum is a bundle of nerve fibers that lies immediately caudal to the cavum septum pellucidum and connects the two cerebral hemispheres. Agenesis of the corpus callosum (ACC) is now known to occur far less frequently than originally presumed. The relative rarity of this malformation, and the fact that it is commonly associated with other chromosomal or structural malformations, gives it a guarded prognosis.

The corpus callosum is not visualized from the standard views used in assessment of the intracranial anatomy. It is best identified from midline coronal or midline sagittal sections of the fetal head, where it can be visualized immediately anterior to the body of the lateral ventricles (Fig. 10.11). Agenesis of the corpus callosum should be suspected if the cavum septum pellucidum cannot be identified, there is enlargement of the posterior ventricle and/or the

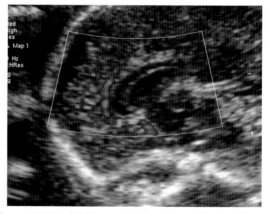

Figure 10.11 Midline sagittal section of the head at 22 weeks' gestation demonstrating the normal corpus callosum.

anterior horns of the lateral ventricles are displaced laterally and are 'tear-drop' in shape (Fig. 10.12).

Hydranencephaly

This is a congenital absence of the cerebral hemispheres and is recognized by the complete absence of echoes from within the cerebral vault

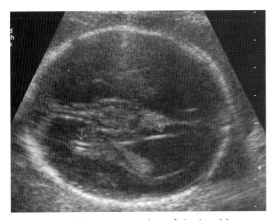

Figure 10.12 Transverse section of the head in a case of agenesis of the corpus callosum at 24 weeks' gestation. Note the absent cavum septum pellucidum, the mild posterior ventriculomegaly (arrow) and the abnormal appearance and position of the anterior horn (arrow) of the lateral ventricles. Compare this appearance with that of the normal fetus shown in Fig. 7.3.

(Fig. 10.13). Theoretically, it is possible to distinguish it from severe ventriculomegaly (as shown in Fig 8.9B) because in the latter the middle cerebral artery can be seen pulsating at the site of the Sylvian fissure. As hydranencephaly is due to bilateral carotid occlusion, no pulsations are seen. However, distinguishing the conditions is academic as both have a very poor prognosis.

Holoprosencephaly

This is a rare spectrum of three abnormalities: alobar, semilobar and lobar holoprosencephaly that result from incomplete division of the forebrain. Alobar holoprosencephaly is the most severe of the three types and is characterized by a single ventricle and fusion of the thalami. The ultrasound appearance is thus effectively of a fluid-filled skull surrounded by a small rim of cortex (Fig. 10.14). The semilobar type demonstrates partial division of the forebrain with partial fusion of the thalami. Both alobar and semilobar holoprosencephaly are associated with typically midline facial defects, including cyclopia, proboscis and midline clefts, and with chromosomal abnormalities, principally trisomy 13. The cavum septum pellucidum is absent in lobar holoprosencephaly but there is normal development of the ventricles and thalami. This type is rarely detected prenatally.

Porencephalic cyst

A porencephalic cyst is a cyst found in the cerebral hemisphere and is the result of liquefaction of an intracranial hemorrhage. The most common cause is hypoxic rupture of the small vessels of the germinal matrix that surround the ventricles. Porencephalic cysts are usually single and unilateral. They are distinguishable from choroid

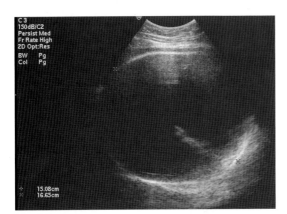

Figure 10.13 Transverse section of the head of a 34-week fetus demonstrating hydranencephaly. Compare this appearance with that of severe ventriculomegaly shown in Fig 8.9B.

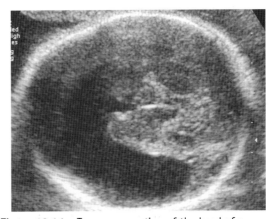

Figure 10.14 Transverse section of the head of a 24-week fetus demonstrating alobar holoprosencephaly. Note the sickle-shaped single ventricle and the unusual appearance of the thalami. Compare this appearance with that of hydranencephaly shown in Fig. 10.13.

plexus cysts because they are extraventricular and extend from the ventricle into the cerebral hemisphere (Fig. 10.15). The prognosis depends upon the size and the location, but it is generally grave.

Abnormalities of the posterior fossa

These are rare but often have a very poor prognosis; many are associated with chromosome anomalies. The most commonly described is the Dandy–Walker malformation, which consists of a posterior fossa cyst and a hypoplastic or absent cerebellar vermis (Fig. 10.16). Anterior displacement of the vermis by larger posterior fossa cysts in

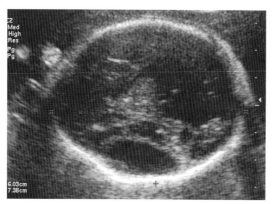

Figure 10.15 Oblique section through the head of a 32-week fetus demonstrating a large porencephalic cyst.

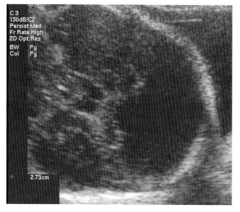

Figure 10.16 Occipitobregmatic view of the posterior fossa of a 26-week fetus demonstrating the Dandy–Walker malformation. Note the absent cerebellar vermis, hypoplastic cerebellar hemispheres and enlarged posterior fossa due to the dilated fourth ventricle.

the absence of cerebellar abnormalities is called a Dandy–Walker variant (Fig. 10.17). Both can be associated with various degrees of ventriculomegaly. The Dandy–Walker variant is generally regarded to have a better prognosis than the malformation, once other associated structural and chromosomal problems have been excluded.

Abnormalities in the shape of the fetal skull

These can be diagnosed by ultrasound. The experienced sonographer will be aware of the long, narrow head (dolichocephaly) that the fetus presenting by the breech might have. Craniostenosis is a very rare condition in which the skull sutures fuse prematurely, and is diagnosable ultrasonically. In these cases the cephalic index can be useful (see Chapter 7). In dolichocephaly the index is reduced and in brachycephaly it is increased. In craniostenosis, the BPD and the cephalic index are persistently low.

Sacral agenesis (caudal regression syndrome)

This is an extremely rare abnormality that is seen almost exclusively in infants born to mothers with insulin-dependent diabetes mellitus (Fig. 10.18).

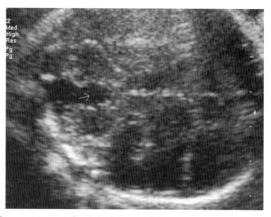

Figure 10.17 Occipitobregmatic view of the posterior fossa of a 26-week fetus demonstrating the Dandy–Walker variant. Note the enlarged posterior fossa due to the dilated fourth ventricle (arrow) in association with the normal appearance of the cerebellar hemispheres and vermis.

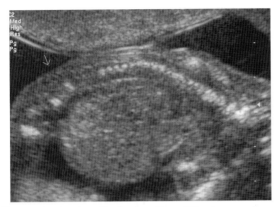

Figure 10.18 Longitudinal section of the lower spine showing agenesis of the lumbar vertebrae and sacrum (arrow).

It ranges in severity from absence of the sacrum with short femora to complete fusion of the lower limbs – the mermaid syndrome (sirenomelia).

REFERENCES AND FURTHER READING

Bernard J P, Moscoso G, Reneir D, Ville Y 2001 Cystic malformations of the posterior fossa. Prenatal Diagnosis 21:1064–1069

Chervenak F A, Kurjak A, Comstock C H (eds) 1995 Ultrasound and the fetal brain. Parthenon Publishing Ltd, Carnforth

Levene M, Chervenak F, Whittle M 2001 Fetal and neonatal neurology and neurosurgery, 3rd edn. Harcourt Brace, Edinburgh

MRC Vitamin Study Research Group 1991. Prevention of neural tube defects: results of the Medical Research Council vitamin study. Lancet 338(8760):131–137

Pilu G, Visentin A, Valeri B 2000 The Dandy–Walker complex and fetal sonography. Ultrasound in Obstetrics and Gynecology 16:115–117

Chapter 11

Other fetal abnormalities

CHAPTER CONTENTS

ABNORMALITIES OF THE FETAL CHEST

Diaphragmatic hernia

Congenital diaphragmatic hernia occurs in approximately 1 in 4000 births. As discussed in Chapter 8, defects in the diaphragm are themselves rarely identified on ultrasound, but can be assumed from the abnormal position of one or more fetal organs. In cases of congenital diaphragmatic hernia (CDH), the defect in the diaphragm is left-sided in approximately 80% of cases. This means that the stomach and bowel are the abdominal organs that most commonly enter the fetal chest. The absence of the normally situated stomach below the diaphragm, in association with a cystic mass in the fetal chest, is strongly suggestive of CDH (Fig. 11.1). In left-sided CDH, the heart is often pushed into the right side of the chest – another suspicious finding in itself – making it difficult to determine if the major vessels are correctly connected.

In right-sided CDH, the fetal liver is the organ most likely to herniate through the defect into the chest. Right-sided cases are less amenable to prenatal ultrasound diagnosis because of the normally positioned stomach and the similarity of the echotexture of the liver and lung. Abnormal positioning of the heart in the left chest might provide the only diagnostic clue in such cases.

It is probable that there are times when neither the stomach nor the bowel are in the fetal chest, so that the effects of the diaphragmatic hernia will not be apparent. This restricts the sensitivity of

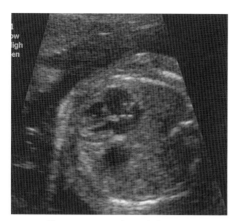

Figure 11.1 Transverse section of the fetal chest demonstrating a left-sided diaphragmatic hernia. Note the cystic mass of the stomach in the left chest displacing the heart from its normal position. Compare these appearances with those of the normal fetal chest as shown in Fig. 8.18.

ultrasound in the detection of CDH and can explain why cases with obvious findings in the third trimester were not diagnosed in the second trimester. A 'swan-neck' bend in the fetal descending aorta is a useful diagnostic clue and, if present, should initiate a detailed and/or repeated examination.

Antenatally, the pregnancies are usually not complicated, although impaired absorption of amniotic fluid by the fetal gut can cause polyhydramnios in the late second and third trimesters. If much of the bowel is in the fetal chest this can result in a reduced abdominal circumference (AC) measurement, giving the impression of asymmetrical growth restriction. Serial measurements, however, usually demonstrate normal growth velocity.

Approximately 50% of cases of CDH are associated with chromosomal abnormalities, principally trisomies 13 and 18. Diagnosis of CDH should therefore always prompt discussion of invasive testing with the parents. Although the defect in the diaphragm is readily amenable to surgery, up to 50% of chromosomally normal neonates will die from associated pulmonary hypoplasia. Poor prognostic indicators in cases of isolated CDH include evidence of early (i.e. at or before 20 weeks) herniation of the liver into the chest, early left

ventricular compression, polyhydramnios or an increased nuchal translucency measurement at 11–14 weeks.

Cystic adenomatoid malformation

Cystic adenomatoid malformation (CAM) occurs in approximately 1 in 4000 births. This malformation is readily diagnosed on ultrasound but its features are often confused with those of diaphragmatic hernia. At prenatal presentation the lesion is usually unilateral and can be one of three types:

- *Type I (macrocystic)*: this type has large cysts (usually more than 10 mm in diameter) and is usually confined to a single lobe.
- *Type II (mixed)*: this type has a mixed appearance of small and large cysts and again might be confined to a single lobe (Fig. 11.2).
- *Type III (microcystic)*: this involves microcysts such that the individual cysts are not resolved on ultrasound examination giving a uniformly bright appearance to the affected tissue (Fig. 11.3).

A wide spectrum of outcomes has been reported, ranging from fetal hydrops, intrauterine death, postnatal surgical intervention to total prenatal or postnatal resolution. This makes counseling at the time

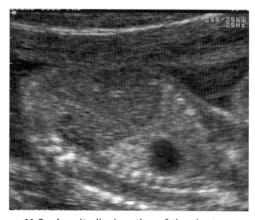

Figure 11.2 Longitudinal section of the chest demonstrating type II cystic adenomatoid malformation. Note the cystic appearance of the mass occupying part of the left chest. Compare these appearances with those shown in Fig. 8.17.

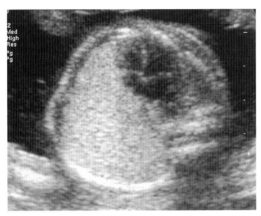

Figure 11.3 Transverse section of the chest demonstrating type III cystic adenomatoid malformation. Note the echogenic appearance of the mass, in contrast to the cystic appearance shown in Fig. 11.2.

of diagnosis difficult in many cases. The prognosis depends on the degree of involvement of the lung tissue and is worst in the presence of the associated findings of mediastinal shift and hydrops. Polyhydramnios is a common finding and is thought to be due either to esophageal compression causing a reduction in fetal swallowing or excess fluid production from the abnormal lung tissue.

Appearances identical to type III CAM, but which resolve, have been reported. It is thought that such cases are due either to transient or intermittent tracheal occlusion. Although this cause for the ultrasound appearances has a far better prognosis than true CAM, it only contributes further to the difficulty in providing an accurate prognosis at the time of diagnosis.

ABNORMALITIES OF THE FETAL ABDOMEN

From early in the second trimester most of the amniotic fluid is fetal urine. Amniotic fluid is therefore effectively all produced by the fetal kidneys and removed by fetal swallowing and subsequent absorption by the fetal bowel. Disruption of this pathway will cause an abnormal reduction (oligohydramnios) or increase (polyhydramnios) in amniotic fluid volume. Polyhydramnios is associated with atresia or obstruction of the upper gastrointestinal tract and with swallowing disorders, whereas oligohydramnios is associated with lower or bilateral upper urinary tract abnormalities.

Bowel atresia or obstruction

Upper gastrointestinal tract obstruction is frequently associated with polyhydramnios that is progressive with increasing gestation. It is not unusual for the amniotic fluid volume to be within normal limits in cases of gastrointestinal tract obstruction in the second trimester.

Bowel that is proximal to the obstructed or atretic segment becomes filled with fluid and is, therefore, easily recognized. Although bowel atresia can be seen at 20–22 weeks, the gastrointestinal appearances are frequently normal at this gestation and the condition is only suspected in the late second or third trimester. Polyhydramnios is a typical finding of upper gastrointestinal tract obstruction in the third-trimester fetus and its finding is frequently the reason for ultrasound referral. However, it should be remembered that normal amniotic fluid volume is the typical finding in such cases in the second trimester. As polyhydramnios is associated with proximal bowel obstruction owing to the disruption in the absorption process, amniotic fluid volume is often normal in cases of distal bowel obstruction.

A stomach bubble that can be linked to a second cystic area in the fetal abdomen is suggestive of duodenal atresia (Fig. 11.4A). Although the lesion is surgically correctable, approximately 30% of cases of duodenal atresia are associated with trisomy 21. Karyotyping should therefore be considered. The main differential diagnosis is with the much rarer condition of a choledochal cyst. In cases of duodenal atresia it should be possible to make the bubbles join up at the pylorus (Fig. 11.4B). The stomach bubble is usually equal in size or larger than the duodenal bubble. Choledochal cysts are often bigger than the stomach bubble, do not connect with the stomach and are not associated with polyhydramnios (Fig. 11.5). They are rarely associated with chromosome abnormalities but should be removed soon after birth because they cause obstructive jaundice.

If no stomach bubble can be identified, rescanning in 20 min should demonstrate fluid in the stomach. Esophageal atresia should be suspected

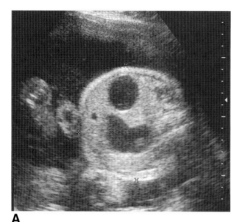

A

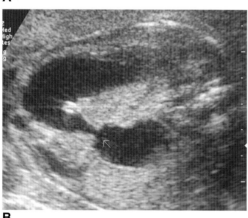

B

Figure 11.4 A. Transverse section of the fetal abdomen at 28 weeks demonstrating the double bubble appearance of duodenal atresia. Note the presence of polyhydramnios. B. An oblique view in a different case demonstrating the connection between the stomach and the duodenum (arrow).

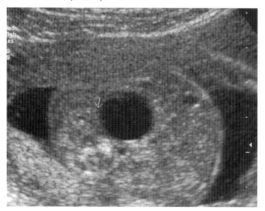

Figure 11.5 Transverse section of the fetal abdomen demonstrating a choledochal cyst (arrow). Note the normal amniotic fluid volume.

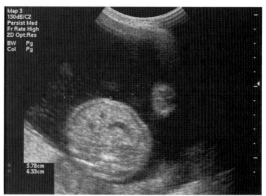

Figure 11.6 Transverse section of the abdomen at the level of the abdominal circumference in a 30-week fetus. Note the abnormally small stomach bubble and accompanying polyhydramnios, the combination of which raises the possibility of esophageal atresia.

either in the persistent absence of the stomach bubble or in the persistent presence of an abnormally small stomach bubble, and especially when polyhydramnios is also present (Fig. 11.6). Esophageal atresia is not associated with trisomy 21 but *is* described in association with trisomy 18. Approximately 90% of cases of esophageal atresia are associated with tracheo-esophageal fistula. The fistula allows amniotic fluid to enter the stomach via the trachea – making the diagnosis of esophageal atresia problematic in the majority of cases.

High small bowel obstruction should be suspected if two or more cystic areas (excluding the gall bladder) are present in the fetal abdomen at approximately the same level as the stomach. Small bowel obstruction should be suspected if the internal diameter of the bowel measures 7 mm or greater. Care should be taken to exclude urinary tract abnormalities or intra-abdominal cysts. Active peristalsis within the mass confirms a gastrointestinal origin.

The normal colon is visible in late pregnancy and a normal range for transverse colonic diameter has been established. Haustrations within the colon can be seen from about 30 weeks (Fig. 11.7) and peristalsis can be frequently observed. Large bowel obstruction should be suspected if its internal diameter measures 20 mm or more (Fig. 11.8).

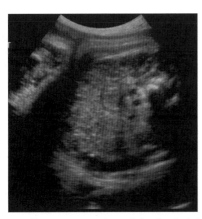

Figure 11.7   Transverse section of the fetal abdomen demonstrating the normal appearance of the colon at 32 weeks. Note the diameter and shape of the normal bowel.

Anterior abdominal wall defects

Both these conditions arise because of defects in the anterior abdominal wall and are amenable to diagnosis from 12 weeks of gestation. They are both associated with raised maternal serum alphafetoprotein (MSAFP) and have a similar incidence of about 1 in 4000 births.

Monitoring fetal growth and estimating fetal weight in the presence of either an omphalocele or gastroschisis are problematic because a significant proportion of the abdominal contents lie outside the abdomen.

Omphalocele

The anterior abdominal wall arises from the fusion of four embryonic body folds – the cephalic, caudal and two lateral folds – during the third week of gestation. If the two lateral folds fail to fuse, the gut fails to return into the abdominal cavity after its physiological herniation into the base of the umbilical cord between 8 and 10 weeks. This results in an omphalocele or exomphalos. This is a midline defect in the abdominal wall through which a peritoneal sac containing liver, small bowel, stomach and occasionally colon protrudes. Figure 11.9 illustrates the ultrasound appearances of an omphalocele. The mass is covered by a protective layer of peritoneum and amnion. The contents of the sac vary, liver and liver and bowel are most commonly described. The umbilical cord inserts into the apex of the defect, making this diagnosis straightforward providing the site of the cord insertion is evaluated routinely. This diagnosis should not be attempted until after 11 weeks of gestation.

Omphalocele is surgically repairable after birth and the survival rate depends largely on the presence of other abnormalities. Up to 50% of cases are associated with chromosomal abnormalities, principally trisomies 18 or 13, or cardiac lesions. Before offering a prognosis, therefore, the fetus should be karyotyped and a detailed cardiac scan should be performed. If the pregnancy continues, vaginal delivery can be considered because the omphalocele

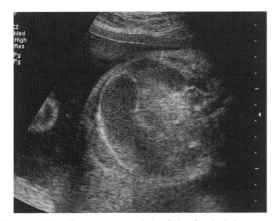

Figure 11.8   Transverse section of the fetal abdomen at 34 weeks' gestation demonstrating dilated bowel. The maximum transverse diameter of the bowel is 22 mm.

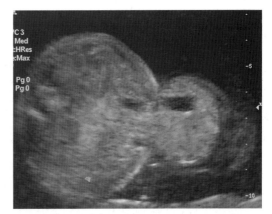

Figure 11.9   Transverse section of the fetal abdomen demonstrating an anterior abdominal wall defect of an omphalocele at 19 weeks. Note that the umbilical vein inserts into the apex of the defect.

rarely causes dystocia and the toughened peritoneal sac is rarely ruptured during delivery. When the condition is isolated, postoperative survival rates of 90% can be expected.

During the maldevelopment of the anterior abdominal wall, if the cranial fold also fails to fuse, the midline defect can extend into the chest such that the fetal heart is outside the body cavity resulting in ectopia cordis. If the caudal fold also fails to fuse, the defect can extend down into the pelvis so that the bladder is involved resulting in ectopia vesicae.

Gastroschisis

Gastroschisis is a condition in which the body folds develop and fuse normally but a small defect arises in the abdominal wall, usually below and to the right of the cord insertion. This is thought to be due to vascular compromise of either the right umbilical vein or the omphalomesenteric artery. The umbilical vein therefore inserts normally into the abdominal wall making the differentiation of gastroschisis from omphalocele relatively easy. The abdominal wall defect is smaller than that of an omphalocele and allows only the small bowel to escape into the amniotic cavity (Fig. 11.10). The bowel is not usually covered by peritoneum, allowing it to float freely in the amniotic fluid. This cauliflower-like appearance is characteristic of free-floating bowel and aids further in the differentiation from omphalocele. Gastroschisis is usually an isolated abnormality and its association with chromosomal anomalies is rare. About 25% of cases are associated with other abnormalities of the gut such as malrotation and atresia due to vascular impairment. Gastroschisis is surgically repairable after birth and postoperative survival rates of 90% can be expected. Postnatal morbidity depends on the quantity of non-functioning bowel that is removed and the problems resulting from short gut syndrome.

Urinary tract anomalies

The methods for imaging and measuring the kidneys and renal pelves are described in Chapter 8.

Renal agenesis

In the normal fetus, the kidneys lie immediately cephalad to the bifurcation of the aorta and can be identified from 14 weeks transabdominally. Using color Doppler, the renal artery can be imaged branching at an angle of 90° off the aorta before entering the kidney. Orientating the fetal aorta in the horizontal plane and applying color Doppler will thus reveal the renal artery of the more anterior kidney in red and of the more posterior kidney in blue (Fig. 11.11). In renal agenesis the renal artery (together with the ureter) is absent (Fig. 11.12). The adrenal glands are present in renal agenesis but might be enlarged, and thus can be mistaken for normal renal tissue. Unlike the kidney, the adrenal gland does not have a collecting system and thus will not demonstrate 'pelvic' echoes.

Bilateral renal agenesis is always associated with anhydramnios. Where anhydramnios is present the differential diagnosis includes bilateral renal agenesis, urethral atresia, severe intrauterine growth restriction and premature rupture of membranes. The fetus is often severely flexed when anhydramnios is present and this further compounds the difficulties of making the correct diagnosis. If the fetal bladder is seen to fill, this effectively excludes the diagnosis of bilateral renal agenesis. Unfortunately, fetal bladder filling is

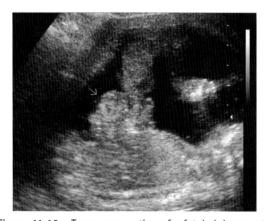

Figure 11.10 Transverse section of a fetal abdomen at 20 weeks demonstrating the free-floating loops of bowel of a gastroschisis. Note the normal insertion of the umbilical cord.

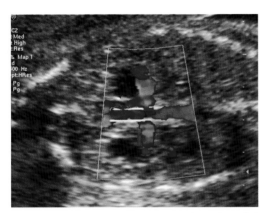

Figure 11.11 Coronal section of the bifurcation of the fetal aorta. The kidneys lie immediately cephalad to the bifurcation in the normal fetus. Application of color Doppler enables both the renal arteries to be seen as they enter the kidneys.

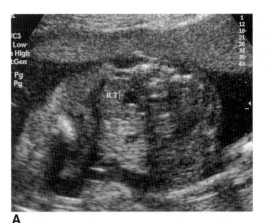

A

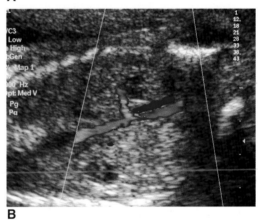

B

Figure 11.12 A. Transverse section of the fetal abdomen in a case of left-sided renal agenesis showing compensatory hydronephrosis in the right kidney. B. Color flow Doppler showing a unilateral right renal artery in a case of left-sided renal agenesis.

usually absent in both bilateral renal agenesis and growth restriction.

Regardless of the cause, the prognosis in cases of anhydramnios or severe oligohydramnios is poor because of the resulting pulmonary hypoplasia. Unless you are certain of the diagnosis we recommend to err on the side of caution, by refuting the diagnosis of renal agenesis, and to allow nature to take its course.

Congenital cystic disease of the kidney

Potter made the original pathological classification of cystic diseases of the kidney in 1972. She described four types of disease: type I describes the kidneys seen in infantile polycystic kidney disease (IPCK). Types II and III describe multicystic disease and type IV describes obstructive disease. Type II involves the nephrons and type III involves the collecting tubules as well as the nephrons. Type II is subdivided into IIA (multicystic and large) and IIB (multicystic and small). Type II disease is also described as multicystic renal dysplasia or multicystic dysplastic kidney disease (MCKD). Type III disease is also described as renal dysplasia or type III renal dysplasia. Type III kidneys are found in autosomal dominant or adult polycystic kidney disease (APKD), Meckel–Gruber syndrome (autosomal recessive) and tuberous sclerosis (autosomal dominant).

It is important to be aware that inconsistencies of definition are occasionally apparent in the literature and this can cause confusion to the reader. It should also be remembered that the terms 'polycystic' and 'multicystic' describe specific and different ultrasound appearances and they should therefore not be used interchangeably. Unfortunately, the ultrasound literature has not always adopted this rigorous approach.

Many centers have adopted a classification based on ultrasound findings of laterality, cyst number, cyst size, appearance of the cortex, bladder size, thickness of the bladder wall and amniotic fluid volume.

Infantile polycystic kidney disease (IPCK)

This is a rare condition with an incidence of about 1 in 30 000 births. It affects the kidneys bilaterally and the liver and has an autosomal recessive inheritance pattern. The condition is amenable to prenatal diagnosis because the gene responsible lies on chromosome 6. Four types of the disease are described (prenatal, neonatal, infantile and juvenile), based on the age at presentation and the degree of renal involvement. The perinatal type is the most common and it is this type that can be diagnosed prenatally, but not always with ease. The condition is always bilateral, with cysts that can vary in size from microscopic to several millimeters. The appearance of the renal cortex depends on the size of the cysts. Microcysts cannot be resolved by ultrasound but the multiple interfaces caused by the cysts return multiple echoes, producing the characteristic hyperechogenic appearance of this condition (Fig. 11.13). Slightly larger cysts can be resolved by ultrasound, producing the second characteristic 'spongy' appearance of this

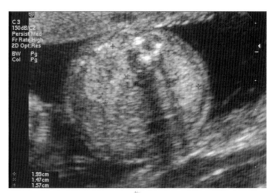

Figure 11.14 Transverse section of a fetus with polycystic kidneys at 22 weeks. Small cysts can be identified in these kidneys and can be compared to the microcysts producing the appearances shown in Fig. 11.13.

condition (Fig. 11.14). The differential diagnosis of enlarged hyperechogenic kidneys includes ADPK.

As IPCK is an abnormality of tubular development, the calyceal system and renal pelvis are present and can be identified. Oligo or anhydramnios is frequently present but not invariably so, suggesting that some degree of renal function is retained in some cases.

The gestational age at which these findings become apparent varies and not all are therefore amenable to second trimester diagnosis. It is possible to identify, and record, normal renal appearances at 20–22 weeks with subsequent examination in the third trimester demonstrating the typical features of IPCK (Fig. 11.13). Women carrying a fetus at risk of IPCK should therefore be offered serial ultrasound examinations throughout pregnancy.

Multicystic dysplastic kidney disease (MCDK)

This encompasses a spectrum of renal appearances that reflect the size of the cysts and the degree of renal involvement. The condition is thought to arise either as a consequence of early obstruction to the ureter or bladder or as a failure in the development of the nephrons. It can be bilateral,

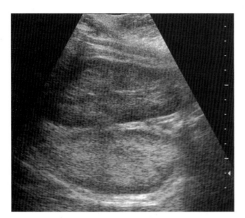

Figure 11.13 Longitudinal section of a fetus with infantile polycystic kidneys at 34 weeks. Microscopic kidney cysts make the kidney much more echogenic than the fetal lungs. Note the anhydramnios. Note that the renal pelves can be identified. Compare the echogenicity and size of these kidneys with the normal kidney shown in Fig. 8.29.

unilateral or segmental, affecting only part of one kidney. The presence of the renal artery and/or ureter is variable. The unilateral condition can be accompanied by agenesis of the contralateral kidney.

The affected renal tissue is replaced by non-communicating cysts of varying size. The kidney might therefore be enlarged or small (Fig. 11.15). In cases where the kidney is enlarged it is important to differentiate between MCDK and severe renal pelvic dilatation. In the latter condition, the cystic areas, representing dilated calyces, intercommunicate. Bilateral MCDK is always associated with severe oligo or anhydramnios and has a poor prognosis irrespective of the presence of other abnormalities. Conversely, isolated unilateral MCDK carries a good prognosis.

Multicystic dysplastic kidneys tend to involute over time. This can occur prenatally or in infanthood. Nephrectomy might be indicated if the affected kidney remains grossly enlarged. The recurrence risk of MCKD is low because the condition is generally sporadic. Because the renal ultrasound appearances of MCKD and renal dysplasia (see below) can be very similar, it is important to be aware of the association of the latter with Mendelian disorders, which therefore have recurrence risks of 1 in 2 or 1 in 4.

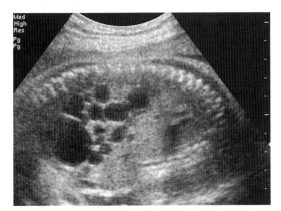

Figure 11.15 A presentation of multicystic renal dysplasia. Unilateral enlarged kidney containing multiple cysts of varying size. Note the oligohydromnios.

Renal dysplasia

The ultrasound appearances of renal dysplasia cover a wide spectrum and include findings that are indistinguishable from IPCK or bilateral MCKD. Renal dysplasia is characterized by enlarged kidneys that contain cysts of varying sizes. Microcysts will produce an appearance indistinguishable from IPCK whereas larger and/or more variably sized cysts will produce appearances similar to those of MCDK. The condition tends to be bilateral, with both kidneys being equally enlarged. As discussed above, MCKD has a low recurrence risk. A number of the conditions amenable to prenatal diagnosis and which are associated with renal dysplasia are autosomal dominant (APKD) or autosomal recessive conditions (Meckel–Gruber syndrome), with recurrence risks of 1 in 2 or 1 in 4, respectively. The characteristic association with other abnormal findings in some of these conditions provides an important aid in the differential diagnosis of enlarged cystic kidneys and thus the recurrence risk of this condition for future pregnancies.

Adult polycystic kidney disease

The finding of large cysts in the fetal kidney, especially in the presence of a normal amniotic fluid volume, should raise the possibility of the antenatal expression of APKD. The prenatal diagnosis of APKD has been reported sporadically and it is associated with a spectrum of appearances. No, single and multiple cysts are described in association with either normally sized or enlarged kidneys, which are of normal or increased echogenicity. The differential diagnosis of enlarged, hyperechogenic kidneys includes IPCK (see above).

APKD is an autosomal dominant condition that is usually asymptomatic until the third or fourth decade of life. The condition is amenable to prenatal diagnosis because the gene responsible lies on chromosome 16. Because of inheritance pattern of this condition, scanning the kidneys of the parents should be considered after suitable discussion has taken place.

Meckel–Gruber syndrome

Meckel–Gruber syndrome is an autosomal recessive condition characterized by Potter's type III renal dysplasia, encephalocele and polydactyly. An occipital encephalocele is the most common neural tube defect found in this condition, although anencephaly, hydrocephalus and microcephaly are also reported associations. Detection of enlarged kidneys should therefore always prompt the search for the other abnormal findings characterized by Meckel–Gruber syndrome. As bilateral renal disease is frequently associated with oligohydramnios, such an examination might be difficult. Although both bilateral renal dysplasia and Meckel–Gruber syndrome carry a poor prognosis for the index pregnancy, it is important that the parents are made aware of the potential difficulties for future pregnancies from a suboptimal examination.

Renal cysts

Unilateral isolated cysts of the fetal kidney are rare and harmless. Isolated renal cysts arise from the renal cortex and should be distinguished from dilatation of the renal pelvis. Cases of isolated renal cyst should be reviewed in the third trimester so as to ensure that the AC is not so large as to prevent safe vaginal delivery.

OBSTRUCTIVE UROPATHY

This is the name given to a range of conditions in which there is dilatation of some or all of the urinary tract due to an obstruction. The obstruction might be intermittent, partial or complete. The ultrasound appearances produced depend on the site and severity of the obstruction. The prognosis depends on the degree of renal compromise and the pulmonary hypoplasia associated with prolonged anhydramnios or oligohydramnios.

Urethral obstruction

In this condition, flow of urine from the bladder to the amniotic fluid via the urethra is blocked. The most common cause of urethral obstruction is posterior urethral valves (PUV), although urethral atresia is a less likely cause. Posterior urethral valves are folds of mucosa at the bladder neck that act as a one-way valve and prevent urine leaving the bladder. They occur in the male fetus exclusively. In

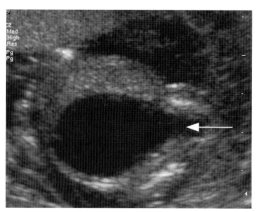

Figure 11.16 Transverse section of the fetal abdomen demonstrating a grossly dilated bladder. Note the associated oligohydramnios and distended proximal urethra (arrow).

both PUV and urethral atresia, renal function is initially preserved – producing the features characteristic of urethral obstruction, namely a markedly distended bladder and severe oligohydramnios (Fig. 11.16). Back pressure from the site of the obstruction causes dilatation of the upper urinary tract and progressive renal dysplasia. It is difficult to determine the degree of dysplasia, although increased cortical echogenicity is taken as indicative by some authors. The longer and/or the more severe the obstruction is, therefore, the greater is the likelihood of renal dysplasia and thus the poorer the prognosis. In the most severe cases, the only organ that can be identified below the diaphragm is the fetal bladder. Intrauterine death is common and, for those fetuses that survive, the prognosis is poor because of pulmonary hypoplasia in addition to the severe renal compromise.

Urethral valves can also be associated with other anomalies, such as chromosomal abnormalities, bowel atresias and craniospinal defects. Although the postnatal removal of PUV is a straightforward procedure, the prenatal challenge is to identify those fetuses that have sufficient renal function and that might therefore benefit from vesicoamniotic shunting. Such shunting involves insertion of a suprapubic catheter into the fetal bladder under ultrasound control to bypass the obstruction caused by the urethral valves. Even with careful selection of fetuses thought to be suitable for such treatment, only about 25% will survive. However, such treatment is now falling out of favor because of the long-term morbidity associated with these cases.

Renal pelvic dilatation

As discussed in Chapter 8, controversy remains as to what constitutes normal renal pelvic size in the fetus (see Figs 8.28 and 8.31). An AP diameter of 5 mm is commonly taken as the upper limit of normal renal pelvic size in the second trimester and 10 mm in the third trimester. The definition of mild renal pelvic dilatation (RPD) also varies between authors. Some use quantitative criteria to distinguish between mild, moderate and severe RPD whereas others use qualitative criteria such as calyceal dilatation. Moderate second trimester RPD is commonly defined as an AP pelvis of 10 mm or more (Fig. 11.17A). Alternatively, it is defined as a dilated renal pelvis associated with calyceal dilatation (Fig. 11.17B).

Prenatal RPD is associated with postnatal uropathies including pelviureteric junction obstruction (PUJO), duplex kidney and reflux. It is traditionally included in the spectrum of obstructive uropathies, although this is a misnomer in the majority of cases because, for most fetuses, RPD resolves before delivery. Fetuses demonstrating moderate RPD in the second trimester, and those fetuses in which initial mild dilatation exceeds 10 mm during gestation, should be followed up with renal ultrasound after delivery because this is the group demonstrating the highest association with postnatal uropathies and subsequent surgery.

Second-trimester RPD will resolve before delivery in up to 80% of cases and in the majority of cases has no postnatal sequelae. However, postnatal urinary tract pathology is present in approximately 10% of fetuses with mild second trimester RPD and approximately 4% of fetuses with mild second trimester RPD will require postnatal surgery.

FETAL HYDROPS

Hydrops fetalis or fetal hydrops describes the combination of edema and ascites. Edema is the

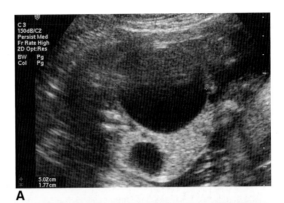

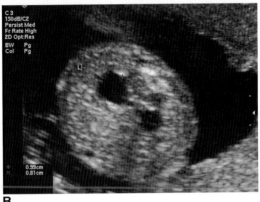

Figure 11.17 Moderate and severe renal pelvic dilatation. A. The AP pelvis of the lower kidney measures 17.7 mm and demonstrates moderate RPD. The AP pelvis of the upper kidney measures 50.2 mm – most authors would classify this as severe RPD. B. Although both renal pelves measure less than 10 mm (9.9 mm and 8.1 mm respectively) calyceal dilatation is present. These appearances can be compared to the normal renal pelvis and mild RPD shown in Figs 8.28 and 8.31, respectively.

accumulation of fluid in the skin whereas ascites is accumulation of fluid within the peritoneal cavity of the abdomen (Fig. 11.18). The normal fetal skin is barely resolved with ultrasound, appearing simply as a bright edge to the underlying organs. Distention of the skin tissue in edema produces a characteristic ultrasound appearance that can be readily recognized. Abnormal collections of fluid within the fetal body are also readily recognized because they produce a characteristic hypoechoic rim, of varying depth, which surrounds the heart, lung(s) and/or abdominal organs.

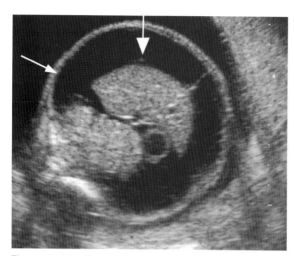

Figure 11.18 Transverse section of the fetal body demonstrating fetal hydrops. Gross ascites (large arrow) is present, outlining the fetal liver. Mild skin edema (arrow) is also present.

Hydrops is traditionally divided into two groups: immune (due to maternal antibodies) and non-immune. The majority of cases are now due to non-immune causes, which are many and varied. These include conditions that cause alterations in cardiac output, venous and lymphatic drainage and membrane permeability. Structural abnormalities involving mediastinal compression, such as some skeletal dysplasias, cystic adenomatoid malformation and diaphragmatic hernia, and abnormalities causing cardiac compromise including tachyarrhythmias, are associated with hydrops. It is associated with trisomy 13, 18 and 21, Turner syndrome (45XO) and triploidy. Fetal infections and anemia are also important causes.

In cases of fetal hydrops it is important, first, to exclude a structural abnormality as the underlying cause. Maternal antibody and infection status can be evaluated from maternal blood sampling and the fetal status from fetal blood sampling. Despite the range of diagnostic tools currently available, the cause of many cases of hydrops remains unproven.

SKELETAL ABNORMALITIES

Many syndromes involve the limbs, and they do not fit into a simple classification. Limbs can be absent or abnormal in length, shape and/or degree of mineralization.

Absent limbs

A limb can be wholly or partially absent. The specific abnormality is described as follows:

- complete absence (amelia)
- partial absence of a limb or segment of a limb (meromelia)
- absence of long bones with the hands and/or feet attached to the body (phocomelia).

Skeletal dysplasia

When suspicion of a skeletal dysplasia is raised it is important to examine not only all the long bones but also the hands, feet, skull, chest and spine if the correct diagnosis is to be reached. For the purposes of ultrasound examination three criteria aid in the differential diagnosis:

1. *Shortening of the long bones of the*:
   - entire limb (micromelia)
   - humerus and/or femur (rhizomelia)
   - radius and ulna and/or tibia and fibula (mesomelia or acromesomelia).

2. *Defective mineralization and/or fracture*: abnormal mineralization might be evident in the skull and/or limbs and/or vertebral bodies, depending on the specific condition. Fractures of the long bones and/or ribs might be present, with healed fractures of the ribs detectable as 'beading'.

3. *Additional features*: abnormalities in appearance of the thorax, ribs, skull, hands and feet, together with polyhydramnios, aid in reaching a specific rather than a differential diagnosis. The severity of the shortening, together with subsequent growth rates are also important pointers towards a specific diagnosis.

Skeletal dysplasias are rare and usually arise as new mutations. The most common lethal dysplasias are thanatophoric dysplasia (Fig. 11.19) and osteogenesis imperfecta (type II) (Fig. 11.20), which have an incidence of 1 in 30 000 and 1 in 55 000 births, respectively. The final arbiters in making the final diagnosis are frequently the post mortem and/or a postnatal radiographic skeletal survey. Both these examinations are invaluable when attempting to counsel the parents on the

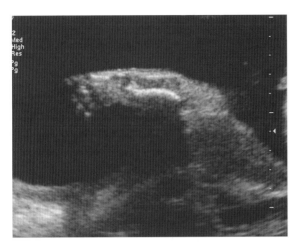

Figure 11.19 Thanatophoric dysplasia. The radius is extremely short and bowed, producing the characteristic 'telephone receiver' shape.

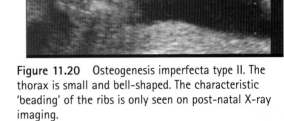

Figure 11.20 Osteogenesis imperfecta type II. The thorax is small and bell-shaped. The characteristic 'beading' of the ribs is only seen on post-natal X-ray imaging.

recurrent risks of the condition in subsequent pregnancies.

The ultrasound features of the most common skeletal dysplasias are given in Table 11.1.

Table 11.1   Ultrasound features of common skeletal dysplasias

Condition	Amniotic fluid volume	Long bones	Femoral bowing	Mineralization of spine	Thorax	Mineralization of head, shape	Hands/feet
Achondrogenesis type I	Polyhydramnios	Extreme micromelia		Poor	Small	Poor	
Achondrogenesis type II	Polyhydramnios	Severe micromelia		Poor	Small	Normal	
Short rib polydactyly	Polyhydramnios	Severe micromelia					Postaxial polydactyly
Osteogenesis type IIa	Polyhydramnios	Micromelia	Yes		Short beaded ribs	Poor, brachy-cephaly	
Hypophosphatasia		Micromelia	Yes			Poor	
Thanatophoric dysplasia	Polyhydramnios	Severe micromelia	'Telephone receiver' shaped	Flat vertebral bodies	Small	Frontal bossing, clover leaf	Trident hand
Campomelic dysplasia		Femur, tibia, fibula moderate shortening	Yes	Flat vertebral bodies	Small clavicles	Macrocephaly, micrognathia	Severe talipes
Diastrophic dysplasia		Rhizomelia, flexion deformities					Hitchhiker thumbs, severe talipes
Achondroplasia		Rhizomelia				Frontal bossing, flattened nasal bridge	Trident hand
Asphyxiating thoracic dystrophy/Jeune's syndrome		Rhizomelia			Long, narrow		+/- poly-dactyly
Chondroectodermal dysplasia/Ellis van Creveld syndrome		Variable mesomelia, tibial hypoplasia			Small (50%)		Postaxial polydactyly
Chondrodysplasia punctata rhizomelic type		Rhizomelia especially humerus, joint contractures					

REFERENCES AND FURTHER READING

Chudleigh T 2001 Mild pyelectasis. Prenatal Diagnosis 21:936–941

Goldstein I, Lockwood C, Hobbins J C 1987 Ultrasound assessment of fetal intestinal development in the evaluation of gestational age. Obstetrics and Gynecology 70:682–686

Jones K L 1997 Smith's recognizable patterns of human malformation, 5th edn. WB Saunders, Philadelphia

Potter E L 1972 Normal and abnormal development of the kidney. Year Book, Chicago p 141–208

Chapter 12

Fetal growth

Abnormalities of fetal growth are encountered far more frequently in clinical practice than fetal abnormalities. Fetal growth restriction, whatever the cause, is associated with a wide variety of adverse outcomes, from minor neonatal morbidity to intrauterine fetal death. The most common reason for fetal growth restriction is uteroplacental insufficiency. Chromosome abnormalities, some fetal abnormalities and fetal infection can be associated with a reduction in growth velocity of varying severity. It is therefore important to be aware of the ultrasound features that aid in distinguishing between uteroplacental insufficiency, fetal abnormality and fetal infection as possible causes for fetal growth restriction.

Many ultrasound features are associated with uteroplacental insufficiency, and these will vary depending on the severity and duration of the problem. Early features include a reduction in growth velocity and oligohydramnios followed by a reduced biophysical profile, mild cardiomegaly (Fig. 12.1A), hyperechoic bowel and bowel dilatation (Fig. 12.1B) Doppler studies typical of uteroplacental insufficiency include uterine artery notches, absent/reversed end-diastolic flow in the umbilical artery and arterial redistribution.

Similar features are seen in fetal abnormality or infection, but usually the uterine artery Doppler values and the amniotic fluid volume are normal (unless the urinary tract is involved). In these situations, consideration should be given to prenatal diagnosis of chromosomal abnormality or congenital viral infection.

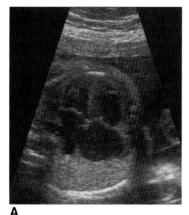

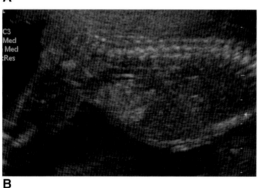

A

B

Figure 12.1 A. Mild cardiomegaly. B. Hyperechoic small bowel in a 30-weeks fetus with severe intrauterine growth restriction.

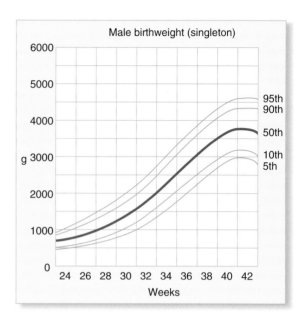

Figure 12.2 Chart of birthweight against gestational age showing 95th, 90th, 50th, 10th and 5th centiles for singleton male. Using this chart, a fetus is defined as growth restricted if its predicted birthweight is on or below the 10th centile for gestation (Hadlock et al 1985).

The relative frequency of fetal growth restriction and the understandable anxiety it causes in both parents and medical carers necessitates a thorough understanding of the differential diagnosis and management of this condition.

DEFINING GROWTH RESTRICTION

Intrauterine growth restriction (IUGR) is often defined as birthweight less than the 10th centile for gestation (Fig. 12.2) However, this simple definition has many drawbacks. First, 10% of the normal population will be identified by this classification. Second, despite being growth-restricted, the majority of fetuses affected by uteroplacental insufficiency have biometry measurements that plot above the 10th centile.

It would seem better to use individualized growth charts to determine whether a fetus is growth restricted (Fig. 12.3). These are based primarily on the mother's height, weight, parity and the birthweights of her previous children. For example, a fetus that weighs 2.9 kg at 39 weeks is probably growth restricted if the mother is 6 feet tall, weighs 65 kg and has had a previous child weighing 4.2 kg at birth. Unfortunately, such individualized or customized antenatal growth charts are not in common usage, and they remain to be validated in large prospective studies.

A simpler alternative would be to use growth velocity to determine the effect of uteroplacental function. For example, a fetus with a falling growth velocity that is crossing centile lines is likely to be compromised, whereas another that has a consistent growth rate on the 5th centile is probably constitutionally small (Fig. 12.4). However, this still remains a subjective assessment because there is no agreed rate of fall or threshold for determining pathologic from physiologic pregnancies.

Before growth restriction can be diagnosed by any of the methods described above, correct pregnancy dating is required. Incorrect or unknown pregnancy dating will result in an increased diagno-

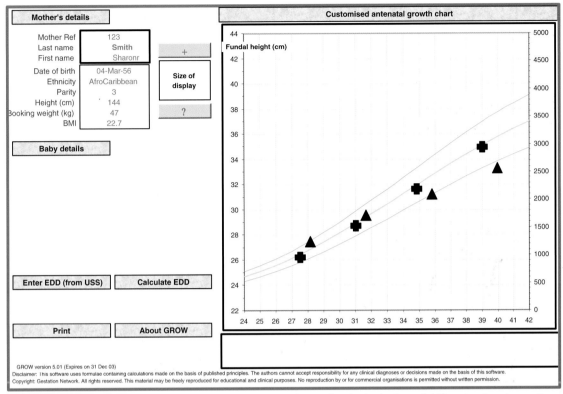

Figure 12.3 Customized growth chart demonstrating normal growth velocity in fetus A (✚) and reduced growth velocity in fetus B (▲).

sis of growth restriction and post-term pregnancy, both of which lead to unnecessary pregnancy intervention.

PREGNANCY DATING

Rationale for ultrasound dating of pregnancies

Several randomized, controlled studies have shown that ultrasound dating, compared to menstrual dating of pregnancies, reduces the inappropriate diagnosis of fetal growth restriction and post-term pregnancy. A detailed description of ultrasound dating is given in Chapters 3 and 7. When fetal growth restriction is suspected on ultrasound, a review of early pregnancy dating should be undertaken to eliminate this simple error. When available, the crown–rump length (CRL) should be used as the preferred measurement for pregnancy dating.

Problems of ultrasound dating

Serial redating

Every effort should be made to avoid redating pregnancies on more than one occasion. If there are several ultrasound measurements, the CRL should be used to date the pregnancy, providing the correct sections were obtained and the measurements were taken accurately by an experienced operator. Any subsequent fetal biometry should be taken to represent true fetal growth velocity, providing the same operator quality criteria are applied.

Parental attitude

Redating of pregnancies concerns many parents. This is understandable, because the hidden meaning of this process to them is that we do not believe them or that the pregnancy was conceived when they were not together. As discussed in Chapter 7,

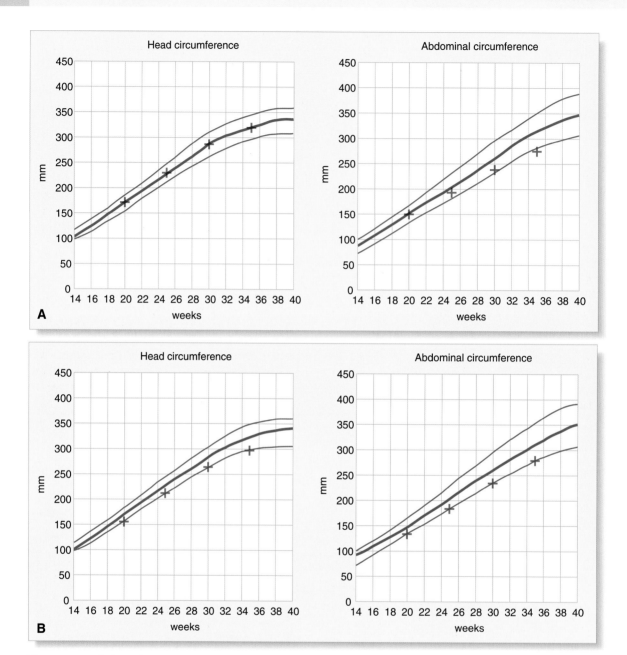

Figure 12.4 A. Growth pattern in asymmetric IUGR. The growth of the HC follows the 50th centile and is therefore normal. The growth rate of the AC can be seen to be slowing as the values obtained plot against falling centiles. B. Growth pattern in symmetric IUGR. The growth of the HC and the AC follow the 5th centile.

the reliability of the menstrual history should be carefully reviewed before reassigning the EDD. If the date of conception is irrefutable or the menstrual history is reliable, it is unwise to reassign the EDD.

SYMMETRIC GROWTH RESTRICTION

Symmetric growth restriction is the description given to the equivalent reduction in growth velocity of both the fetal head circumference and abdominal circumference. In the vast majority of cases, the H:A ratio would be in the normal range and this picture would represent a constitutionally small fetus. In a very small number of pregnancies, symmetric growth restriction occurs in pathological pregnancies. In the latter case, the insult or injury has occurred in early pregnancy and results in severe growth restriction and very poor pregnancy outcome (Fig. 12.5).

Distinguishing between normal and abnormal pregnancies

Constitutionally small fetuses

Typically, the growth velocities in these pregnancies continue along the same centile (see Fig. 12.4B). There is an absence of ultrasound features of uteroplacental insufficiency or fetal abnormality. Additionally, uterine, umbilical and fetal Doppler values remain in the normal range.

Pathologically small fetuses

The growth velocity in these pregnancies continues to fall and progressively cross lower centiles (see

Fig. 12.5) The majority of these pregnancies have severe early-onset uteroplacental insufficiency or fetal abnormality, typically triploidy.

Problems with symmetric growth restriction

Equivocal findings

If unsure as to whether the pregnancy is constitutionally or pathologically small, refer to a fetal medicine specialist. Should the latter be undesired or not be possible, a repeat scan to check growth velocity in 2–3 weeks should reveal the diagnosis.

ASYMMETRIC GROWTH RESTRICTION

Asymmetric growth restriction is the description given to differential reduction in growth velocity of the fetal head to abdominal circumference (see Fig. 12.4A). In the vast majority of cases, asymmetric fetal growth restriction is a consequence of uteroplacental insufficiency.

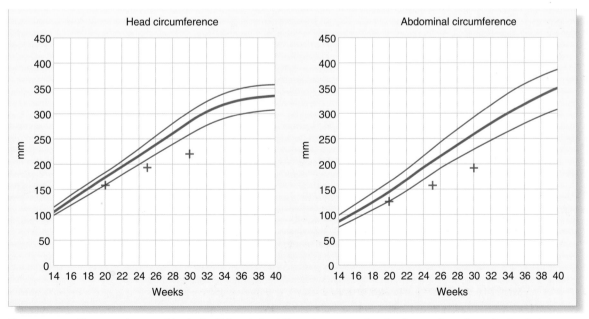

Figure 12.5 The growth rate of both the HC and the AC can be seen to be slowing as the values obtained plot against falling centiles. This growth pattern suggests either severe early onset uteroplacental insufficiency or a chromosomal abnormality, most commonly triploidy.

Ultrasound features of fetal growth restriction

Ultrasound features of uteroplacental insufficiency include placental abnormality (lakes, calcification, jelly-like consistency) and reduction in amniotic fluid volume. Fetal features include mild cardiomegaly, hyperechoic bowel and small bowel dilatation (see Fig. 12.1). The presence of these features would support the diagnosis of uteroplacental insufficiency.

Doppler assessment

Doppler findings typical of uteroplacental insufficiency include: uterine artery notches, absent/reversed end-diastolic flow in the umbilical artery and arterial redistribution. Fetal Doppler studies are discussed in detail in Chapter 16.

Fetal biophysical profile

Biophysical profile scoring is a formalization of fetal behavioral assessment. For instance, it would be easy to distinguish, by observation, a long distance runner who has just finished a marathon from one who is yet to start. Biophysical profile scoring allows sonographers to formalize that assessment process. Healthy fetuses would demonstrate good tone, general movement, breathing movement, amniotic fluid volume and heart rate pattern. Biophysical profile scores are usually given on a scale of 0–10. Typically, scores of 6 or below are considered frankly abnormal, and scores of 7 and 8 are considered suspicious.

Various biophysical profiles have been published, which differ slightly from each other. A typical example is given in Table 12.1. Each criterion is assigned a score from 0 to 2, depending on the ultrasound findings.

Fetal heart rate patterns can be subjectively classified as reactive or non-reactive. Computerized assessment provides an objective score for the fetal heart rate pattern. The grading of the latter is outside the scope of this text. Within an ultrasound unit, this part of the assessment is often omitted and the overall score given out of 8, rather than 10. Other units prefer to replace this score with Doppler assessment of the umbilical artery.

Recommendations

Typically, reduced biophysical profile scores are found in growth restricted pregnancies that already demonstrate abnormal umbilical and fetal Doppler findings. The finding of abnormal biophysical scores should prompt the clinician to consider immediate delivery.

GROWTH IN MULTIPLE PREGNANCY

Many multiple pregnancies are diagnosed as being growth restricted. Indeed, the majority of neonates delivered from multiple pregnancies are small.

Table 12.1 The biophysical profile

Criterion	Score 2	Score 1	Score 0
Fetal tone (assessed over 30 min)	At least 1 motion of limb and spine from flexion to extension and back	At least 1 motion of limb or spine from flexion to extension and back	No movements
Fetal movements (assessed over 30 min)	3 or more gross body movements	1 or 2 movements	No movements
Breathing movements (assessed over 30 min)	At least 1 episode of breathing of at least 60 s	At least 1 episode of breathing lasting 30–60 s	<30 s breathing
Amniotic fluid volume	Largest pocket of fluid > 2 cm in depth	Largest pocket 1–2 cm in vertical depth	Largest pocket of fluid < 1 cm
Fetal heart rate (assessed over 20 min)	At least 5 accelerations of 15 bpm, lasting 15 s	2–4 accelerations of 15 bpm, lasting 15 s	No accelerations

However, most of these fetuses are constitutionally small, and are not suffering from uteroplacental insufficiency.

Assessment of growth

Abdominal palpation is of little value in multiple pregnancy. It is appropriate for multiple pregnancies to have serial ultrasound scans for assessment of fetal growth. These should be scheduled every 4–5 weeks if the pregnancy is dichorionic, or more frequently (2–3 weekly) if the pregnancy is monochorionic or if one or both twins is affected by growth restriction.

Labeling of twins

The labeling of twins was discussed in Chapter 3. It is very important that a consistent approach is developed to the labeling and consequent identification of each fetus in a twin pregnancy. Problems will be rarely encountered where there is normal growth of both twins or where there is an obvious and prolonged size difference between the twins. Difficulties will arise in those pregnancies where a differential growth rate becomes apparent during pregnancy. A worsening of the growth velocity in one twin can be overlooked if the same twin is not consistently identified at each examination irrespective of its presentation and its position relative to its sibling.

Inter-twin growth discrepancy

An inter-twin growth discrepancy of 20–25% is considered to be significant. As twins act as 'internal controls', the latter finding suggests a pathologic cause. Efforts should be made to exclude uteroplacental insufficiency (see above) or twin-to-twin transfusion syndrome (TTTS) on ultrasound. The ultrasound finding of an inter-twin growth discrepancy should necessitate a referral to a fetal medicine unit.

Twin-to-twin transfusion syndrome

Twin-to-twin transfusion syndrome (TTTS) describes a wide range of problems that can occur in monochorionic twins as a result of unequal sharing of placental blood through inter-twin vascular anastomoses. Usually, due to a paucity of inter-twin

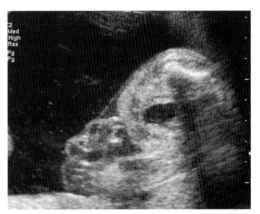

Figure 12.6 Appearance of the donor or 'stuck twin' in severe TTTS. The characteristic features are the lack of amniotic fluid in the sac and severe growth restriction. Note the membrane lying over the cramped fetal abdomen and umbilical cord.

vascular connections in the monochorial placenta, there is net transfer of blood from one fetus (donor) to the other (recipient). Twin-to-twin transfusion syndrome is thought to occur in about 10–15% of monochorionic twins and is not usually detectable before 16 weeks of gestation.

Ultrasound features in the donor include intrauterine growth restriction, an empty bladder and anhydramnios. The lack of amniotic fluid in the amniotic sac of the donor causes the amnion to surround the fetus as if it is wrapped in cling film. This sac commonly lies immediately adjacent to the anterior uterine wall. These features are described as those of the 'stuck twin' (Fig. 12.6). By contrast, the recipient usually has normal growth velocity, a large bladder and severe polyhydramnios. In cases of severe TTTS, the recipient twin develops hydrops (Fig. 12.7). Color Doppler findings in the donor are usually typical of uteroplacental insufficiency (increased placental vascular resistance and fetal arterial redistribution), whereas the donor might have abnormal venous Doppler findings because of high-output cardiac failure.

Depending on the severity and gestation at diagnosis, management options include amniodrainage to prevent premature labor, selective fetocide by cord occlusion to protect the healthier twin in utero and fetoscopic laser ablation of the interconnecting vessels.

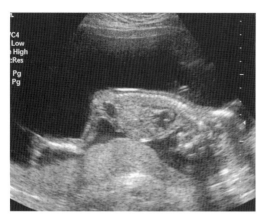

Figure 12.7 Appearance of the recipient twin in severe TTTS. The characteristic features are the polyhydramnios and an enlarged fetal bladder. Note the extended fetal position with polyhydramnios.

Problems with growth in multiple pregnancy

Sudden catch-up growth

If a growth-restricted twin shows sudden catch-up growth (or conversely fall-off in growth), the fetal measurements and labeling should be rechecked. Either the labeling of the twins has been changed or the wrong fetus has been measured during the ultrasound procedure.

Monoamniotic twins

Treat the diagnosis of monoamniotic twins with caution. Note that monochorionic diamniotic twins with TTTS are far more common than monoamniotic twinning.

REFERENCES AND FURTHER READING

Baschat A A, Harman C R 2001 Antenatal assessment of the growth restricted fetus. Current Opinion in Obstetrics and Gynecology 13:161–168

Creasy R K, Resnik R 1999 Intrauterine growth restriction. In: Creasy R K, Resnik R (eds) Maternal–fetal medicine, 4th edn. W B Saunders, Philadelphia, p 569–584

Gembruch U, Gortner L 1998 Perinatal aspects of preterm intrauterine growth restriction. Ultrasound in Obstetrics and Gynecology 11:233–239

Kingdom J C, Baker P (eds) 2002 Intrauterine growth restriction. Springer, New York

Chapter **13**

Discussing the findings

CHAPTER CONTENTS

An ultrasound examination includes two equally important components: performing the examination and disseminating its findings. Performing an ultrasound examination to the highest level of competence is of little value if its results are not disseminated in a way that can be readily understood by all those concerned.

The findings of an examination should be reported verbally and in writing by the individual who has performed the examination, both to the woman and to other healthcare professionals involved in her care. At the current time, the accepted role of the non-medical sonographer is to describe the findings of an ultrasound examination; it is the role of the clinician responsible for the care of the woman to make a diagnosis based on those findings.

There can be very few health professionals who are fully conversant with the jargon of a discipline that lies outside their expertise. An ultrasound report should therefore be written in a way that its recipient can understand. Descriptive ultrasound terminology such as transonic, hypoechogenic, hyperechogenic or acoustic shadowing can provide useful additional information to your ultrasound colleagues but are unlikely to provide the general practitioner or consultant gynecologist with useful information on which to base further management decisions.

The sonographer should also be aware that there might be more than one interpretation of a word or phrase – describing echogenic foci of the fetal heart as 'golf balls' is an example. Conversely, it is important that bad news is given in a way that the mother is unlikely to misinterpret, as is discussed later.

Discussing the findings in such a way that the receiver of the information can assimilate that information provides a variety of challenges to the sonographer. The majority of the lay public does not have an indepth appreciation of, for example, assessing risk in pregnancy. So information relating to nuchal translucency screening or invasive testing must be delivered in such a way that the parents can understand it and can make an informed choice based on the received information.

Few individuals can find it easy to give unanticipated abnormal findings. You will need to be able to explain the findings clearly and to act in a professional and supportive manner while remaining detached from the emotion of the situation. Every case of abnormal findings is different because each incorporates a unique combination of ultrasound findings and patient reactions. You will inevitably feel that you handled some situations better than others, and this will not necessarily relate simply to the severity of the problem or problems you identified. As a professional, with a duty of care to the women you scan, it is important that you reflect on each case and try to analyze how you handled that case. This will help you to further develop those skills that resulted in positive contributions and to address those that were less effective.

It is clear that the sonographer needs a range of skills to disseminate results appropriately. Some of these skills are relatively easy to learn – entering data into a database and printing off a report that relates to a selected examination are not usually difficult. Finding the right words to explain that you have detected a fetal abnormality is much more difficult. You must be able to communicate your findings in a range of situations, from the woman on her own to a woman accompanied by a fractious toddler and a partner who expresses his anxiety through aggression. Such skills improve with reflection, experience and learning from one's peers. Listening to others discussing findings with parents and colleagues will, hopefully, suggest what to say and how to say it. It is also worth remembering that listening to others can help you learn what *not* to say and how *not* to say it.

MANAGING THE EXAMINATION

Gathering the information that will constitute the final report begins with your introduction at the start of the examination. Individual professionalism together with the requirements of the departmental protocol should ensure that every examination is performed to an agreed level of competence. As discussed elsewhere in this book, the quality of the examination you perform is related to your expertise and experience. Other factors, including the suitability and quality of the equipment and patient size, are also important. However, the way in which you approach the examination is also influenced by the rapport you develop with the woman and her attenders. The sonographer is much more likely to perform a thorough examination in a relaxed and friendly room than in one with a hostile and suspicious atmosphere. Equally, the woman will feel more able to express any concerns she might have if she feels welcomed and informed about the ensuing examination.

As it is your responsibility to perform the ultrasound examination, assimilate its findings and report them, then it is your responsibility to ensure you are able to discharge those functions correctly. If you prefer to scan in silence until you have made a preliminary assessment then it is important that you should be allowed to do this. However, you should appreciate that the majority of women and their attenders will interpret your silence as suggesting that you have found a problem, unless you explain *before* you start the examination that that is your preferred method of working.

If you find the frequent questioning of an individual (or the activities of accompanying children and/or attenders) distracting then you must politely ask that individual to desist in their questioning or the distracting attenders to wait outside so that you can concentrate properly on the examination for which you are responsible. Alternatively, you must develop strategies to cope with these potential distractions while maintaining your concentration.

Invasion of personal space either by an attender (or an observer allocated to you by your department) might also undermine your ability to concentrate. Again you must politely ask the individual to observe the examination from a different area of the room, or develop strategies to cope in such a situation.

GATHERING THE INFORMATION

It should be remembered that the most important role of the sonographer when performing an ultrasound examination is to distinguish between findings that are normal and findings that are not normal. Further interpretation of such findings might be the responsibility of that sonographer or a colleague to whom the woman is referred. This will depend on the working practices of the department as laid down in its protocols.

Routine ultrasound screening requires two significant skills that are frequently less fundamental to the healthcare professionals to whom a woman might subsequently be referred. The first is to detect findings that are both unanticipated and not normal and the second is to communicate this fact to the woman, who is usually unprepared to receive such information.

As an examination proceeds it will become apparent to you whether its results will be normal. In the majority of both gynecological and routine obstetric examinations your findings will be normal and, in the majority of situations, reporting such results will be straightforward. This will not, however, be the case in all examinations you perform. In some cases you will be unsure of your findings and will need to seek a second opinion. In others you will detect findings that are clearly abnormal. In others the consequences of your findings might be less severe but they are still 'not normal'. Such 'not normal' findings are often the most difficult to evaluate, first, because of lack of published data from unselected populations, and second, because their interpretation might vary depending on other factors. For example, the implications of a minor marker of aneuploidy will differ depending on the age of the woman. It will also vary depending on whether nuchal translucency or serum screening has already been performed. Similarly, a reduction in amniotic fluid normally has less severe clinical implications when associated with a normally grown fetus than with a growth-restricted fetus showing evidence of vascular redistribution.

The sonographer should also be aware that there might be more than one interpretation of a word or phrase. As mentioned previously, the use of ultrasound jargon is open to misinterpretation.

When having difficulty in finding a fetal limb due to fetal movement, fetal position or poor technique for example it is advisable to avoid using phrases such as 'I can't find the leg' because this will cause understandable anxiety to the pregnant woman. It is better to state what you actually mean, i.e. that you 'will be looking at both legs, one is easy to see but the other is more difficult to see because of the position of the fetus at the moment'.

In the majority of cases you, the sonographer, will identify a potential problem some time before the woman whom you are examining is aware of your concerns. Attempting to gauge the likely reaction of the woman can be helpful before you start to explain your findings. This will enable you – hopefully – to deliver those first crucial sentences in a way that is attuned to the woman's levels of expectation and understanding. From a practical point of view, what might be helpful is to continue scanning while concentrating equally on talking to the woman about other aspects of her pregnancy or relevant matters. This might enable you to gauge better the reaction she will have to what you are about to say. It also allows you time to prepare mentally the most appropriate way of explaining your findings to her.

DISCUSSING THE FINDINGS

The first issue that you need to consider is where to discuss your findings. You might consider that the correct procedure is to explain your findings immediately after you have completed the examination. However, this very natural decision could result in the woman receiving information for which she is unprepared, lying on the couch with her abdomen exposed and covered in scanning gel or, if she has had a transvaginal scan, with her legs in stirrups and her underwear removed. Anyone who has been in such a situation, or a comparable situation, will appreciate the feelings of vulnerability and lack of control that accompany such positions. These feelings will be accentuated by your relative positions – although you are sitting beside the woman you are not communicating with each other at the same height because you are talking down to her and she talking up to you. Conversely, inviting the woman to get dressed and taking her to a separate room before telling her your findings (or asking her to wait while you find a colleague to impart them on your behalf) seems, to many, to prolong the agony unnecessarily.

Possibly the best compromise is to ask the woman to dress and sit down on a chair or on the couch in the scanning room. Wait until she is sitting down, and can therefore give you her full attention, before you begin speaking. Do not be tempted to start talking while she is still getting dressed. Imagine yourself at your own doctor's surgery. You are getting dressed after an examination that has been conducted by a locum whom you have never met before. You are probably embarrassed and anxious. Would you prefer the findings to be given to you while you are struggling with the zip of your trousers that has stuck in your shirt, or would you rather receive them sitting fully clothed on the chair beside the doctor's desk?

Some women will already be anticipating bad news because of findings prior to the examination. Other women, especially those attending a routine screening examination, will be anticipating normal findings and be unprepared for results that suggest otherwise. Every 'not normal' situation is different, and is made so by the combination of the implications of the ultrasound findings and their interpretation by the woman. Finding the correct words for the first sentence of the discussion that must follow the completion of such an examination is arguably one of the most difficult tasks that a sonographer faces. Unfortunately, there is no verbal formula that can be applied successfully to all problems in all situations, but there are certain strategies that might be of help.

It is important that bad news is given in a way that the mother is unlikely to misinterpret. If the fetus is dead then it is preferable to say 'I'm afraid I have to give you some bad news, there is no heart beat. I am very sorry to have to tell you that the fetus is dead' than 'I can't find the fetal heart'. The latter can be interpreted as meaning that the fetus is alive but that you are unable to demonstrate the fetal heart beating because of some technical difficulty.

In a situation where you have identified a serious abnormality, such as spina bifida, a major cardiac defect or severe ventriculomegaly, you could try an opening phrase such as 'I am afraid I have to give you some bad news. I think the baby's spine/heart/brain is abnormal'.

The above are situations where it might be preferable to break the news to the woman as soon as you are certain of your findings, i.e. while she is still lying on the couch. This position is also easier for all concerned because you might need to seek confirmation of your findings from a colleague who is elsewhere in the department but who wishes to scan the woman. Before beginning your discussion you might want to take a memento-type image that can be recorded on hard copy and filed in the notes, to be given to the woman at a later date should she so wish.

Mild renal pelvic dilatation, echogenic foci or choroid plexus cysts have a higher prevalence than major structural abnormalities and you will invariably first detect them early in your scanning career. It is much more likely, therefore, that you will need to explain one or more of these findings and their implications to a woman than a spina bifida or a cardiac defect. There is currently a lack of consensus over the significance of these and other 'minor markers' of aneuploidy, both with and in the absence of prior screening. The literature indicates that a single minor marker produces a small increase in the age-related risk of aneuploidy. This increase is not significant. This is not the same as no increase in risk. Moreover, the current literature does not support the interpretation of these appearances as 'normal findings'. For these reasons, we recommend that such findings should not be ignored but should be discussed with the woman and recorded in the case notes. The challenge for the sonographer is to impart the correct information without causing the woman anxiety.

The assumption is that these findings, although outside the range of normal appearances, are very unlikely to indicate anything other than a normal outcome for the pregnancy. Your body language, the tone of your voice and the eye contact you make with the woman should all emphasize this fact. Opening the discussion on choroid plexus cysts with words such as 'I'm afraid I have to tell you that your baby has cysts in its brain but they are nothing to worry about. We'll arrange to rescan you later in the pregnancy to make sure they have disappeared' is unlikely to reassure the woman that these findings are insignificant. It would be preferable to introduce the subject slowly, starting off with words such as 'I've performed a thorough examination of the baby and there are some findings that I want to discuss with you. Adults, children and babies have several glands in the brain that produce fluid in order to 'lubricate' the brain. Occasionally one of these glands can get temporarily blocked. We can see this on ultrasound and call this blockage a choroid plexus cyst. The vast majority of glands that become blocked become unblocked on their own by 28 weeks and so the cyst disappears'. Finding the right words to explain other 'not normal' findings, and delivering them appropriately is frequently easier because their implications are less emotive than 'cysts on the brain'.

It is important to speak slowly and pause frequently to give the woman time to take in what you are saying to her. She must be given the opportunity to ask questions and might need to have the information repeated or explained in a different way. If she becomes upset do not feel you must comfort her by continuing to talk. In such situations silence can be more supportive than well-meaning chatter.

Irrespective of whether the findings are normal, not normal or abnormal, the information you impart should always be representative of the findings of your examination. It is always better to be honest and truthful. Your responsibility is to have sufficient, accurate and up-to-date knowledge of the range of findings that you are likely to identify in your current role, and their implications. It is unrealistic to assume that you will have the answer to every question a woman might ask you and you should not feel inadequate if you are unable to answer questions that are outside your range of expertise. If you are uncertain or do not know there are always other people to whom you can refer the woman for information and advice. It is important, however, to develop ways of explaining that you are unable to provide the required information. Using a phrase such as 'that is something that you need to discuss with Dr X or your midwife' is more helpful for the woman, and is a more professional response, than simply saying 'I don't know' or 'I'm not sure, I'll go and ask'.

These skills might not come easily but are an essential component of your role as a sonographer. Providing you learn from every new situation, your communication skills will continue to develop as your expertise and experience grows.

WRITING THE REPORT

The written report is an integral part of the ultrasound examination. Irrespective of whether the report is handwritten or computer generated, it should include the:

- woman's full name
- woman's date of birth
- woman's hospital or reference number
- reason for performing the examination
- date of examination
- measurement (in mm) of relevant structures
- additional text to describe other findings
- interpretation of findings
- actions taken or recommendations for follow-up
- name and status of sonographer performing the examination.

Reports of obstetric examinations should also include the:

- gestational age
- fetal position/presentation
- placental position relative to the internal os
- evaluation of amniotic fluid volume
- graphical representation of relevant biometry.

A tick-list format for all the fetal and other structures that are to be evaluated is recommended for the routine anomaly scan. It is essential that the proforma identifies clearly how a tick should be interpreted, i.e does it signify 'seen' or 'normal in appearance' or 'normal in appearance, size and position'?

The report should address the reasons for the examination in addition to recording other relevant findings.

Where the EDD, as calculated from the LMP, has been reassigned by prior ultrasound examination, the gestational age should be calculated from the ultrasound assigned EDD. This should be clearly stated in the report.

One of the sonographer's roles is to interpret the ultrasound findings for the referring clinician. With respect to biometric data this is best done by plotting the data on the relevant charts. As fetal size and/or growth is evaluated relative to the gestational age, your interpretation should relate to the fetus as a whole rather than to individual biometric parameters. Consider a pregnancy of 20 weeks' gestation. The BPD is equivalent to 20 weeks, the head circumference to 20+ weeks, the abdominal circumference to 19+ weeks and the femur length to 20 weeks. Evaluation of these measurements when plotted on the relevant charts indicates that they are within the normal range for gestational age (Fig. 13.1). There is no significant disparity between any of them to indicate the need for follow-up. The correct interpretation of these measurements is therefore 'within normal range for dates' or 'equivalent to dates'. It is unhelpful to report these findings as individual gestational age equivalents, i.e. BPD = 20 weeks, HC = 20+ weeks, AC = 19+ weeks, FL = 20 weeks' and unaccompanied by further interpretation.

Similarly, when evaluating fetal growth with serial scans it is essential that the serial measurements are represented graphically. It is helpful to the referring clinician to report the findings of a disparity in size between a graphically represented head circumference and abdominal circumference as 'abdominal circumference 5th centile while head circumference remains on 50th centile, suggestive of intrauterine growth restriction'. It is less helpful to the referring clinician to report the same findings as 'head circumference = 32 week size, abdominal circumference = 29 week size' with no graphical representation. It is unprofessional to expect the clinician to assimilate correctly the information from this and previously written reports and to decide whether the growth rate is normal or not.

CONTACTING RELEVANT HEALTHCARE PROFESSIONALS

A member of the team of healthcare professionals involved in the care of the woman should be informed of any clinically significant findings from the examination as soon as possible, preferably before the woman leaves the ultrasound department. This is your responsibility and you must therefore either make contact yourself of entrust a colleague to do this on our behalf.

It is inappropriate and unprofessional to provide the woman with a written report and assume that

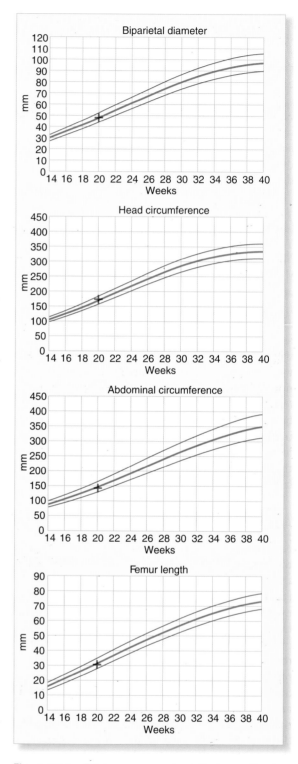

Figure 13.1 Fetal measurements plotted according to gestational age of 20 weeks 0 days, as calculated from the LMP (Snijders & Nicolaides 1994).

the relevant individuals will receive this information following her next contact with her care team.

Less clinically significant findings require a value judgment on your part. Your departmental protocol should outline the recommended action pathway in such situations. If you are unsure then it is better to err on the side of caution, make contact with a member of the woman's care team and act on that person's decision. This should be done before the woman leaves the ultrasound department.

ARRANGING FOLLOW-UP

Your departmental protocol should identify the findings that require ultrasound follow-up and the gestational age at which the follow-up appointment(s) should be made. You must ensure that the necessary appointment is made with the appropriate staff member, it is not appropriate to assume that someone else, or even the woman, will do this on your behalf. It is important that the arrangement of any further appointments is noted on the report and that the woman is aware that a further ultrasound scan appointment has been made for her. It is also important to ensure that the woman understands that she is to return to the ultrasound department on that date, rather than to the antenatal clinic on the hospital or at her GP's surgery.

AUDIT OF FINDINGS

Any information that women are given concerning the quality of the ultrasound service that your department provides should be based on the regular audit of your department's results. Such audit might identify the sensitivity of your nuchal translucency programme or your cardiac screening programme at the 20 week scan. It might identify the accuracy of estimated fetal weight or the reporting of placenta previa in the third trimester. Such results can be used to identify the successful areas of the service and to highlight those areas that produce poor results. Once the reasons for these poor results have been identified, improving this area of service can be addressed.

The expectations of the routine anomaly service should be directly related to the results of the departmental audit. If your audit reveals that all scanned cases of spina bifida and anencephaly were detected prior to 24 weeks then it is reasonable for your departmental literature to state that the majority of such cases will be detected. If only 30% of major cardiac abnormalities and 20% of facial clefts were detected prior to 24 weeks, it is equally important to state that the majority of such cases will not be identified.

DEPARTMENTAL PROTOCOL

Every department should have a protocol that provides the following information:

- the objectives of each type of examination that is offered
- the structures that will be sought and evaluated
- a description of what constitutes normal/abnormal findings in those structures
- the measurements that will be taken
- a description of when a measurement or a combination of measurements will be considered abnormal
- the procedures that will be undertaken when a problem is identified
- by what means the findings of normal examinations will be recorded and what images will be recorded
- by what means the findings of abnormal examinations will be recorded and what images will be recorded
- how examinations will be reported and to whom
- the type of follow-up, and its frequency, following the detection of specified findings.

The protocol should be dated and reviewed on a regular basis. Once a protocol is superseded it should be kept on file and should not be destroyed.

In the first instance, the protocol should reflect the level of service provided by the department. All members of staff, including all new staff members, should be familiar with the contents of the protocol and should ensure that their scanning abilities encompass its requirements. If they do not, this should be addressed urgently by further training followed by assessment.

The protocol should accurately describe, for each type of examination, what will be undertaken, how it will be interpreted and how it will be reported. It should therefore be possible for an individual from outside the department to read the protocol and form an accurate impression of what each examination includes and the level of expertise being applied. The content of the protocol should be as detailed as is needed to fulfill these requirements. As discussed earlier, a tick-list proforma can be used in all routine anomaly ultrasound examinations. The protocol must identify clearly how a tick should be interpreted, i.e does it signify 'seen' or 'normal in appearance' or 'normal in appearance, size and position'? These details should be addressed clearly in the protocol.

MEDICOLEGAL ISSUES

The increasing reliance that is placed on ultrasound examinations increases the expectations of parents that normal prenatal ultrasound findings equate to a normal baby at delivery. Sadly, this is not always the case, leading to an increasing number of parents seeking litigation. In many instances the problems evident postnatally could not have been detected prenatally and there would therefore be no case to answer. In other cases, the problem would have been amenable to prenatal detection but the relevant structure was not sought, in accordance with the departmental protocol. In these cases it is unlikely that there would be a case to answer. In still other cases, an abnormal finding is overlooked, or its appearance is misinterpreted, despite the departmental protocol requiring evaluation of that structure. In such cases it might indeed be the case that the sonographer was negligent and there is therefore a case to answer.

For the majority of sonographers, litigation will only be a distant anxiety. However, it is your responsibility as a sonographer to ensure that your actions do not leave you open to litigation. The way to do this is to ensure that every examination you undertake is performed to a standard appropriate to, or above, that required by your departmental protocol. The range of abnormalities that you should detect, and therefore should not overlook, will be evident from the contents of your departmental protocol. This information is relevant both to you, the sonographer, and to the woman you are scanning.

In some circumstances it might not be possible to perform an examination to the standard required by your protocol, e.g. in cases of maternal obesity or a persistently difficult fetal position. If this is the case you should state this fact in your report.

Taking hard-copy of a specified number of standard images of a normal examination is good practice because it provides a visual record of the examination. This should be seen as positive evidence of the quality of the examination you have performed. It can also endorse the technical difficulties, such as maternal obesity, described in your report. Should you feel threatened by having to record images then you should question why this is and ensure that this matter is addressed satisfactorily.

The majority of medicolegal cases never reach the courts either because there is no case to answer or because the matter is settled out of court. However, this is likely to be of little comfort when it is first brought to your attention that parents have decided to issue proceedings against your employer and that you were responsible for performing the ultrasound examination(s) of their fetus that subsequently was born with an abnormality. Your departmental protocol should provide the evidence required to support you providing it can be demonstrated that you acted within its requirements. You must be aware, however, that if you do *not* perform an ultrasound examination to the standard required by your departmental protocol and this results in a fetal abnormality being missed, then your actions can be interpreted as negligent because you have breached the duty of care you owe to the woman.

REFERENCES AND FURTHER READING

Joint Working Party of the Royal College of Obstetricians & Gynaecologists and the Royal College of Paediatrics and Child Health 1997 Fetal abnormalities: guidelines for screening, diagnosis and management. RCPCH and RCOG, London

Snijders RJM, Nicolaides KH 1994 Fetal biometry at 14–40 weeks gestation. Ultrasound in Obstetrics and Gynecology 4:34–48

The Royal College of Obstetricians and Gynaecologists 1997 Ultrasound screening for fetal abnormalities: report of the RCOG working party. RCOG, London

The Royal College of Obstetricians and Gynaecologists 2000 Routine ultrasound screening in pregnancy: protocol, standards and training. RCOG, London

United Kingdom Association of Sonographers 2001 Guidelines for professional working standards: ultrasound practice. United Kingdom Association of Sonographers, London

Chapter **14**

Invasive procedures

CHAPTER CONTENTS

AMNIOCENTESIS

Amniocentesis means the removal of amniotic fluid. The indications for its use in both early and late pregnancy are given in Box 14.1. All invasive procedures are now performed under direct ultrasound control. This means that the person performing the amniocentesis also performs the preliminary scan to locate the most ideal spot and inserts the needle under direct ultrasound visualization.

Amniocentesis is usually performed at about 16 weeks' gestation, with the full karyotype result being available about 3 weeks later. Although it is technically possible to perform amniocentesis before this gestation, several studies have demonstrated that early amniocentesis is associated with a higher miscarriage and culture failure rates, as well as with increased prevalence of talipes equinovarus.

Indications

The most common reason for amniocentesis in early pregnancy is to determine the fetal karyotype. Table 14.1 indicates the maternal-age-specific risks of all chromosomal abnormalities at delivery and Table 14.2 indicates the maternal-age-specific risks of trisomy 21 with gestation. Most obstetric centers offer genetic amniocentesis to mothers of 35 years or over. The risks associated with amniocentesis are identified in Box 14.2.

Box 14.1 Indications for second trimester amniocentesis

For genetic reasons:
  maternal age (see Table 14.2)
  previous history of chromosomal anomaly
  balanced translocation in either parent
  to determine fetal sex if history of sex-linked
    disorders
  following detection of a fetal cardiac lesion,
    omphalocele or obstructive uropathy
  a history of three or more first-trimester
    abortions
  following an abnormal maternal serum triple
    test
The presence of markers of aneuploidy
For inherited disorders of metabolism:
  previous or family history
  racial group

Table 14.1 Maternal age-specific risks of all chromosome anomalies at delivery (from Ferguson–Smith, Yates 1984 with kind permission of the editor, authors and publishers)

Age (years)	Incidence	Percentage risk
35	1 in 250	0.4
36	1 in 143	0.7
37	1 in 125	0.8
38	1 in 111	0.9
39	1 in 83	1.2
40	1 in 71	1.4
41	1 in 63	1.6
42	1 in 43	2.3
43	1 in 30	3.3
44	1 in 22	4.6
45	1 in 12	8.2

Table 14.2 Risk of trisomy 21 in relation to maternal age and gestation birth (adapted from Snijders et al 1999 with kind permission of the publishers).

Maternal age (years)	Gestational age		
	12 weeks	16 weeks	40 weeks
20	1 in 1068	1 in 1200	1 in 1527
25	1 in 946	1 in 1062	1 in 1352
30	1 in 626	1 in 703	1 in 895
35	1 in 229	1 in 280	1 in 356
36	1 in 196	1 in 220	1 in 280
37	1 in 152	1 in 171	1 in 218
38	1 in 117	1 in 131	1 in 167
39	1 in 89	1 in 100	1 in 128
40	1 in 68	1 in 76	1 in 97
41	1 in 51	1 in 57	1 in 73
42	1 in 38	1 in 43	1 in 55
43	1 in 29	1 in 32	1 in 41
44	1 in 21	1 in 24	1 in 30
45	1 in 16	1 in 18	1 in 23

Box 14.2 Risks of amniocentesis

Maternal:
  damage to bladder, uterus or bowel
  rectus sheath hematoma
Fetal:
  damage to a fetal organ
  fetomaternal hemorrhage
  orthopedic deformities
  increased incidence of respiratory distress
    syndrome

All women should have a preliminary anomaly scan. If a structural anomaly is diagnosed on the preliminary scan then the woman might opt for a termination. Serious thought should be given to proceeding with the amniocentesis in such cases, because the structural abnormality could represent a chromosomal problem and karyotyping post-abortal fetal tissue often fails. The diagnosis of a sporadic chromosomal abnormality could influence the risk of recurrence in future pregnancies.

Method

A pool of amniotic fluid should be located away from the fetus and the placenta. An anterior placenta rarely covers the entire anterior uterine wall and there is often a 'window' available for a lateral approach. If no window is found then the needle might be put through the anterior placenta, aiming to avoid the placental edge and the site of the cord insertion.

Having located a pool of amniotic fluid away from the fetus, the ultrasound transducer is moved slightly away from the spot, but angled to keep the pool in view. The skin over the spot is cleansed with antiseptic and the needle is introduced rapidly through the woman's skin and rectus sheath, directed towards the pool. As the needle enters the uterus it is visualized on the ultrasound screen and is advanced under direct ultrasound vision until it can be seen entering the pool. If there is an anterior wall fibroid it should be avoided because pushing the needle through it can cause pain.

An assistant should then remove the stilette and aspirate 20 mL of amniotic fluid. The technique of holding the transducer in the operator's left hand while visualizing an advancing needle held in the operator's right hand is used in amniocentesis, cordocentesis and transabdominal chorion villus sampling.

At the end of the procedure, ultrasound should be used to check the fetal heart is still beating and to demonstrate this to the woman. The amniotic fluid sample should be sealed in a suitable container for cytogenetic studies. This jar should be labeled with patient identification name and number. It is good practise to show the sample and labeling to the patient.

Check the maternal blood group. If she is rhesus negative, give 1250 IU of anti-D gammaglobulin intramuscularly. Ideally, this should be given immediately following the procedure, but to be effective it must be given within 72 h. The woman should be advised to avoid strenuous physical exercise for 48 h.

Problems

Maternal obesity

This is rarely sufficient to prevent the use of a standard 18- or 20-gauge spinal needle. However, if you are concerned that the needle is going to be too short then measure the depth from the skin surface to the centre of the chosen pool on the ultrasound monitor screen. If it is more than 5 cm then use a long spinal needle.

Failure to aspirate fluid

If you feel that the needle has entered the amniotic cavity then rotate the syringe through 180° and aspirate again. If this fails, use the ultrasound transducer to locate the end of the needle. The needle can be located by the acoustic shadow it produces and by the characteristic echo pattern of its tip (Fig. 14.1). If the needle is not in the amniotic pool then withdraw or advance it until the pool is reached.

If the needle appears to be in an amniotic pool, first check this by scanning in two planes at 90° to each other. If you are convinced it is in an amniotic pool, then it is likely that either the needle is blocked or you have stripped the chorion from the amnion and the needle is between the membranes. If you have used a needle with a stilette then you can clear a blocked needle by reintroducing the stilette. If this fails then withdraw the needle and start afresh.

Aspirating blood

Stop aspirating and look at the fluid carefully to determine if it is pure blood or if it is blood-stained amniotic fluid. If it is pure blood, remove the needle and check the fetal heart. If it is amniotic fluid stained with old blood then remove 20 mL for examination. If it is fresh blood staining, then locate the tip of the needle with the transducer and move the needle into a pool of amniotic fluid. Change the syringe and remove 20 mL of fluid. All blood-stained specimens should be sent to the cytogenetics laboratory as soon as possible because

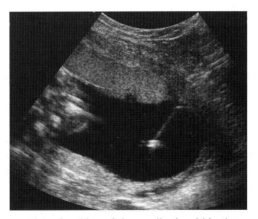

Figure 14.1   Location of the needle tip within the amniotic sac during amniocentesis. Note the characteristic high level echoes and the posterior acoustic shadowing produced from the needle tip.

red blood cells are highly toxic to desquamated fetal cells.

Failure to obtain amniotic fluid

If you have had two attempts and you have been unable to obtain amniotic fluid, you should abandon the procedure. Rescan the woman to check the fetal heart and, should she wish to proceed with prenatal diagnosis, she should be referred to a specialist center for further management.

TWIN AMNIOCENTESIS

The finding of twins prior to amniocentesis poses counseling and technical problems. The risks of a chromosomal abnormality in one or both twins differ depending on the zygosity of the twin pair. It is important, therefore, to attempt to try and establish zygosity, but this will only be possible in a dizygotic twin pair and if the fetuses are of different sex. The less preferable, but more commonly possible, option is to establish the chorionicity of the pregnancy. Ideally, chorionicity should have been determined by identifying either the lambda sign or T sign by ultrasound examination in the first trimester. As described in Chapter 3, the lambda sign is demonstrated by a dichorionic pregnancy whereas the T sign is demonstrated by a monochorionic pregnancy.

Prior to amniocentesis, the parents should be informed of the difficulties in establishing zygosity and the resulting implications, including the possibility of discordance for aneuploidy and the risks of selective fetal reduction (p. 204).

If the twins are monochorionic (and hence monozygotic), the chances that one twin has a chromosomal abnormality is equivalent to the maternal-age-related risk. As both individuals are genetically identical, the chance of both monozygotic twins having the chromosomal abnormality is also equivalent to the maternal-age-related risk. If the twins are dizygotic, the risk of one fetus having a chromosomal abnormality is twice that of the maternal-age-related risk. The risk of both fetuses being affected is the maternal-age-related risk squared.

With skill, it is possible to aspirate fluid from each sac separately during amniocentesis. Some workers used to inject methylene blue into the first sac after aspiration to ensure that the same sac was not tapped twice. With improvements in ultrasound technology, we feel this is no longer indicated. In theory, it should only be necessary to take one sample from a monozygotic twin pregnancy, but we prefer to take fluid from behind each fetal back. This is because it is not possible confidently to diagnose monozygotic twins using ultrasound.

CORDOCENTESIS

The increasing resolution of the newer ultrasound machines has allowed accurate placement of the needle within the uterus. Under ultrasound guidance, fetal skin can be biopsied but the most common procedure performed is percutaneous umbilical blood sampling (PUBS), also known as cordocentesis. The indications are given in Box 14.3 with risks similar to those of amniocentesis. Additional risks of cordocentesis are tamponade or tearing of an umbilical cord vessel.

Method

This is usually a single-operator technique but it can be carried out by two people, one of whom scans the woman while the other performs the needling.

Locate the placenta and the cord insertion. Visualize the cord about 1 cm away from the placenta in both the longitudinal and transverse planes. Cleanse the skin with antiseptic solution. As the 15 cm 20-gauge needle is whippy, it needs to be steadied during its insertion by grasping the hub and shaft in a sterile, gloved hand. Once the needle has passed the rectus sheath, however, it can usually be guided by the operator's right hand while the left hand holds the ultrasound transducer. The needle is moved forward until it punctures the umbilical cord (Fig. 14.2). The tip of the needle should be visualized within the cord in two scanning planes 90° apart and then the stilette should be withdrawn.

A 1-mL syringe is attached and blood is aspirated for the appropriate studies. Firm pressure needs to be applied to the syringe to aspirate because of the fine bore of the needle. If it is necessary to know whether the needle is in the umbilical vein or the artery, a small amount of normal saline can be flushed down the needle and the

Box 14.3   Indications for cordocentesis

Early pregnancy (20 weeks):
   chromosomal analysis:
      women who present too late for
         amniocentesis
      fetuses with a structural abnormality or
         marker suggestive of a chromosome
         anomaly
   viral-specific IgM, e.g. toxoplasmosis, rubella,
      cytomegalovirus
   genetic disorders that require fetal blood, e.g.
      fragile-X syndrome, Menke's disease
   assessment and treatment of rhesus disease
   exclusion of fetal hemoglobinopathies, e.g.
      sickle-cell disease and thalassemias. This
      can also be performed by chorionic villus
      sampling

Late pregnancy:
   karyotyping:
      fetuses with a structural abnormality or
         marker suggestive of a chromosome anomaly
      severely growth-restricted fetuses
      fetuses with an abnormal fetal circulation but
         a normal uteroplacental circulation (see
         Chapter16)
   blood gas analysis – in fetuses with absent
      end-diastolic frequencies (see Chapter 16)
   assessment and treatment of rhesus disease

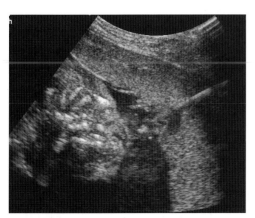

Figure 14.2   Cordocentesis. The small arrows indicate the track of the needle through the placenta into the cord close to its insertion.

direction of the subsequent turbulence observed. Turbulence that flows in the direction of the placenta indicates that the needle is in the umbilical artery. It is also usual practise to send 20 mL of amniotic fluid at the same time.

Problems

Failure to aspirate blood from the cord

Visualize the tip of the needle in two planes 90° apart. Often, the needle that appears to be in the cord in one plane has completely missed the cord in the opposite plane. This usually results in amniotic fluid being aspirated. If the needle appears to be in the cord and blood is not aspirated, this suggests that the needle has not entered a cord vessel, and it should be advanced or withdrawn until it enters a vessel. If the tip appears to be within a vessel, the needle should be flushed with 1 mL normal saline because fine-bore needles commonly block.

Fetal bradycardia

A bradycardia as slow as 60 bpm is not uncommon when the cord is first punctured, especially with fetuses around 20 weeks. They usually recover within 60 s; if not, the needle should be removed and the procedure repeated at a later date.

Unfavorable cord insertion

If the cord insertion into the placenta is not accessible then the intrahepatic portion of the umbilical vein can be used. In this case, the needle is directed to pass through the fetal skin and liver. Many operators prefer this approach because the needle is fixed within the fetus and is therefore less likely to be dislodged as a result of fetal movement.

CHORION VILLUS SAMPLING

This is usually performed at 10–14 weeks' gestation, although it can be carried out transabdominally at any stage in pregnancy. It can be performed transabdominally or transcervically. It is usually a single operator technique but can also be performed as a two-operator procedure.

Both methods should be preceded by an initial scan performed with an abdominal or a vaginal probe to demonstrate fetal cardiac pulsations, confirm gestational age, check placental site and to determine the presence of any other abnormalities, such as fibroids.

The risk of chorion villus sampling is quoted as a 3% chance of losing a normal pregnancy following the procedure. At 10–14 weeks, approximately 2% of women will spontaneously lose a pregnancy after a viable fetus has been seen on ultrasound and therefore the increased risk is of the order of 1% (equivalent to 16-week amniocentesis). The major advantage of chorion villus sampling is that the results are known sufficiently early in the pregnancy to allow a vaginal termination if an adverse result is obtained.

Amniocentesis is the method of choice in twin prenatal diagnosis. Currently, the role of chorion villus sampling in twin pregnancy is reserved for cases where fetal abnormalities (i.e. increased nuchal translucency or exomphalos) are detected in the first trimester. It is difficult to be certain on ultrasound as to the placental domains of each twin when there is a fused dichorionic or suspected monochorionic placenta. Hence, the operator cannot be certain that the placentae of both twins have been sampled, rather than the same placenta twice.

TRANSCERVICAL CVS

Method

Ideally, the woman should be positioned on a gynecological examination couch with her legs in low stirrups, but she must be in the lithotomy position with her legs supported. The vulva and vagina are cleansed with antiseptic solution and the operator then passes a sterile Cusco's speculum to visualize the cervix. In most cases, the cervix does not need to be grasped with a tenaculum but if it is high in the vagina this might be necessary. After warning the woman that she might experience some low abdominal pain the cervix is grasped and gentle traction applied. In either case, the cervix is then cleansed with antiseptic solution and dried.

The position of the uterus (anteverted, axial or retroverted) is then determined by ultrasound and the aspiration cannula is bent into the required shape. Under ultrasound guidance, the cannula is passed through the cervix and directed into the placental site such that it lies directly beneath the cord insertion. Suction is then applied by means of a 20-mL syringe that contains about 5 mL of culture medium and 1 mL of heparin. While maintaining the suction, the needle is then moved to and fro, so as to shear off some of the trophoblastic villi. The needle is then removed and the entire contents of the syringe and needle are squirted into a Petri dish. The sample is examined under the microscope and should contain villi with visible blood vessels. If these are not present, the procedure is repeated.

Single-operator techniques require the use of a suction catheter attached to a suction apparatus and the use of a tissue trap. The operator inserts the cannula through the cervix, while holding the ultrasound transducer in the other hand. The introducer is then withdrawn and the cannula is attached to the suction apparatus. When the cannula is in the correct position, occlusion of the hole on the suction tubing allows a continuous negative pressure of 400–500 mmHg to be applied while moving the cannula to and fro as above. A popular alternative is the use of 20-gauge biopsy forceps to obtain an adequate specimen.

Following the procedure, the fetal heart is checked and the woman is advised to avoid physical exertion or sexual intercourse for the next 72 h. If she is rhesus negative, 1250 IU of anti-D gammaglobulin should be given intramuscularly.

Problems

The presence of vaginal infection

If a vaginal infection is suspected when the speculum is introduced, high vaginal swabs should be taken and the procedure abandoned. The choices are then to perform a transabdominal chorion villus sample or to treat the infection and repeat the procedure at a later date.

Inability to obtain sufficient villus material

Ideally, some 20–40 mg of tissue can be obtained and it should contain visible blood vessels, as this improves the chances of successful culture. If this is not obtained, the technique should be repeated again. If insufficient material is still not obtained then the procedure should be abandoned, after checking the fetal heart.

TRANSABDOMINAL CVS

The technique for this approach is similar to that involved in amniocentesis or cordocentesis. A good sector scanner is required to demonstrate the pelvic organs. At 10–14 weeks' gestation the uterus tends to be anteverted or retroverted and so presents the placental site as upper or lower to the abdominal operator (Fig. 14.3). Most workers use a double needle technique.

Method

Scan the uterus to determine the placental site. Cleanse the skin of the abdomen with antiseptic solution. Insert the 18-gauge needle as far as the edge of the placenta. This can usually be done without local anesthetic but, for anxious women or operators, the proposed track can be infiltrated with 10 mL of 1% plain lignocaine. Aim for a site toward the center of the placenta, preferably directly beneath the cord insertion. The placental edge should be avoided because the villi from this site can be hydropic and degenerative, and hence might not culture. Remove the stilette and pass the 20-gauge needle attached to the 20 mL syringe. Draw the plunger back as far as is comfortably possible to create some negative pressure and then gently move the needle to and fro within the placenta two or three times. While maintaining the negative pressure, withdraw the needle and squirt the contents of the syringe into a Petri dish containing culture medium. As with transcervical sampling, a 20-gauge biopsy forceps could be used instead of the suction technique.

Flush the syringe out with the culture medium. The contents of the Petri dish are then examined under the microscope to determine if sufficient villi have been obtained. If not, the 20-gauge needle can be reintroduced through the 18-gauge needle, which should be left in position until an adequate sample has been obtained.

Check the fetal heart and demonstrate it to the woman. If the woman is rhesus negative she should be given 1250 IU anti-D gammaglobulin intramuscularly.

LABORATORY PROCEDURES

Chromosome analysis

Rapid tests

Chromosome analysis from chorionic villi can be by direct preparation or by villus culture. Direct preparation gives a result within 2–3 days and is accurate for the exclusion of aneuploidy (abnormal number of chromosomes). However, as direct preparations produce fewer mitoses than culture, the technique is less accurate for detecting minor chromosomal changes and is therefore usually backed up by villus culture.

Fluorescent in situ hybridization (FISH) involves the use of fluorescent-labeled probes to the chromosomes involved in common aneuploidies (21, 18, 13, X and Y). This technique allows rapid reporting of aneuploidies from amniocentesis

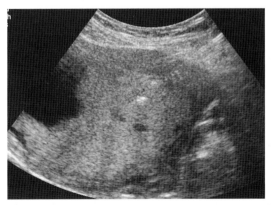

Figure 14.3 Transabdominal chorion villus sample. Longitudinal section of the uterus at 12 weeks demonstrating the needle tip within the posterior placenta.

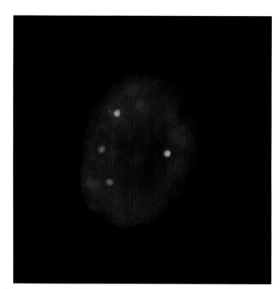

Figure 14.4 Fluorescent in situ hydridization demonstrating two fluorescent signals in this CVS sample. The probes used are specific for chromosomes 21 and 18 confirming a normal karyotype.

samples (Fig. 14.4) It is, however, an expensive and labor-intensive process with a significant failure rate (1–2%). Newer, much safer techniques, such as polymerase chain reaction (PCR) and comparative genomic hybridization, can allow similar rapid reporting at a much faster and cheaper rate.

Cell culture

Results from amniocytes (fetal fibroblasts) and villus culture are usually available in 10–14 days. Contamination from decidual cells can lead to an overgrowth of maternal cells and hence give a false result in villus culture. This does not happen with the direct preparation, so ideally both techniques should be employed. As amniocytes are of fetal origin, amniocyte culture is taken to be the gold standard for the investigation of the fetal karyotype.

In villus culture, as the tissue being tested comes from the placenta (trophoblast), it might not demonstrate the same karyotype as the fetus in about 1% of cases. In most of these cases, this results in a trisomy 2, 16 or 20 being reported, and although these would be lethal to the fetus they do not appear to affect the placenta. In such cases, an amniocentesis can be performed in later pregnancy to determine the fetal karyotype.

DNA analysis

Placental tissue and fibroblasts can be used for gene probing. This can be performed by a direct gene probe or by a more complex method involving restriction enzymes. If the technique requires large quantities of DNA, chorion villus sampling would be the prenatal test of choice, as placental tissue is much richer in DNA than desquamated fetal skin fibroblasts. DNA analysis can be used to identify conditions such as β-thalassemia, in which a gene is missing, or for conditions such as sickle-cell anemia and cystic fibrosis where the gene is damaged.

In cystic fibrosis, gene probes exist for about 95% of mutations known to cause the disease. Investigation of the parents will provide information regarding the accuracy of prenatal diagnosis. For example, if the parents carry known, identifiable mutations, certainty regarding prenatal diagnosis can be achieved.

Unfortunately, direct gene probes are only available for a limited number of conditions that are caused by a single gene mutation. Some conditions, for example β-thalassemia, can be caused by multiple mutations. In such cases, family studies, involving an affected child and its parents, are necessary to determine whether the gene is informative. DNA from each member of the family is broken down into short lengths by specific enzymes, and a specific segment (known as a restriction fragment length polymorphism, or RFLP) that is attached to the gene in question is sought. If an RFLP is found in the affected child and one or both of its parents, then this can be sought by DNA analysis of chorionic villi in the next pregnancy.

Enzyme analysis

Most inborn errors of metabolism are autosomal recessive, carrying a 1 in 4 chance of affecting the next pregnancy. Increasingly, they are being detected by direct assay of culture of chorionic villi or amniocytes, although great care must be taken to avoid maternal contamination.

EMBRYO REDUCTION

An adverse effect of the widespread introduction of assisted reproductive technology has been the increased prevalence of multiple pregnancy (Fig. 14.5). Higher-order pregnancies, in particular, have much higher rates of cerebral palsy and perinatal mortality. Scientific data supports the selective reduction of quadriplets and higher-order pregnancies down to twins to improve pregnancy outcome.

Technique

The high spontaneous embryo loss rate in the early first trimester (the 'vanishing twin syndrome') dictates that embryo reduction is performed at 11–13 weeks' gestation. Additionally, this allows the determination of chorionicity, increased nuchal translucency and fetal abnormality, all of which can significantly influence the procedure.

As with other transabdominal procedures, a single-operator ultrasound-guided technique is used to introduce a needle into the fetal heart or thorax. At this gestation, the injection of 1–2 mL of strong potassium chloride solution (20 mM/10 mL) is enough to produce fetal asystole. The procedure is normally covered with a short course of oral, broad-spectrum antibiotics. Over the next few months, the reduced fetuses are gradually reabsorbed, until at delivery, they are usually delivered as part of the placenta. Rarely a fetus papyraceous (mummified) can be barely recognized at delivery.

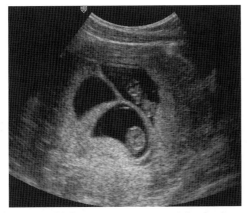

Figure 14.5 Triplet pregnancy at 8 weeks' gestation.

Problems

Miscarriage

The miscarriage risk for the entire pregnancy is approximately 6–8% at 11–13 weeks' gestation. This rate is increased the later it is performed (up to 15% at 20 weeks) and proportionately with the number of fetuses needing to be reduced.

Chorionicity

Reduction of only one monochorionic fetus should be avoided. The poor outcome of surviving monochorionic twins dictates either that both should be reduced or both allowed to continue in the pregnancy. In the latter situation, the parents should be warned about and monitored for the development of twin-to-twin transfusion syndrome, which occurs in 15% of these pregnancies.

Selection

The term 'selective reduction' is being abandoned because it implies that a choice has to made by the parents or the operator as to which fetuses to terminate. The fetuses positioned in the fundus are reduced, because this is associated with a lower miscarriage rate compared to reduction of fetuses positioned lower in the uterus.

Fetal abnormality

At 11–13 weeks, a fetal abnormality or increased nuchal translucency might be diagnosed. These fetuses should be reduced selectively. The position and chorionicity of these fetuses can, however, influence the subsequent risk of miscarriage.

Psychological effects

The long-term psychological trauma parents suffer when faced with embryo reduction is well documented. The effect of losing a pregnancy achieved by fertility treatment alone cannot be underestimated. If successful, parents will always have siblings to remind them of the fetuses they terminated.

Ethical dilemmas associated with embryo reduction

The ethical and moral arguments for and against termination of pregnancy aside, embryo reduction itself produces certain unique ethical dilemmas. Although reduction of quadruplets and higher-order pregnancies is scientifically justified, embryo reduction of triplets to twins has not been shown to significantly reduce perinatal morbidity or mortality. This procedure would seem to revolve around the ability of obstetric/pediatric services to care for premature triplets and the parents to provide financially for the children in the long term. This argument poses equally difficult dilemmas when parents request reduction of a twin pregnancy to a singleton.

FETOCIDE

Detection of serious fetal abnormality and aneuploidy is often delayed until the anomaly scan at 20–22 weeks' gestation. Termination of pregnancy is an option for parents when the risks of physical and mental handicap to the fetus are significant. The process of termination of pregnancy at this gestation is induction of labor with prostaglandin and oxytocics. It is distressing for parents who have decided to terminate the pregnancy to be faced with the delivery of a child with signs of life, which can occur in 10–15% of cases. The likelihood of the latter occurrence obviously increases the later the termination is performed.

It can be equally distressing for the parents to comprehend that the majority of fetuses die during the process of premature, induced labor, presumably through hypoxia-mediated events. In many countries, obstetricians are advised to precede induction of labor with fetocide, a procedure that causes intrauterine death of the fetus. This is especially important for termination of pregnancy carried out after 22 weeks' gestation, when the premature neonate might actually survive.

Technique

A single-operator ultrasound-guided technique is used to introduce a needle into the fetal heart, preferably the left ventricle. A 1-mL syringe is attached and blood is aspirated for any appropriate studies. If amniotic fluid is required for any specific tests, it should be aspirated *before* the fetocide, because potassium chloride can affect laboratory tests such as cell culture. Once the position of the needle in the fetal heart has been confirmed, 2–4 mg of diazepam is injected to cause heavy fetal sedation. Strong potassium chloride solution (20 mM/10 mL) is then injected in 2-mL aliquots until fetal asystole is seen. At 20–22 weeks' gestation, the injection of up to 10 mL potassium chloride solution is usually enough to produce fetal asystole. The later the gestation of fetocide, the more potassium chloride solution is required.

Problems

Failed access to the fetal heart

In certain situations it can be difficult to achieve access to the fetal heart: maternal obesity, polyhydramnios and persistent fetal back anterior position, where the fetal spine and ribs hinder access to the thorax. Under these circumstances, access to the fetal circulation will be easier by cordocentesis, especially with an anterior placenta. Cordocentesis is performed as detailed above, and after confirmation of needle position in the umbilical vein, strong potassium chloride solution is injected in 1-mL aliquots until asystole is achieved. With direct access to the umbilical vein, often much smaller volumes of potassium chloride are required to achieve fetal asystole.

Failure to achieve fetal asystole

If the needle is positioned in the pericardial space or thorax, fetal asystole is unlikely to occur with small volumes of potassium chloride. Attempts should be made to reposition the needle in the cardiac ventricle and then proceed as before. If the latter is not possible, it might be possible to produce fetal asystole by cardiac tamponade, but we would advise against the use of large volumes of potassium chloride solution. Sterile water could be used as an alternative to produce cardiac tamponade and asystole.

Fetal survival

Recovery from fetal cardiac asystole is a rare occurrence. Because of the enormity of the consequences of such a complication, it is recommended practise to check fetal asystole approximately 10–20 min after the procedure.

INTRAUTERINE THERAPY

There is a small, but growing area for invasive procedures in the delivery of intrauterine therapy. Although detailed descriptions of many of these procedures are beyond the scope of this text, brief overviews of the more common ones follow.

Intrauterine blood transfusion

This procedure is usually carried out for fetal anemia secondary to fetal alloimmunization or parvovirus infection. The blood bank must be given notice prior to the procedure going ahead so that specially cross-matched blood can be prepared for fetal transfusion. A blood-giving set and three-way extension is primed with the donor blood, ensuring that there is no air collection. A 5-mL or 10-mL syringe is attached to the three-way tap, the size used depends on the gestation and the amount likely to be required.

Access to the fetal circulation is achieved in an identical manner to cordocentesis (see above). When the first fetal blood sample is obtained, the hemoglobin (Hb) concentration is immediately determined using a Heamocue (desktop Hb monitor). With the donor and fetal Hb known, a simple calculation can predict the required amount of blood to be transfused. The three-way connection with the blood-giving set is attached to the needle and the transfusion commenced at a rate of 5–10 mL/min (Fig. 14.6). Once the transfusion is complete, the three-way extension connection is removed and several 1-mL samples are taken from the needle. The first two are discarded; the third is taken as a reflection of the post-transfusion fetal Hb concentration.

Fetoscopic laser for twin–twin transfusion syndrome

Ultrasound mapping of the site of the placenta and of the donor and recipient umbilical cord insertions should be performed before the procedure.

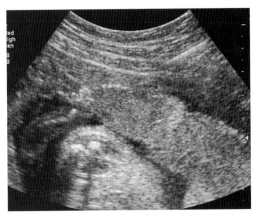

Figure 14.6 Intrauterine blood transfusion.

The entry site should be located so that the recipient sac can be entered without injury to the mother, fetuses or placenta and so that the placental geographic equator can be visualized. The latter is marked as lying midway and perpendicular to an imaginary line running between the donor and recipient cord insertions (Fig. 14.7). Tocolytic antibiotic prophylaxis is usually given periopera-

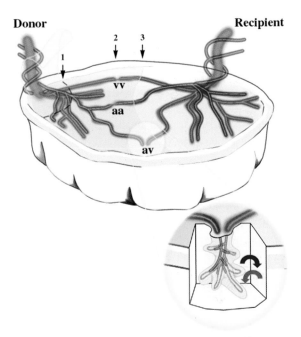

Figure 14.7 Identifying the placental geographic equator prior to fetoscopic laser of interconnecting vessels in a case of twin–twin transfusion. aa, artery to artery anastomosis; av, artery to vein anastomosis; vv, vein to vein anastomosis.

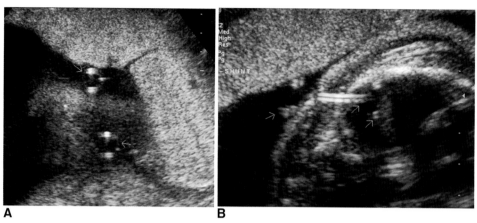

A   **B**

Figure 14.8   A. Insertion of a thoracoamniotic shunt into the left chest to drain the pleural effusion. The catheter produces characteristic high level echoes. B. The position of the catheter within the chest can be confirmed at the end of the procedure.

tively. Local anesthesia (1% lignocaine) is injected from skin to myometrium and intravenous maternal sedation (5 mg diazepam) might be required.

A rigid, 2 mm diameter 0° fetoscope in a 2.8 mm operating sheath is introduced into the recipient sac under continuous ultrasound guidance. A laser fiber 400 or 600 μm in diameter is passed down the operating channel until the tip is just visible through the fetoscope. Ultrasound and direct vision can then be used to identify the placental vascular equator. All vessels that are judged to cross the vascular equator should be identified and coagulated. At the end of the procedure, amniotic fluid is drained until the amniotic fluid index in the recipient is normalized.

Fetal shunting procedures

Although fetal shunting procedures were adopted with vigor in the past, the indications for these are now limited and fetal primary/congenital chylothorax (using thoracoamniotic shunting) is one of the few that is generally accepted. Fetal bladder outflow obstruction is now a debatable indication for fetal vesicoamniotic shunting, with the arguments for and against this procedure being beyond the scope of this text.

The aim of thoracoamniotic shunting is to decompress the fetal thorax (Fig. 14.8A), thereby decreasing the risk of pulmonary hypoplasia and cardiac failure. Shunting is usually a single-operator,

ultrasound-guided technique, with many different kits available for the delivery of a double pig-tailed catheter between the amniotic cavity and thorax.

The entry site of the shunting catheter is chosen so that the chest and pleural effusion can be entered from the fetal lower back without injury to the mother or placenta. Local anesthesia (1% lidocaine) is injected from skin to myometrium. Intravenous maternal sedation (5 mg diazepam) might be required. Once the position of the shunt needle is confirmed on ultrasound, the trocar is removed and the catheter-dispensing device is introduced. One end (the smaller) is deployed in the fetal chest, the needle is then withdrawn into the amniotic cavity before the remainder of the catheter is deployed. At the end of the procedure, the position of the catheter can easily be confirmed on ultrasound (Fig. 14.8B). Tocolytics and antibiotic prophylaxis are usually necessary immediately after the procedure.

REFERENCES AND FURTHER READING

Canadian early and mid-trimester amniocentesis trial (CEMAT) group 1998 Randomized trial to assess safety and fetal outcome of early and mid-trimester amniocentesis. Lancet 351:242–247

Ferguson-Smith M, Yates J W R 1984 Maternal age-specific rates for chromosomal aberrations and factors influencing them: report of a collaborative European study on 52,965 amniocenteses. Prenatal Diagnosis 4:5–44

Milunsky A 1979 Genetic disorders and the fetus: diagnosis, prevention and treatment. Plenum, New York

Snijders R J, Sundberg K, Holzgreve W 1999 Maternal age-and gestation-specific risk for trisomy 21. Ultrasound in Obstetrics and Gynecology 13:167–170

Tabor A, Philip J, Madsen M et al 1986 Randomised controlled trial of genetic amniocentesis in 4606 low-risk women. Lancet 88:559–562

Wilson R D 2000 Amniocentesis and chorionic villus sampling. Current Opinion in Obstetrics and Gynecology 12:81–86

Chapter **15**

The physics of Doppler ultrasound and Doppler equipment

The Doppler effect was first described by Christian Johann Doppler (1803–1853), who discussed the apparent change in the color of the light emitted by stars caused by their motion relative to the Earth. He later investigated the closely related phenomenon that occurs with moving sources of sound and recorded a remarkable experiment in which a brass band was commissioned to play a series of notes while sitting on a moving train and observers at the track side were asked to identify the notes being played! There are many such examples in the world around us today, including the apparent change in the sound of a racing car or a train coming toward us compared with the same car or train seconds later, when it has passed us and is moving away; people on board the moving car or train do not perceive any change in the sound it makes as it passes an observer standing at the side of track. We can generalize this as follows:

- the Doppler effect is an apparent change in the pitch or frequency of a wave due to relative movement between the source and the receiver
- it can be demonstrated for any type of wave, including light, sound and ultrasound
- it is direction dependent.

THE DOPPLER PRINCIPLE

The situation in which the source is stationary and the receiver is moving differs slightly from that in which the receiver is stationary and the source is moving. Let us consider the first case and assume for the moment that the receiver is moving directly toward the source (Fig. 15.1). The receiver will detect more waves per second than are actually being sent out. In other words, the receiver will detect an increase in the frequency relative to the source. If the receiver is moving in the opposite direction, then it will receive fewer waves per second than are being generated, and hence detect a lower frequency. Note that an independent observer would conclude that it is the receiver that is 'wrong', i.e. the Doppler shift is introduced by the receiving device.

The situation is slightly different if the source is moving and the receiver is stationary. In this case, the actual wave traveling through the material is altered. If we take the case in which the source is moving towards a stationary receiver (Fig. 15.2), the physical distance between the waves is reduced by the motion. In a sense, the wave is being compressed. In other words, its wavelength is reduced. As there is a relationship between wavelength and

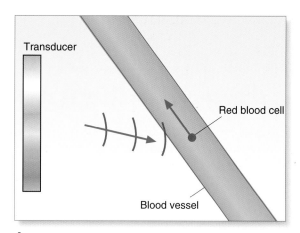

A

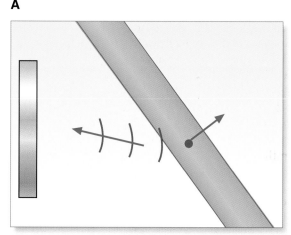

B

Figure 15.3 A. A stationary source insonates a moving target. In this case, the target is a single blood cell. B. A blood cell scatters sound back towards the transducer. This is then a moving source and the transducer is a stationary receiver.

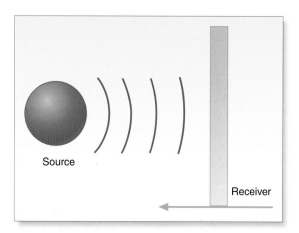

Figure 15.1 A receiver moving towards a stationary source detects waves more rapidly than they are being generated. Hence an increased frequency is perceived.

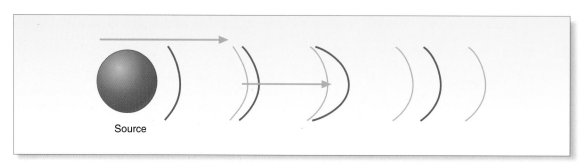

Figure 15.2 A source moving towards a stationary receiver. The wave fronts are positioned ahead of where they would otherwise be. This is a reduced wavelength and hence an increased frequency is detected.

frequency, then we would predict that this reduction in wavelength corresponds to an increase in frequency. This increase is detected by the receiver. Unlike the previous case, an independent observer would judge that the receiver is 'correct' and that it is the source that has created the change.

The importance of this is that both effects occur in medical Doppler applications. The original wave is sent out from the stationary transducer at the skin surface and arrives at some moving target or interface. The target might be an erythrocyte in a blood vessel intersected by the beam (Fig. 15.3). The fact that the target is moving means that it will experience a slightly different frequency from that which was sent out. This target will then scatter or reflect the sound and so act as a moving source. Some of this movement will be detected at the surface by the transducer and so, on the return path, we have the moving source and the stationary receiver. Although the two Doppler shifts can be calculated and described separately, it is convenient to combine them into a single expression. In a round trip such as this, the change or Doppler shift in the frequency f_d can be shown to be given by

$$f_d = 2f_0 v \cos\theta/c$$

where f_d is the Doppler shift in the frequency; f_0 is the frequency of the emitted ultrasound; v is the velocity of the moving target; θ is the angle between the ultrasound beam and the direction of movement of the target; and c is the speed of sound in tissue (Fig. 15.4).

Note that the angle θ is important. The maximum value of $\cos\theta$ is 1, and this occurs when θ is

zero. Thus the greatest shift in frequency will be found when the sound is traveling in the same direction as the target. If the target is moving toward the transducer then the value of f_d will be positive and there will be an increase in the frequency, but if it is moving away from the target the shift will be the same but negative, and so the received frequency will be less than the transmitted frequency. On the other hand, if the target is moving at right angles to the beam, θ will be 90 or 270 degrees and $\cos\theta$ will have the value zero. We conclude that this will result in there being no Doppler shift under these circumstances. The speed of sound in this calculation is normally assumed to be 1540 m s^{-1}, as for imaging, despite the fact that the speed of sound in blood is known to differ from this value.

For example, a 4MHz Doppler beam that is directly in line with blood moving with a velocity of 1.54 m s^{-1} will detect a Doppler shift frequency of

$$f_d = 2 \times 4 \times 10^6 \times 1.54/1540$$
$$= 8 \times 10^6/10^3 \text{ Hz}$$
$$= 8 \text{ kHz}$$

Doppler shifted frequencies obtained from flowing blood in the uteroplacental and fetal circulation with angles of insonation of 20–60° are typically in the audible range (up to 12 kHz). This is convenient because it means that the signals can be monitored by loudspeakers and stored on magnetic audio tape for later off-line analysis.

THE DOPPLER FREQUENCY SPECTRUM

The strength of the signal from a single blood cell is too low to be detected at the surface; its level is less than the size of the noise signal. It is thought that the signals used clinically arise from the multiple scattering from groups (or ensembles) of cells, although the erythrocytes are the major contributors. However, at any time the blood cells along a length of blood vessel (of, say, a few millimeters) will have a range of velocities. The simplest model is that of a fluid flowing in a long, straight, smooth-sided, non-branching tube. In this case, the distribution of velocities is radially symmetrical about the centre of the tube. The velocities are greatest at the centre and tail off radially, following a parabolic law, to end with zero velocity at the tube walls. This velocity distribution is known as laminar or parabolic flow

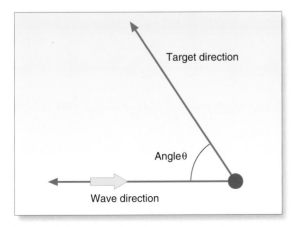

Figure 15.4   The angle between wave and target movement.

and is shown in Fig. 15.5. An important characteristic of parabolic flow is that the maximum velocity, which occurs at the center, is twice the mean velocity. This implies that a reliable estimate of mean velocity can be obtained simply by measuring the peak velocity at the center of the vessel and halving it. This will, of course, vary throughout the cardiac cycle but if it is averaged over several cycles, an estimate of volume flow in the vessel can be made, assuming that the cross-sectional area of the vessel, A, is measured by ultrasound or other means

$$V = (V_{max})_{ave} \, A/2$$

where V is the volume flow in ml s^{-1}; $(V_{max})_{ave}$ is the maximum velocity at the vessel center in cm s^{-1} averaged over several cardiac cycles and A is the cross-sectional area of the vessel in cm^2.

Laminar flow of this type is rare in practice, although it is often a sufficiently good approximation to be of practical clinical value. Another, slightly idealized profile is plug flow, which theoretically can be found close to the inlet to a vessel. In this case, the flow is assumed to be more or less the same at all radii, reducing to low values very sharply close to the vessel walls. This is shown in Fig. 15.6. If the profile of velocities is traced along

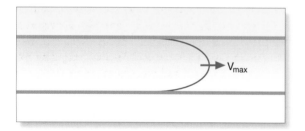

Figure 15.5 Velocity profile associated with laminar or parabolic flow. Note that the peak velocity is at the centre, reducing parabolically to zero at the vessel walls.

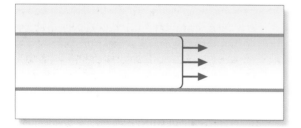

Figure 15.6 Velocity profile for plug flow. The velocity is uniform over most of the vessel radius.

a vessel, the tendency is for it to begin as plug flow and gradually move to a more parabolic profile. The main reason for the transition is viscous drag at the interface between the vessel walls and the blood in close contact with them. In practice, the mean velocity will normally lie between the two extremes, i.e. it will be more than half of the maximum measured velocity. The pattern will be disrupted by branching, twisting and pulsatility.

In the fetal circulation, the descending aorta normally demonstrates plug flow during systolic acceleration and parabolic flow during diastole. The umbilical artery normally demonstrates parabolic flow throughout the cardiac cycle.

The consequence of the above is that any ultrasound beam irradiating a volume that includes a blood vessel will create a range of Doppler shifts in the returning echoes, as opposed to the single value of f_d that might be expected from the basic Doppler shift equation. At any point in time, this range or spread of Doppler frequencies can be described and displayed as a Doppler spectrum. The nature of the spectrum at any location will be subject to change throughout the cardiac cycle. If all of the blood cells were moving at the same speed all of the time, then the spectrum would simply consist of a single line. The factors listed above give rise to a range of Doppler frequencies that result in a band rather than a line. This is known as spectral broadening. In fact, the scanner itself, as we will see, adds further broadening to the spectrum, which is undesirable and is a misleading artifact, and this additional factor is known as intrinsic spectral broadening.

The spectrum is further complicated by the fact that the frequency shift signal at some frequencies will be stronger (i.e. have a greater amplitude) than that at others. If there is a large number of blood cells moving at one speed and a smaller number moving at another then the strength of the Doppler signal will also be stronger at the first frequency. The spectral display therefore needs to be three dimensional if it is to show all of the available information. It needs to show:

• time
• frequency shift
• Doppler signal strength.

This is shown diagrammatically in Fig. 15.7. The horizontal axis represents time, the vertical axis is

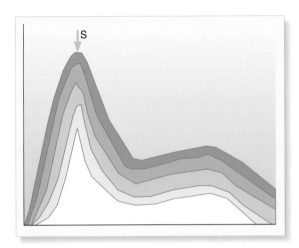

Figure 15.7 Doppler spectrum. The horizontal axis represents time; the vertical axis is Doppler shift frequency. The shade of gray is related to the strength of the signal received at that frequency. Peak systole (S) is often chosen as a reference point.

Doppler shift or velocity and the gray level shows the strength of the signal at any time and frequency.

Plug flow can be recognized in the Doppler spectrum by all the frequencies being clustered close to the maximum frequency waveform, whereas parabolic flow shows frequencies evenly distributed from the level of the vessel wall filter to the maximum frequency, thus filling the waveform (Fig. 15.8).

Yet more spectral broadening originates from factors such as divergences of the ultrasound beam as it travels through different tissues, or slight spectral distortion due to differences among the velocity directions of dispersing erythrocytes. These components of contamination, however, are minor, but the most important additional source of con-

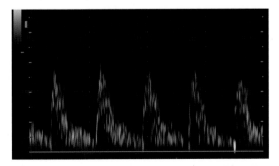

Figure 15.8 Spectrum from the fetal aorta. Note the change from parabolic flow within each cardiac cycle.

tamination is caused by Doppler shifts attributable to the pulsatile movements of the vessel walls.

The vessel wall filter

Doppler shifts due to vessel walls are low in frequency but high in intensity. They have an amplitude that is many times higher than the echoes from the erythrocytes because the acoustic mismatch between the vessel wall and blood is much greater than that between the red-cell–plasma interface. To remove these low-frequency Doppler signals generated by the vessel walls, a high-pass filter (or wall-thump filter) can be used. Filters of 50–200 Hz are common. The most important error caused by high-pass filters is to eliminate low velocities occurring at the end of diastole. Nevertheless, manufacturers use high-pass filters for very good reasons and whenever Doppler frequencies are substantially above 200 Hz there is nothing to be gained by switching the filter to 50 Hz because vessel motion signals might contaminate an otherwise good signal. High-pass filters should therefore be used at their highest value and only switched to 50 Hz when necessary.

DOPPLER FLOWMETERS

These are instruments for acquiring, displaying and analyzing Doppler waveforms. They can be relatively cheap stand-alone instruments or part of more sophisticated imaging systems.

The continuous wave flowmeter

The simplest Doppler device is the continuous wave (CW) flowmeter, the basic elements of which are illustrated in Fig. 15.9. One important feature of this device it that it requires two transducers. However, only one is needed for imaging because once each short pulse has been generated there is no more transmission work to do and the transducer can be used as a receiver. For a CW device, the transducer must transmit all the time and hence a separate receiver is required. In fact, it is common to house both transducers in the same cover (often as concentric rings or back-to-back D shapes) and the user can be unaware that two separate transducers are involved.

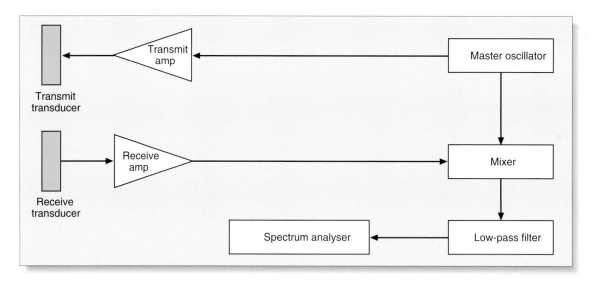

Figure 15.9 Block diagram of a simple continuous wave flowmeter

The master oscillator produces a steady, continuous, sinusoidal waveform that is amplified and used to drive the transmitting transducer at its resonating frequency. The consequent ultrasonic beam hits the moving targets (erythrocytes) that produce reflected and back-scattered echoes, some of which will eventually return to the receiving transducer. It also hits stationary targets, which can produce much stronger echoes, although they will not have any Doppler shift. All of these echoes are mixed together in the received signal that is amplified and presented to the Doppler demodulator. The demodulator therefore has to perform two tasks. It must identify the echoes from moving targets and reject the stationary target echoes that will be unshifted. In addition, it needs to measure the size of the Doppler shift, i.e. how large a deviation has there been from the original frequency? It does this by comparing the incoming signal with a reference signal that is in fact simply the original unshifted frequency. In one simple version the demodulator simply mixes the received signal with the reference. The outcome of this is a combination of sum and difference frequencies. At first sight this would seem to be a retrograde step because we now have an even greater variety of signals than before. However, the difference frequency will be at a much lower frequency than the rest and this is the component that is wanted. After the demodulator it can be readily identified by using a low-pass filter that will eliminate all the unwanted higher frequency signals. The signal after low-pass filtering contains only the desired Doppler shifted frequencies and can be processed and presented to the user in a variety of ways.

Display options

All of the available data can be presented to the user in the form of a spectral display. However, the clinical application might not require that level of complexity. It is possible to calculate a mean velocity as a function of time and to display this on a screen or meter. Alternatively, the maximum velocity alone can be calculated and displayed.

To give some idea of the required capabilities of Doppler flowmeters it is useful to examine the properties of the Doppler shift spectrum. Using a 5 MHz ultrasound probe to insonate the fetal aorta with an angle of about 40°, the Doppler spectrum would be expected to extend up to a frequency of about 12 kHz, corresponding to a peak velocity of about 1.6 m s^{-1} during the maximum systolic phase. Furthermore, the blood would accelerate from almost complete rest at the end of diastole up to this peak velocity in a time interval of less than 0.1 s. The Doppler signal frequency analyzer must therefore be able to accommodate frequencies up to 12 kHz and must be capable of updating the analysis at a rate of at least 100 spectra per second. However, if lower ultrasonic frequencies are used to investigate more slowly moving venous blood it would be better to use lower range analysis frequencies placed closer together to maintain the required frequency (and therefore velocity resolution). Thus a variable frequency analyser is useful where multiple purpose instrumentation is needed.

Simple continuous wave flowmeters are not limited by the maximum velocity that can be measured and, as they do not usually use real-time imaging, they are relatively cheap. Their major disadvantage, however, is their inability to discriminate in range. All targets within the beam are producing echoes all the time and so the receiving transducer cannot use time to distinguish echoes from different depths as it does in imaging systems. In clinical use it is sometimes impossible to separate signals from vessels at different depths.

Pulsed Doppler flowmeters

Pulsed Doppler combines the range discriminating capabilities of a pulsed echo system with the velocity detection properties of a Doppler system.

A block diagram of a pulsed Doppler system is shown in Fig. 15.10. The key differences between this and the CW system are that there is now a second transducer and that it uses long pulses rather than continuous waves.

The system is essentially an extended version of the CW system. There is still an oscillator, demodulator and filter. However the pulsed Doppler system needs some form of sample and hold device. A clock is started when the initial long pulse is transmitted. The operator stops the clock at a time that is selected to be the arrival time for the echoes from the depth of interest. When this happens, an electronic 'gate' is opened; this is called the range gate. It admits echoes for a short time and then closes. It is this short burst of signal that is processed, thereby excluding echoes from all other depths. The pulsed Doppler arrangement can be readily combined with an imaging system. The B-scan image can then be made to show precisely where the Doppler signals are to be sampled. In this way, ambiguity arising from uncertainty in the anatomy or proximity of other vessels can be avoided. A typical pulsed Doppler display is shown in Fig. 15.11.

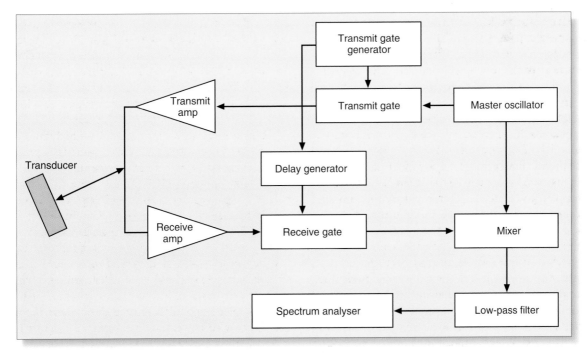

Figure 15.10   Block diagram of a pulsed Dopper flowmeter

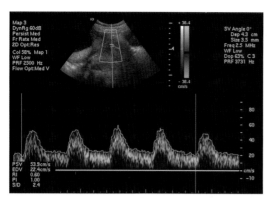

Figure 15.11 Scan showing the range gate of the pulsed Doppler system and the spectrum arising from the selected depth.

The sample volume

The sample volume can best be visualized as a region at some distance in front of the transducer and from which all returning echoes must have originated. The dimensions of the sample volume are defined axially by the pulse length and laterally by the beam width of the ultrasonic beam (see Chapter 1).

Limitations of pulsed Doppler

In practice, pulsed Doppler has two important limitations. The first is that there is a maximum flow velocity that it can reliably detect. The second is that because Doppler information is only collected from one sample volume, it will fail if the operator is unable to identify the correct location at which to position it.

Sampling limitations. The upper limit of frequency shift that can be detected by the pulsed Doppler flowmeter is determined by the sampling process. In pulsed Doppler mode, the sample volume is interrogated every time a pulse is sent down that specific scan line. The sampling rate can be increased by freezing the displayed image and ceasing to fire along the length of the array. Even then, the Doppler waveform has to be reconstructed from a series of samples taken at regular intervals and the maximum Doppler frequency that can be detected is one-half of the pulsed repetition frequency (Nyquist criterion). If higher-frequency

signals are present then the sampled waveform cannot be reconstructed correctly and a phenomenon known as aliasing occurs (Fig. 15.12). This is the same effect that causes wagon wheels to appear to rotate backwards on the cinema or television screen.

Range–velocity limitations. Pulsed Doppler systems are subject to maximum range and maximum velocity limitations. The range restrictions occur because it is necessary to wait for the returning echo to have been received from the most distant target before a further pulse of ultrasound is transmitted. This affects the maximum velocity because the deeper the target, the lower the pulse repetition frequency (PRF) and the lower the maximum detectable blood velocity. Major fetal vessels are generally located within 15 cm of the surface of the maternal abdomen and the peak systolic velocities recorded from the descending aorta can approach 1.5 m s^{-1}, so that with angles of insonation from 45 to 55° the optimum PRF is 5–7.5 kHz with ultrasound frequencies of 2–3 MHz. For pulse repetition frequencies of up to 2.5 kHz it is possible to interlace Doppler and real-time ultrasound such that a simultaneous real-time image can be displayed (duplex, pulsed Doppler ultrasound). To achieve higher PRF values, the real-time screen has to be frozen to record the Doppler signals. Most systems have a means of updating the real-time picture about once every second, although some modern scanners utilize ingenious techniques that allow the simultaneous presentation of real-time images and Doppler signals, albeit with a frame rate penalty. For optimum

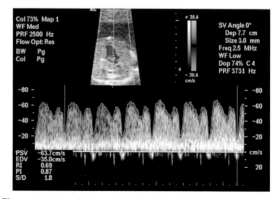

Figure 15.12 Image showing the effect of aliasing.

Doppler signals, however, the real-time image must always be frozen.

Real-time spectrum analysis

A real-time spectrum analyzer measures the power at each frequency contained in the Doppler signal, as described above. Furthermore, it separates forward (that is blood flowing towards the transducer) and reverse signals. The Doppler signal is digitized and scanned rapidly (200 times per second) by a sweeping filter that measures the power of each individual frequency. The method most commonly employed is known as the Fast Fourier Transform (FFT), the details of which are beyond our scope here. The characteristics of an analyzer that are important to the user are the speed of operation and the number of separate frequencies that can be resolved. For obstetric use, a sampling time of 5 ms (200 per second) is desirable, with a frequency resolution of at least 64 bins per channel, although most analyzers offer at least 128 frequency bins.

Real-time spectral analysis is essential in obstetrics use because the Doppler signals are often complex and contain frequencies emanating from more than one vessel. Providing the user can see the spectrum displayed in real time, these artifacts can be detected. More importantly, as most analyzers now perform automatic calculations, the user must be able to judge whether the signal selected by the analyzer is valid or whether the reading should be discarded because of artifact.

Automatic calculations performed by the analyzer are mostly carried out on the maximum frequency outline. To recognize this, the analyzer inspects each of the frequency bins in turn and determines the highest frequency at which there is a signal. This simple approach only works on near perfect waveforms with a high signal-to-noise ratio, so in practise the analyzer's software imposes several conditions, which must be satisfied before it validates the maximum frequency. The maximum frequency is usually superimposed upon the spectral display so that the user can judge whether it is a true representation. Of course, they are still prone to error if there is too little gain to make the highest velocity components detectable, and this is an important source

or error and inconsistency in obstetric Doppler measurements.

Calculations performed using the maximum frequency outline

When the vascular system is subject to pulses from the heart, its behavior is very similar to mechanical springs that are subject to a weight and some kind of damper. Everyday examples are car suspension springs and guitar strings, which perform some kind of damped oscillation in response to being disturbed, and blood velocity waveforms exhibit similar characteristics. The spring is represented in blood vessels by their compliance, and dampening by factors such as blood viscosity, vessel length and luminal diameter. Thus a typical blood velocity waveform will have a maximum at the peak of systole followed by diastolic frequencies that might, in one extreme, oscillate to the reverse flow direction before falling to zero, or in the other extreme could fall gently until the next systole. Several indices attempt to describe these variations in the waveforms and the most commonly used are illustrated in Fig. 15.13. All these indices are independent of the angle between the Doppler beam and the vessel.

The pulsatility index (PI) was originally described as the difference between the most positive (or highest) value and the most negative (or

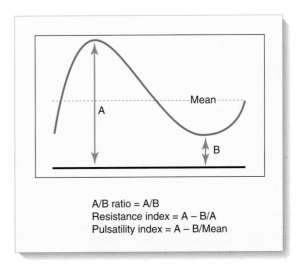

A/B ratio = A/B
Resistance index = A − B/A
Pulsatility index = A − B/Mean

Figure 15.13

lowest) value over one cardiac cycle, divided by the mean value. In bidirectional waveforms the most negative value is found in the reverse channel. The mean (or time-averaged mean, TAM) is the mean frequency averaged over one cardiac cycle. The concept of this index is that the more pulsatile the waveform, the greater the difference between the positive and negative peaks and the higher the value of the PI. Flow velocity waveforms from the uteroplacental circulation are rarely (if ever) bidirectional and reverse flow in the umbilical artery occurs only when the fetus is in extremis, so simple indices have been more widely applied to such waveforms.

The A:B (or S:D) ratio is simple and describes the rate at which flow velocities fall away during diastole. This closely corresponds to the peripheral resistance to blood flow beyond the measurement point.

The resistance index (RI) makes use of the same two points as the A:B ratio but expresses the values in a more convenient form.

Peripheral resistance cannot be measured directly by means of Doppler waveforms but increasing peripheral resistance causes a diminution and then a loss of frequencies in end-diastole. In vessels that supply vascular beds of muscles, increasing peripheral resistance causes an increase in pulsatility and consequently a rise in the PI. In obstetric practice, reverse flow rarely occurs and, as peripheral resistance is further increased, the systolic peak decreases in amplitude, thus giving a decrease in the PI. If the values of the PI are considered in isolation, this worsening situation can result in a false sense of security. Furthermore, calculation of the PI requires a complete and accurate maximum frequency waveform to calculate the time-averaged mean frequency.

As end-diastolic frequencies disappear, point B becomes zero, so the A:B ratio becomes infinity whereas the RI becomes unity. In all situations where end-diastolic frequencies are lost it is best to describe this in words rather than using indices.

Frequency calculations

The maximum frequency waveform is relatively simple to derive from the Doppler spectrum and describes the variation in the fastest moving red blood cells, which occupy the centre of the vessel. To calculate blood flow, an estimate of the mean of all the velocities recorded throughout the cardiac cycle is needed. This parameter is known as the intensity weighted mean frequency (IWMF). The IWMF is the sum of the product of the square of the amplitude of each frequency (a) and that frequency (f), divided by the sum of the square of the amplitudes

$$IWMF = \frac{\sum\limits_{0}^{max} a^2 f}{\sum\limits_{0}^{max} a^2}$$

The amplitude of the signal must be squared when making this calculation because the power or intensity of each frequency is proportional to the square of the signal amplitude or voltage. Contamination by signals from other vessels invalidates IWMF because the mean of all signals is calculated, whereas the maximum frequency waveform is much more reliable in this respect.

Velocity calculations

If the angle between the Doppler beam and the blood vessel is known then the frequency can be converted into actual blood velocity (see p. 211). Velocity measurements have not achieved popularity in obstetric use because of the difficulty of obtaining accurate measurements of the angle of insonation. In obstetric practice, velocity measurements can be reliably obtained only from the descending fetal aorta.

Volume flow calculations

To calculate volume flow accurately, estimation of the IWMF, the angle of insonation and the vessel diameter are required. Measuring the vessel diameter is difficult because:

- Diameter measurements are usually made by means of onscreen calipers to the nearest millimeter.
- The diameter has to be squared to derive the cross-sectional area of the vessel, hence any error in measurement will be squared.

- The cross-section of the vessel is not necessarily round, e.g. the descending fetal aorta tends to be flattened in an anteroposterior direction.
- The cross-sectional diameter of the vessel can change between systole and diastole.

Overall, errors in the vessel diameter measurements, measurements of angle and calculation of IWMF result in errors of up to 30% in volume flow calculation in the obstetric field.

COLOR FLOW DOPPLER ULTRASOUND

Color flow Doppler is an attempt to overcome some of the limitations of pulsed Doppler. It was introduced in the 1980s and is now a common feature on ultrasound scanners.

The key feature is that the search for Doppler shifts is not restricted to a single volume, as in pulsed Doppler, but rather applies to a large region, possibly even the whole image. Each ultrasound line is divided into blocks (typically 50–100 blocks per line) and the echo signals returning from each block are examined for evidence of Doppler shift. If a shift is detected, then a color (typically blue or red) is superimposed on the underlying image. However, if the Doppler signal arises from a block that is already white (because it originates from a strong reflector), then the color signal is suppressed and the gray level is presented instead. In this way, colors are presented only in regions that would otherwise be black or quite dark.

There is scope for interpretation of the rules governing this selection and this can form an operator option via a front panel control.

The task of searching such a large region for Doppler shifts in real-time is demanding and requires certain compromises. To evaluate each of the blocks or sections in each line, it is necessary to send multiple pulses along each line (typically eight pulses per line). This, not surprisingly, has an effect on frame rate and hence there are further compromises for the operator to consider.

The detection of Doppler shifts is not done using Fourier spectral analysis as in pulsed Doppler. Instead, the successive pulses along each scan line are examined in pairs and evaluated for changes in phase. If we consider a single cycle of a sine wave as corresponding to a trip round a circle, then one cycle corresponds to 360°. Thus the angle of the wave can be thought of as changing from 0 to 360 during each cycle. The rate of change of phase will be greater for higher frequency waves and less for lower frequencies because the time taken for one cycle varies accordingly. Hence we can, in effect, measure frequency and frequency shifts by measuring the rate of change of phase. Of course, if many frequencies are present then this will be more complex and the result will be some kind of mean or average shift. The calculation of the mean rate of change of phase is normally performed using a mathematical tool known as autocorrelation, although other tools have been used with some success. The outcome of each use of autocorrelation is to produce just four pieces of information for each block:

1. the mean Doppler shift
2. the strength of the signal
3. its direction (forward or reverse)
4. its variance, i.e. the amount of spread.

The size of each block is larger than the pixels used for imaging and it would be fair to say the color Doppler has poorer spatial resolution than B-mode imaging for any selected machine.

Although the choice is arbitrary, it has become conventional to use red to designate flow towards the probe and blue for flow away from it. Typically, the shade of red or blue displayed indicates the mean velocity. Hence a deep blue often indicates low mean velocity and a very light blue high velocity. The strength of the signal can be displayed by the luminance or brightness of the color, i.e. the shade of blue or red can remain unchanged but there can simply be more or less of it. Variance is often shown by the introduction of different color, with green and yellow being common choices. The user needs to be aware that these color options vary considerably between scanners and can normally be altered by the operator. It is a mistake to allocate quantitative meaning to the colors displayed unless the color calibration has been conducted previously.

The great advantage of color flow mapping is that the signal relies only upon the presence of a Doppler signal, so that small blood vessels (e.g. those in the fetal circle of Willis) can be visualized even though they are below the spatial resolution of the real-time image (Fig. 15.14). Errors in

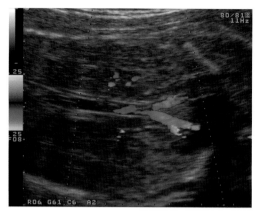

Figure 15.14   Color flow image of the fetal aorta and bifurcation. Flow within the fetal kidneys can also be seen.

interpretation can occur, however, as each color flow pixel in a single scanning line is sampled by transmitted pulses. Hence, the Nyquist theory applies and if the mean Doppler frequency is more than half the pulse repetition frequency then aliasing occurs (see p. 216). The wraparound effect leads to a blue contamination of a red color map in areas of very high flow toward the probe.

The disadvantages of color flow Doppler are the absence of the spectral display that is such a valuable feature of pulsed Doppler and the absence of quantification. Despite the fact that the spectrum is absent, the limitations identified for pulsed Doppler remain. There is a similar trade-off between maximum detectable velocity, frame rate and depth of penetration. Failure to recognize this can lead to aliasing, as for pulsed Doppler. The angle dependence is the same as pulsed Doppler and hence the colors displayed are dependent on the angle of insonation. Blood moving at the same velocity can appear in different colors in differing parts of a curved vessel. Furthermore, absence of color does not necessarily indicate absence of flow as no color will be displayed if the beam is at right angles to the vessel.

POWER DOPPLER

A recent innovation is the introduction of power Doppler. In this mode the Doppler signal is processed differently for different reasons. You will note from the block diagrams of Fig. 15.9 and Fig. 15.10 that the signal emerging from the demodulator contains a mixture of Doppler signals from a variety of targets at each range. In the conventional color flow system, these are then divided into separate frequency slots (or bins) and displayed as a spectrum. In the case of power Doppler, no attempt is made to identify velocities. Instead, the total signal level across all frequencies at each depth is displayed. This gives a crude measure of how much energy or power there is in the local blood flow. It can be altered by changing either the local mean velocity or the total mass of moving blood in the locality. It has been described (wrongly!) as a perfusion map, although it can come close to this on occasions. A typical power Doppler image is shown in Fig. 15.15. Note that there is no longer any angle dependency because velocities are not being measured.

One advantage of power Doppler is its signal-to-noise ratio, which is normally better than that of its color flow counterpart. At a simple level we can see why this is so. In color Doppler, each velocity 'bin' has a signal accumulating in it that depends on the amount of energy that has been found at that frequency. The noise level is more or less fixed by the electronics. If all of the signals from all of the bins are put into the same bin then the total will be many times greater and the noise level will remain the same. This improved signal-to-noise ratio will mean that small vessels can be imaged, which are otherwise invisible to ultrasound.

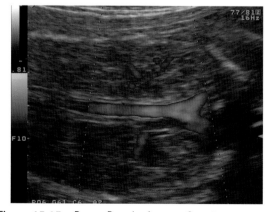

Figure 15.15   Power Doppler image of anatomy demonstrated in Fig. 15.14.

In general terms, the advice often given is to start a scan in B-mode and turn on the color only when the gross anatomy has been identified. Color used at this stage can help to separate blood vessels from other fluid collections, distinguish one vessel from another by virtue of its flow direction and find small vessels that are not seen in B-mode. Detailed hemodynamic information can then be obtained by using pulsed Doppler on selected regions.

REFERENCES AND FURTHER READING

Deane C 2000 Doppler ultrasound: principles and practice. In: Nicolaides K H, Rizzo G, Hecher K (eds) Placental and fetal Doppler. Diploma in Fetal Medicine series. Parthenon Publishing, New York

Evans D H, McDicken W N, Skidmore R, Woodcock J P 1989 Doppler ultrasound: physics, instrumentation and clinical applications. Wiley, Chichester

Chapter 16

Evaluating the pregnancy using Doppler

Doppler ultrasound is now routinely used in obstetric ultrasound practice. A brief description of Doppler techniques is included below and a fuller explanation is given in Chapter 15.

Continous wave Doppler

Most commonly, continuous wave equipment is used without concurrent real-time imaging facilities and its use in obstetrics is therefore limited to acquiring waveforms from the umbilical artery and the uteroplacental vessels. Although waveforms from other vessels, such as the fetal aorta, can occasionally be obtained, they cannot be produced reliably without pulsed Doppler equipment. Hence continous wave Doppler is rarely used in the clinical setting.

Spectral or pulsed wave Doppler

Most modern obstetric and gynecology ultrasound machines use spectral or pulsed wave Doppler to provide detailed information from a small region. Analysis of direction of flow, velocities and indices can be calculated, in addition to examining the waveform.

Ultrasound flow modes

Pulsed wave Doppler is usually used in conjunction with color flow or power Doppler, which allows the user to demonstrate the site and vessels under investigation.

UTEROPLACENTAL WAVEFORMS

Rationale for uteroplacental waveform analysis

Uteroplacental waveforms are acquired from the uterine artery by means of color, pulsed Doppler ultrasound. As it was not always possible to determine whether these waveforms arose from the uterine artery or the arcuate artery by using pulsed wave Doppler alone, they are still commonly referred to as uteroplacental waveforms. With the use of color Doppler, the uterine artery can be reliably identified so that pulsed wave Doppler information can be acquired.

Resistance to blood flow in the uterine arteries falls with advancing gestation due to trophoblastic invasion of the uterine spiral arteries. For example, notched, high-resistance uterine artery waveforms are three times more likely to be present at 20 than at 24 weeks, when they occur in about 5% of pregnancies. Failure or poor trophoblastic invasion is characteristic of pre-eclamptic and growth-restricted pregnancies. Assessment of uterine artery blood flow is an established screening test for these pregnancy problems (Fig. 16.1).

Finding the uterine artery waveform

Ideally, the equipment should be designed specifically for obstetric purposes as cardiovascular equipment has high power output levels. If your machine has a choice of probes, select a 4 MHz probe. Set

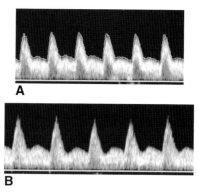

Figure 16.1 A. Normal color Doppler waveform of the uterine artery at 24 weeks. Note the shape of the waveform. B. Abnormal color Doppler waveform of the uterine artery at 24 weeks. Note the presence of a 'notch' at the end of systole and reduced end-diastolic frequencies.

the vessel wall filter (also known as the thump filter) to 50 Hz, the frequency range to 4 KHz and the sweep speed to 5 m s^{-1}. Ensure the balance control is exactly at its midposition and that the gain control is set at about 50% of maximum. Turn the volume control on the loudspeaker up so that on gentle tapping the probe produces a loud noise. If your machine has an automatic maximum frequency follower it should be set to average three waveforms and, ideally, should be turned off until you are happy that the waveforms on the screen are ideal.

Use color flow imaging to identify the bifurcation of the common iliac artery in longitudinal section. Move the probe medially and angle it slightly toward the symphysis pubis to reveal the uterine artery just medial to the bifurcation, as it ascends toward the uterus. It is conventional to place the uterine artery sample gate of the pulsed wave Doppler at the point of maximal color brightness close to the bifurcation (Fig. 16.2 top).

When the waveform is seen, alter the frequency range on the equipment until the waveform fills about two-thirds of the height of the screen. The waveform itself will contain a range of frequencies, represented by a range of differing colors within it (Fig. 16.3A). If the waveform obtained appears very bright, contains few colors and the background is noisy, then reduce the Doppler gain until the optimal balance is obtained (Fig. 16.3B).

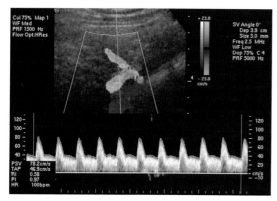

Figure 16.2 Identifying the uterine artery using color Doppler. Top. The uterine artery crosses the iliac artery just medial to the bifurcation of the latter. Bottom. Measurement of the uterine artery waveform using the maximum frequency follower. Both the pulsatility index (PI) and resistance index (RI) are calculated automatically by the machine.

Taking measurements

Having obtained an optimal waveform, turn on the maximum frequency follower, if available, and freeze the image when the automatic calculations are displayed. Examine the three waveforms that the machine has chosen to ensure that they are free from substantial noise and that the machine has correctly chosen the maximum systolic point and the lowest frequency in end-diastole. If the machine does not have a maximum frequency follower then freeze the image and manually measure the Doppler indices. Various measurements of the uterine artery waveform can be calculated, the most commonly used is the resistance index (RI). The systolic/diastolic (S/D) ratio and pulsatility index (PI) can also be used (Fig. 16.2 bottom)

How to report uteroplacental waveforms

Loss of end-diastolic frequencies is extremely rare in the uteroplacental circulation so a simple index of impedance to flow, such as the RI or PI, is sufficient. We recommend that you store at least 10 optimal waveforms in the machine's memory and measure the three with the highest signal-to-noise ratio. A subjective assessment of the flow velocity waveform is also usually performed to note the presence/absence of notches (see Figs 16.1 and 16.3B).

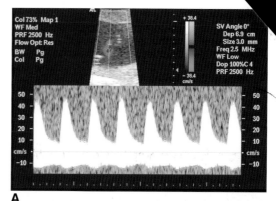

A

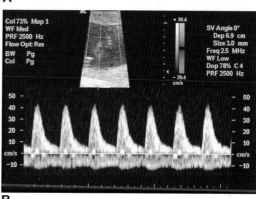

B

Figure 16.3 A. Normal uterine artery waveform at 22 weeks' gestation obtained using a Doppler gain setting that is too high. Note the over-bright waveform with little distinction between the differing frequencies. B. The correct Doppler gain settings. Note the range of frequencies, represented by varying shades of yellow, that can be identified.

Record the waveforms from both sides of the uterus. We suggest that you report them as follows:

- *high resistance pattern*: bilateral notches with mean RI > 0.55 or unilateral notch with mean RI > 0.65.
- *low resistance pattern*: all other situations.

Problems

A signal that is not visualized

Check the machine settings. Restart the signal acquisition process as set out on p. 224. The vessel wall filter, frequency range, sweep speed and gain controls should be rechecked.

...uishing waveforms from the
...from pathological
...forms

...tal waveforms (see Fig. 16.1B)
...phasic deceleration slope in systole, whereas those from the internal iliac artery have a smooth, steep slope (Fig. 16.4).

Indication for, and interpretation of, uteroplacental waveforms

Screening of high-risk populations

Women at increased and/or high-risk for pre-eclampsia and intrauterine growth restriction are usually identified from the maternal history at pregnancy booking. The prevalence of complications in this group of pregnancies is much higher than in the normal population. Uterine artery Doppler screening is a validated screening tool for this group. The sensitivity of uterine artery notches and high RI for an abnormal pregnancy outcome has varied from 45 to 65% in previous studies.

Screening of low-risk pregnancies

Although several studies have used uterine artery Doppler as a screening tool for pre-eclampsia and fetal growth restriction in unselected populations, debate continues as to its value. Varying sensitivities are obtained depending on the type of Doppler used, the sampling site, the definition of abnormal uterine artery resistance, gestation of assessment and different end-points.

Currently, the following statements are supported by at least one published study for two-stage (20- and 24-week) screening, using color pulsed wave Doppler of the uterine arteries:

- The presence of a low resistance pattern is associated with a very low chance of pregnancy complications:
  - less than 1% chance of developing proteinuric hypertension
  - less than 1% chance of a coexisting small-for-gestational-age fetus.
- A high resistance pattern is associated with a higher rate of pregnancy complications:
  - a 70% chance of developing proteinuric hypertension
  - a 30% chance of a coexisting small-for-gestational-age fetus.

Managing pregnancies with high resistance patterns

Doubts over the value of uterine artery Doppler screening is dispelled by the consistent findings of randomized studies on low-dose aspirin therapy (75 mg daily). Most studies demonstrate an average reduction in the prevalence of pre-eclampsia by 15% with the use of low-dose aspirin in women with high-resistance uterine artery Doppler waveforms.

UMBILICAL ARTERY WAVEFORMS

Rationale for umbilical artery waveform analysis

Umbilical artery flow velocity waveforms are thought to reflect 'downstream' placental vascular resistance. Resistance to blood flow in the umbilical arteries falls with advancing gestation due to continuing development of the placental vascular system throughout pregnancy (Fig. 16.5). With uteroplacental insufficiency, the umbilical artery impedence is increased only when a significant proportion of the placental vascular bed is obliterated. Characteristic umbilical artery waveforms have also been correlated to various degrees of fetal hypoxemia and acidemia. Hence umbilical artery Doppler

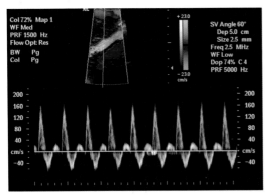

Figure 16.4 Waveform from the internal iliac artery. Note the reverse flow component of this normal waveform and compare it with that shown in Fig. 16.1B.

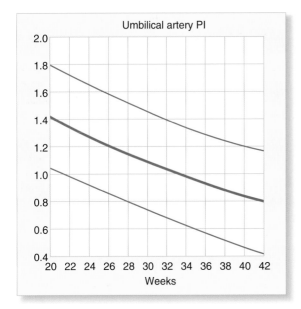

Figure 16.5 Reference range, showing 95th, 50th and 5th centiles, for the pulsatility index for the umbilical artery with gestation.

is now a standard tool in the assessment of the growth-restricted fetus.

Finding the umbilical artery waveform

Set the vessel wall filter to 50 Hz, the frequency range to 4 KHz and the sweep speed to 5 m s^{-1}. Ensure the balance control is exactly at its mid-position and that the gain control is set at about 50% of maximum. Turn the volume control on the loudspeaker up so that on gentle tapping the probe produces a loud noise.

Use color flow imaging to identify the umbilical cord at the placental insertion. This end of the cord is used because the resistance indices are lower here than at the fetal end. Place the sample gate over one of the umbilical arteries with angle-correction (Fig. 16.6 top). When the waveform is seen, alter the frequency range on the equipment until the waveform fills about two-thirds of the height of the screen. If the machine has a maximum frequency follower, turn it on and freeze the image when the automatic calculations are displayed. Examine the three waveforms that the machine has chosen to ensure that they are free from substantial noise and that the machine has

correctly chosen the maximum systolic point and the least frequency in end-diastole (Fig. 16.6 bottom). If the machine does not have a maximum frequency follower then freeze the waveforms on the screen and use the cursors to measure the Doppler indices.

Measuring and reporting the umbilical waveform

The umbilical artery is most commonly reported in terms of the PI. The PI should be derived from the average of at least three, and preferably five, waveforms. We suggest that you plot the PI on a data reference range (see Fig. 16.5). As well as reporting the PI, you should comment if this value lies outside the data reference range. Situations where no frequencies are recorded in end-diastole (Fig. 16.7) are best reported in words, i.e. 'end-diastolic frequencies were absent in the umbilical artery.' Rarely, frequency in end-diastole can be

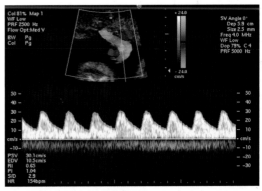

Figure 16.6 Positioning the sample gate over the umbilical cord at its insertion into the placenta is the preferred site for obtaining a recording of the umbilical artery waveform. Note that increasing the size of the sampling gate also allows a recording of the umbilical vein to be obtained. Note also the consistent appearance of the waveform from both the artery and the vein due to sampling during fetal apnea. This factor is helpful in the exclusion of fetal breathing movements that could affect the accuracy of any measurements taken. Measurement of the umbilical artery waveform using the onscreen cursors. Both the PI and RI are calculated automatically by the machine. The PI is more commonly used in reporting umbilical artery waveform measurements.

reversed (Fig. 16.8) and this should also be reported as: 'the umbilical artery demonstrated reversed end-diastolic frequencies'.

The justification for the use of PI and the verbal reporting is that other Doppler indices are of no use when end-diastolic frequencies are lost. As these situations have major significance, you should recheck the signal from another site to avoid artifactual loss of end-diastolic frequencies.

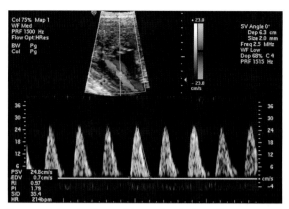

Figure 16.9 Artifactual loss of end-diastolic frequencies in the umbilical artery as the result of a high angle between the ultasound beam and the section of the umbilical artery being interrogated. Compare this image with that of genuine absent end-diastolic flow in Fig. 16.7.

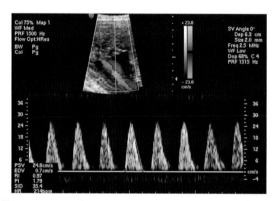

Figure 16.7 Color Doppler umbilical artery waveform demonstrating absent end-diastolic frequencies. Compare these appearances with the normal appearances shown in Fig. 16.6.

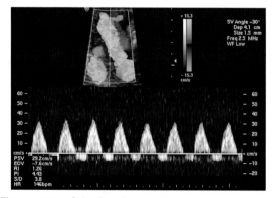

Figure 16.8 Color Doppler umbilical artery waveform demonstrating reversed end-diastolic frequencies. Compare these appearances with the less severe appearances shown in Fig. 16.7 and with the normal appearances shown in Fig. 16.6.

Problems in acquiring and interpreting the waveforms

Artifactual loss of end-diastolic frequencies

A high angle between the ultrasound beam and the vessel results in very low frequencies disappearing below the height of the vessel wall filter (Fig. 16.9). If end-diastolic frequencies appear absent you should reduce the vessel wall filter to its lowest setting, or remove it if possible. Then you should alter the angle of the probe relative to the maternal abdomen to reduce the angle of insonation. If end-diastolic frequencies are still absent you should then attempt to obtain the signal from a different site, because this is likely to result in a different angle of insonation. Do not report the absence of end-diastolic frequencies until this has been demonstrated on two successive days.

Fetal breathing movements

These cause wild fluctuations in the signal from the umbilical artery and are readily recognizable by an inability to demonstrate a steady state in the umbilical arterial signal (Fig. 16.10). The only course of action to take if the fetus is breathing is to wait until this stops.

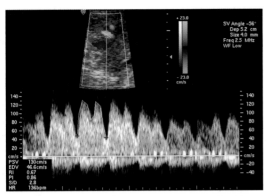

Figure 16.10 Fluctuations in the waveform of the ductus venous due to fetal breathing movements during vessel interrogation.

Fetal heart rate

Fetal bradycardia is associated with decreased end-diastolic frequencies. When reporting Doppler indices, you should check to ensure that the fetal heart rate is in the normal range.

Indications for umbilical artery waveforms

Umbilical artery waveform analysis has been validated only in the assessment and continued monitoring of the fetus that has been demonstrated to be small for gestational age on real-time ultrasound.

Contraindications to umbilical artery waveforms

Although umbilical artery waveforms are invaluable in the management of fetal growth restriction, they are of little or no value as a screening test for the small-for-gestational-age fetus. Additionally, umbilical artery Doppler does not appear to predict unexplained antepartum stillbirths or placental abruption. Despite being commonly requested, umbilical artery Doppler is not of established value in the management of antepartum hemorrhage, preterm rupture of membranes or rhesus isoimmunized, diabetic, post-term or multiple pregnancies, unless these coexist with fetal growth restriction.

Interpretation of the waveforms

Normal umbilical artery waveforms

A growth-restricted fetus with normal umbilical artery waveforms will not be acidemic but has 10% chance of being hypoxemic. The pregnancy is unlikely to develop loss of end-diastolic frequencies within a 7–10-day period, so Doppler monitoring can be performed weekly. It is important to note that normal umbilical artery waveforms after 36 weeks' gestation do not exclude fetal hypoxemia and acidemia.

Absent end-diastolic frequencies

Loss of end-diastolic frequencies occurs only when over 75% of the placental vascular bed has been obliterated. The latter is less likely to occur after 36 weeks' gestation, hence the limitation of umbilical artery Doppler at later gestations. Loss of end-diastolic frequencies is associated with an 85% chance that the fetus will be hypoxemic and a 50% chance that it will also be acidemic. The finding of a symmetrically growth-restricted fetus with absent end-diastolic frequencies in the umbilical artery but with normal uteroplacental waveforms suggests the possibility of a primary fetal cause for the growth restriction (i.e. chromosomal abnormality or congenital viral infection).

Reversed end-diastolic frequencies

Growth-restricted fetuses with reversed end-diastolic frequencies have a ten-fold increase in perinatal mortality compared with those with normal umbilical artery waveforms. Reversed frequencies in end-diastole are observed in only a few fetuses prior to death. This finding should be considered as a preterminal condition. Few, if any, fetuses will survive without delivery.

Current recommendations

There are currently over ten randomized, controlled studies of umbilical artery Doppler monitoring of high-risk pregnancy in the literature. They demonstrate an overall reduction in perinatal mortality of 40% with the use of Doppler compared to cardiotocography. Additionally, significant reductions in antenatal admission, induction of labor and cesarean section with the use of umbilical artery Doppler are reported.

It is probably reasonable for the clinician to deliver growth-restricted fetuses that present with absent or reversed end-diastolic frequencies after 28 weeks of gestation. In units with neonatal intensive care facilities, the perinatal mortality for infants that are more than 28 weeks of gestation is less than 10%, with a less than 5% chance of handicap in the survivors. At less than 28 weeks of gestation, growth-restricted fetuses with absent or reversed end-diastolic frequencies should probably be referred to a regional center for detailed studies of the fetal arterial/venous circulation (see below) and further management.

FETAL ARTERIAL DOPPLER

Rationale for fetal arterial Doppler analysis

Fetal growth restriction

Fetal arterial waveforms are acquired from the thoracic aorta and middle cerebral arteries by means of color, pulsed Doppler ultrasound. With fetal hypoxemia, there is conservation (or increase) of blood flow to the fetal brain, heart and adrenal glands with concomitant decrease in flow to the splanchnic bed and extremities. This phenomenon is termed 'arterial redistribution of blood flow', and serves to deliver oxygen and nutrients to vital organs in the face of impaired placental function. Hence, fetal arterial Dopplers can be used to monitor fetal compensatory responses to progressively deteriorating placental function.

Fetal anemia

There is an established inverse correlation between the degree of fetal anemia and the peak systolic velocity (PSV) of blood in fetal arterial vessels. This is presumably due to decreased blood viscosity with a hyperdynamic circulation, and is most pronounced when assessing the peak systolic velocity in the fetal middle cerebral artery.

Means of acquiring the signal

The machine setup and waveform analysis should be carried out as described previously.

Fetal middle cerebral artery

A transverse view of the fetal brain is obtained at the level of the biparietal diameter (BPD). The transducer is then moved caudally to demonstrate the thalamus clearly. With color flow imaging, the middle cerebral artery (MCA) can be identified as the major anterolateral branch of the Circle of Willis. The pulsed Doppler sample gate should be placed at the junction of the medial third and middle third of this artery (Fig. 16.11). The angle of insonation is invariably small due to the usual occipitotransverse position of the fetal head.

Fetal thoracic aorta

A longitudinal view of the fetal thoracic aorta is obtained with color flow imaging. The pulsed Doppler sample gate should be placed on the linear portion of the descending thoracic aorta, above the level of the diaphragm (Fig. 16.12). You should attempt to keep the angle of insonation below 45°.

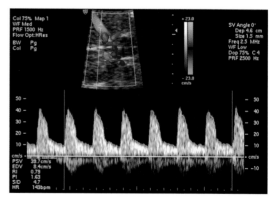

Figure 16.11 Top. Color Doppler waveform obtained from the middle cerebral artery in a normally grown fetus at 34 weeks. Bottom. Measurements are obtained using the maximum frequency follower.

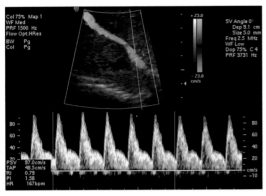

Figure 16.12   Top. Color Doppler waveform obtained from the thoracic aorta in a normally grown fetus at 34 weeks. Bottom. Measurements are obtained using the maximum frequency follower.

How to report fetal arterial Doppler waveforms

The MCA and thoracic aorta flows are most commonly reported in terms of the PI. The PI is derived from the average of at least three and preferably five waveforms. We suggest that you plot the PI values on data reference ranges (Figs 16.13 and 16.14) and also calculate the PI ratio

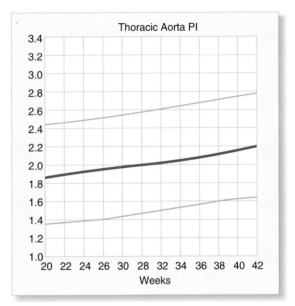

Figure 16.14   Reference range, showing 95th, 50th and 5th centiles, for fetal aorta pulsatility index (PI) with gestation.

of the MCA and thoracic aorta (MCA/TA) or the MCA and umbilical artery (MCA/UA). As well as reporting the PI, you should comment if this value lies outside the data reference ranges.

Fetal arterial distribution

When the ratio of the MCA PI to either the thoracic aorta or umbilical artery PI is increased above the 95th centile, this should be reported as 'evidence of fetal arterial redistribution' (Fig. 16.15). As the reproducibility of umbilical artery Doppler is greater than that of the aorta, the MCA to umbilical artery ratio is preferred for clinical descision making.

Hyperdynamic circulation

When the MCA peak systolic velocity (PSV) is above the 95th centile in pregnancies at risk of fetal anemia, this should be reported as 'Doppler evidence of a hyperdynamic circulation secondary to fetal anemia (Fig. 16.16). When the MCA PSV is above the 66th centile in pregnancies at risk of fetal anemia, this should be reported as 'Doppler suggests that there is a significant risk of fetal anemia'.

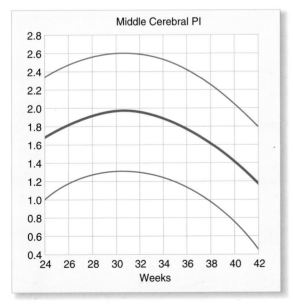

Figure 16.13   Reference range, showing 95th, 50th and 5th centiles, for middle cerebral artery pulsatility index (PI) with gestation.

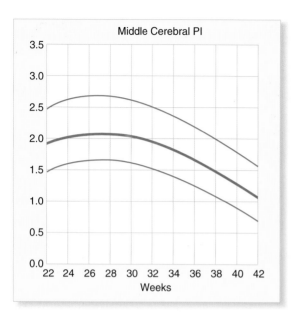

Figure 16.15 Reference range, showing 95th, 50th, and 5th centiles, for ratio of the MCA PI over the umbilical artery PI (cerebroplacental ratio) with gestation (with kind permission of A. Baschat).

Problems

Problems such as occur with umbilical artery waveform analysis (loss of end-diastolic frequencies, fetal breathing and fetal bradycardia effects) should be anticipated and can be dealt with as described earlier (p. 228).

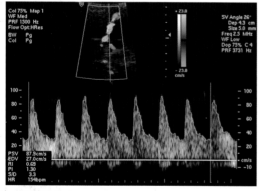

Figure 16.16 Top. Color Doppler waveform of the MCA. Bottom. The maximum frequency follower has been used to calculate the PSV (87.9cm). The value lies above the 95th centile for gestation, making it highly suggestive of fetal anemia.

Variation in MCA PI during the examination

Care must be taken not to use excessive transducer pressure on the fetal head during the examination, as this can cause significant fluctuation of the middle cerebral artery PI.

Variation in MCA PSV during the examination

Care must be taken to angle correct when taking velocity measurements, as this can cause significant fluctuation of the MCA PSV.

Uninterpretable aortic Dopplers

Aortic Doppler signals might be difficult to acquire because of fetal lie, movement or proximity of cardiac structures. It is for this reason that fetal arterial redistribution is often assessed using the MCA/umbilical artery ratio.

Indications for fetal arterial Doppler

Detailed evaluation of the fetal arterial circulation is indicated when absence of end-diastolic frequencies has been demonstrated in the umbilical artery in a growth-restricted fetus but delivery is not considered desirable because of extreme prematurity. Fetal MCA PSV measurements are indicated in fetuses at risk of fetal anemia through maternal isoimmunization or parvovirus infection.

Interpretation of fetal arterial Doppler

Fetal arterial redistribution

A growth-restricted fetus would usually develop abnormal umbilical artery waveforms before developing fetal arterial redistribution. Fetal arterial redistribution is limited to a ceiling of adaptation. When this plateau phase of the response is reached, it is usually termed severe fetal redistribution. Severe fetal redistribution would normally be followed, within 2 weeks, by the development of reduced biophysical profile, abnormal venous Dopplers or suboptimal cardiotocography. Hence, it is usual at this stage to perform one or more of the latter tests on a frequent basis (at least every other day). If the fetus is considered viable, delivery is indicated when one of these tests is found to be abnormal or suspicious. Fetal arterial redistribution can occur in the presence of normal umbilical artery waveforms after 36 weeks' gestation. These fetuses are at a higher risk of complications in labor because of fetal hypoxemia.

Hyperdynamic circulation

When the MCA PSV is below the 66th centile, the fetus is extremely unlikely to be anemic. Use of MCA Doppler can significantly reduce the need for invasive monitoring (cordocentesis) of the fetal hemoglobin concentration. When the MCA PSV is above the 95th centile, the fetus is likely to be anemic. An urgent referral should be made to a fetal medicine specialist. When the MCA PSV is between the 66th and 95th centile in an isoimmunized pregnancy, the fetus is considered to be at risk of mild to moderate anemia and a second opinion should be sought from a fetal medicine specialist.

FETAL VENOUS DOPPLER

Rationale for fetal venous Doppler analysis

Fetal venous waveforms are acquired from the ductus venosus by means of color, pulsed Doppler ultrasound. The ductus venosus is the main vessel through which oxygenated blood returning from the placenta is directed to the fetal heart and circulation. With worsening fetal hypoxemia, abnormal umbilical artery waveforms and severe fetal arterial redistribution develop. In addition, there is also increased redistribution of highly oxygenated umbilical vein blood through the ductus venosus to the fetal heart.

When the fetal condition becomes critical, due to increasing right ventricular afterload and heart failure, abnormal ductus venosus flow waveforms are seen. These changes are reflected in an increase in peak systolic forward flow, and during atrial contraction when there is retrograde flow. Hence, fetal venous Doppler can be used to monitor fetal compensatory responses to progressively deteriorating placental function.

Obtaining the ductus venosus waveform

The machine setup and waveform analysis should be carried out as described on p. 224.

A transverse view of the fetal abdomen is obtained at the level of the intrahepatic portion of the umbilical vein. Rotate the probe slightly to image the entire length of the umbilical vein, from the umbilicus to its anastomosis with the portal sinus. The large right portal vein can be seen as a continuation of the portal sinus, which also gives rise to a smaller left portal vein. The probe is then moved to an oblique transverse position to image this intrahepatic vessel complex (Fig. 16.17). Using color flow imaging, the ductus venosus can be identified as a small vessel running from the portal sinus to the junction of the inferior vena cava and right atrium. This is often best visualized by imaging the full length of the umbilical vein with color Doppler. The ductus can then be identified arising from the intrahepatic vessel complex at the end of the umbilical vein by its higher velocities. The high velocity of blood flow in the ductus venosus is characteristically triphasic and typically produces an aliasing effect on color flow Doppler (Fig. 16.18). The pulsed Doppler sample gate should be placed at the inlet of the ductus venosus from the portal sinus.

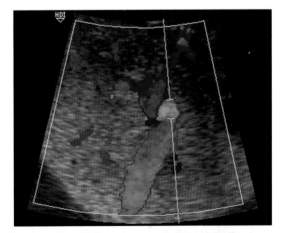

Figure 16.17 Oblique transverse view of the fetal abdomen demonstrating the ductus venosus. Note the relative positions of the umbilical vein, portal sinus, right and left portal veins and ductus venosus.

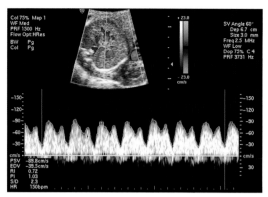

Figure 16.18 Top. Doppler gate placed on ductus venosus in a 30 week fetus. Bottom. Waveform obtained from the normal ductus venosus. Note the triphasic appearance of the normal waveform. Measurements are obtained using the onscreen calipers.

How to report fetal venous Doppler

The ductus venosus flow is reported in terms of the pulsatility index for veins (PIV). The PIV is derived from the average of at least three, and preferably five, waveforms. We suggest that you plot this on a data reference range (Fig. 16.19). As well as report-

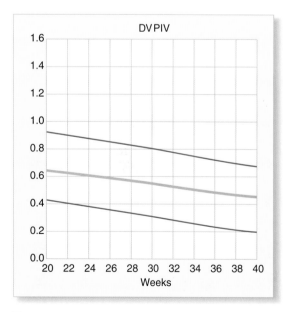

Figure 16.19 Reference range, showing 95th, 50th and 5th centiles, for pulsatility index for veins (PIV) of the ductus venosus (DV) with gestation.

ing the PI, you should comment if there is absent or reversed flow during atrial contraction (a-wave).

Problems

Fetal breathing movements have more pronounced effects on fetal venous than on fetal arterial Doppler. This is presumably due to the negative intrathoracic pressure produced during fetal breathing movements. Ductus venosus Doppler indices should only be measured during fetal apnea.

There is considerable variation in Doppler indices, depending on where the sampling gate is placed. Doppler velocities at the ductus venosus inlet are higher than at the outlet. The pulsed wave gate should be placed at the ductus venosus inlet.

The ductus venosus is part of the subdiaphragmatic venous plexus. Hence, ductus venosus Doppler flow waveforms can be corrupted by signals from nearby vessels. This is a compounding reason for absence/reversal of flow in the a-wave. To avoid this complication, the sample gate should be kept as small as possible and the Doppler indices should be measured several times, until reproducible results are obtained.

Indications for fetal venous Doppler

Detailed evaluation of the fetal arterial circulation is indicated when fetal arterial redistribution is seen in an extremely preterm growth-restricted fetus. In this situation, abnormal umbilical and arterial Dopplers can persist for many weeks, before fetal demise. Absent or reversed flow during atrial contraction occurs when fetal physiological responses fail to prevent the development of fetal hypoxia. Under extreme conditions, pulsatile blood flow can be seen in the umbilical vein because atrial pressure is transmitted through the ductus venosus to the umbilical vein.

Interpretation of fetal venous Doppler

Normal ductus venosus Doppler indices in a growth-restricted fetus suggest that there is adequate fetal compensation. Abnormal ductus venosus Doppler findings are closely allied to poor biophysical profile scores (Fig. 16.20). Arterial redistribution is associated with moderate acidemia,

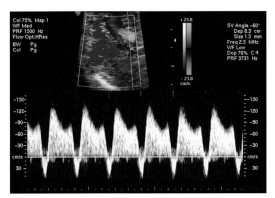

Figure 16.20 Top. Abnormal ductus venosus waveform demonstrating reverse flow and increased PIV in a growth-restricted 32 week fetus. Compare with the normal appearances shown in Fig. 16.18. Bottom. Measurements are obtained using the onscreen calipers.

whereas abnormal venous Dopplers are associated with severe fetal acidemia. Development of pulsations in the umbilical vein occurs just prior to abnormal fetal heart rate patterns. In growth-restricted fetuses, neonatal mortality is at least 60%

under these circumstances, compared to 20% in the absence of venous pulsations.

REFERENCES AND FURTHER READING

Aguilina J, Thompson O, Thilaganathan B, Harrington K 2001 Improved early prediction of pre-eclampsia by combining second trimester maternal serum inhibin-A and uterine artery Doppler. Ultrasound in Obstetrics and Gynecology 17:477–484

Baschat A A, Harman C R 2001 Antenatal assessment of the growth restricted fetus. Current Opinion in Obstetrics and Gynecology 13:161–168

Hecher K, Campbell S, Doyle P et al 1995 Assessment of fetal compromise by Doppler ultrasound investigation of the fetal circulation. Arterial, intracardiac and venous blood flow studies. Circulation 91:129–138

Mari G, Deter R I, Carpenter R L et al 2000 Noninvasive diagnosis by Doppler ultrasonography of fetal anemia due to maternal red-cell alloimmunization. Collaborative group for Doppler assessment of the blood velocity in anemic fetuses. New England Journal of Medicine 342:9–14

Nicolaides K H, Rizzo G, Hecher K 2000 Placental and fetal Doppler. Diploma in Fetal Medicine series. Parthenon Publishing, New York

Appendices

APPENDIX 1: GROWTH OF CROWN RUMP LENGTH WITH GESTATIONAL AGE

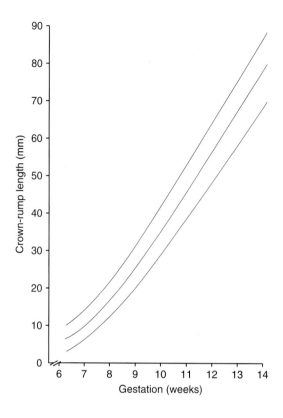

APPENDIX 2: ESTIMATION OF GESTATIONAL AGE FROM CROWN RUMP LENGTH (CRL) (AFTER ROBINSON & FLEMING 1975)

| CRL (mm) | Gestational age | | Error (± 2 SD) |
	Weeks	Days	
4	6	0	
6	6	3	
8	6	6	
10	7	1	
12	7	4	
14	8	0	
16	8	2	4.7 days
18	8	4	
20	8	5	
22	9	0	
24	9	2	
26	9	3	
28	9	5	
30	9	6	
32	10	1	
34	10	2	
36	10	3	4.7 days
38	10	5	
40	11	0	
42	11	1	
44	11	2	
46	11	3	
48	11	4	
50	11	5	
52	11	6	
54	12	1	4.7 days
56	12	2	
58	12	3	
60	12	4	
62	12	5	
64	12	6	
66	13	0	
68	13	1	4.7 days
70	13	2	
72	13	3	
74	13	4	
76	13	5	
78	13	6	
80	14	0	

APPENDIX 3: ESTIMATION OF GESTATIONAL AGE FROM BIPARIETAL DIAMETER (BPD) (OUTER TO OUTER) (AFTER ALTMAN & CHITTY 1997)

BPD (mm)	Estimated GA (weeks + days)	5th centile (weeks + days)	95th centile (weeks + days)
22	12 + 4	11 + 5	13 + 4
23	12 + 6	12 + 0	13 + 6
24	13 + 1	12 + 1	14 + 1
25	13 + 3	12 + 3	14 + 3
26	13 + 4	12 + 3	14 + 5
27	13 + 6	12 + 5	15 + 0
28	14 + 1	13 + 1	15 + 2
29	14 + 3	13 + 3	15 + 4
30	14 + 5	13 + 4	15 + 6
31	15 + 0	13 + 6	16 + 1
32	15 + 2	14 + 1	16 + 3
33	15 + 4	14 + 3	16 + 5
34	15 + 5	14 + 4	17 + 0
35	16 + 0	14 + 6	17 + 2
36	16 + 2	15 + 1	17 + 5
37	16 + 4	15 + 3	18 + 0
38	16 + 6	15 + 4	18 + 2
39	17 + 1	15 + 6	18 + 4
40	17 + 3	16 + 1	19 + 0
41	17 + 5	16 + 3	19 + 2
42	18 + 0	16 + 4	19 + 4
43	18 + 2	16 + 6	19 + 6
44	18 + 4	17 + 1	20 + 2
45	19 + 0	17 + 3	20 + 4
46	19 + 2	17 + 5	20 + 6
47	19 + 4	18 + 0	21 + 2
48	20 + 6	18 + 2	21 + 4
49	20 + 1	18 + 4	22 + 0
50	20 + 3	18 + 5	22 + 2
51	20 + 5	19 + 0	22 + 4
52	21 + 1	19 + 2	23 + 0
53	21 + 3	19 + 4	23 + 2
54	21 + 5	19 + 6	23 + 5
55	22 + 0	20 + 1	24 + 0
56	22 + 2	20 + 3	24 + 3
57	22 + 5	20 + 5	24 + 5
58	23 + 0	21 + 0	25 + 1
59	23 + 2	21 + 2	25 + 4
60	23 + 5	21 + 4	25 + 6
61	24 + 0	21 + 6	26 + 2
62	24 + 2	22 + 1	26 + 5
63	24 + 5	22 + 4	27 + 0
64	25 + 0	22 + 6	27 + 3
65	25 + 2	23 + 1	27 + 6
66	25 + 5	23 + 3	28 + 2
67	26 + 0	23 + 5	28 + 4
68	26 + 3	24 + 0	29 + 0

BPD (mm)	Estimated GA (weeks + days)	5th centile (weeks + days)	95th centile (weeks + days)
69	26 + 5	24 + 2	29 + 3
70	27 + 1	24 + 4	29 + 6
71	27 + 3	25 + 0	30 + 2
72	27 + 6	25 + 2	30 + 4
73	28 + 1	25 + 4	31 + 0

Dating is most accurate when carried out before 24 weeks. It should not be attempted after 28 weeks of gestation.

APPENDIX 4: GROWTH OF HEAD CIRCUMFERENCE (HC) DERIVED FROM BIPARIETAL DIAMETER (BPD) (OUTER TO OUTER) AND OCCIPITOFRONTAL DIAMETER (OFD) (OUTER TO OUTER) WITH GESTATIONAL AGE (AFTER CHITTY ET AL 1994)

Weeks of gestation	Centile					SD
	3rd	10th	50th	90th	97th	
12	55.5	59.6	68.1	76.7	80.8	6.7
13	69.1	73.3	82.2	91.1	95.2	6.9
14	82.6	86.9	96.0	105.2	109.5	7.2
15	95.8	100.2	109.7	119.2	123.6	7.4
16	108.8	113.4	123.1	132.9	137.5	7.6
17	121.6	126.3	136.4	146.4	151.2	7.9
18	134.1	138.9	149.3	159.7	164.6	8.1
19	146.4	151.4	162.0	172.7	177.7	8.3
20	158.4	163.5	174.5	185.4	190.6	8.6
21	170.1	175.4	186.6	197.9	203.2	8.8
22	181.5	186.9	198.5	210.0	215.5	9.0
23	192.6	198.1	210.0	221.9	227.4	9.3
24	203.4	209.1	221.2	233.4	239.1	9.5
25	213.8	219.6	232.1	244.5	250.4	9.7
26	223.8	229.8	242.6	255.3	261.3	10.0
27	233.5	239.7	252.7	265.8	271.9	10.2
28	242.9	249.1	262.5	275.8	282.1	10.4
29	251.8	258.2	271.8	285.5	291.9	10.7
30	260.3	266.8	280.7	294.7	301.2	10.9
31	268.3	275.0	289.2	303.5	310.2	11.1
32	275.9	282.7	297.3	311.8	318.7	11.4
33	283.1	290.0	304.9	319.7	326.7	11.6
34	289.8	296.9	312.0	327.2	334.3	11.8
35	296.0	303.2	318.7	334.1	341.3	12.1
36	301.7	309.0	324.8	340.5	347.9	12.3
37	306.9	314.4	330.4	346.4	354.0	12.5
38	311.5	319.2	335.5	351.8	359.5	12.0
39	315.6	323.4	340.0	356.7	364.5	13.0
40	319.2	327.1	344.0	361.0	368.9	13.2
41	322.1	330.2	347.4	364.7	372.7	13.5
42	324.5	332.7	350.3	367.8	376.0	13.7

APPENDIX 5: ESTIMATION OF GESTATIONAL AGE (GA) FROM HEAD CIRCUMFERENCE (HC) DERIVED FROM BIPARIETAL DIAMETER (BPD) (OUTER TO OUTER) AND OCCIPITOFRONTAL DIAMETER (OFD) (OUTER TO OUTER) (AFTER ALTMAN & CHITTY 1997)

HC (mm)	Estimated GA (weeks + days)	5th centile (weeks + days)	95th centile (weeks + days)
80	12 + 4	11 + 3	13 + 5
85	12 + 6	11 + 6	14 + 1
90	13 + 2	12 + 2	14 + 4
95	13 + 5	12 + 4	15 + 0
100	14 + 1	13 + 0	15 + 3
105	14 + 4	13 + 3	15 + 5
110	15 + 0	13 + 6	16 + 1
115	15 + 3	14 + 2	16 + 4
120	15 + 6	14 + 5	17 + 0
125	16 + 2	15 + 1	17 + 3
130	16 + 4	15 + 4	17 + 6
135	17 + 0	15 + 6	18 + 2
140	17 + 3	16 + 2	18 + 5
145	17 + 6	16 + 5	19 + 1
150	18 + 2	17 + 1	19 + 3
155	18 + 5	17 + 4	19 + 6
160	19 + 1	17 + 6	20 + 2
165	19 + 3	18 + 2	20 + 5
170	19 + 6	18 + 5	21 + 1
175	20 + 2	19 + 1	21 + 4
180	20 + 5	19 + 3	22 + 0
185	21 + 1	19 + 6	22 + 3
190	21 + 4	20 + 2	22 + 6
195	22 + 0	20 + 4	23 + 2
200	22 + 2	21 + 0	23 + 5
205	22 + 5	21 + 3	24 + 2
210	23 + 1	21 + 5	24 + 5
215	23 + 4	22 + 1	25 + 1
220	24 + 0	22 + 4	25 + 5
225	24 + 3	22 + 6	26 + 1
230	24 + 6	23 + 2	26 + 5
235	25 + 3	23 + 5	27 + 1
240	25 + 6	24 + 1	27 + 5
245	26 + 2	24 + 3	28 + 2
250	26 + 5	24 + 6	28 + 6
255	27 + 2	25 + 2	29 + 3
260	27 + 5	25 + 5	30 + 0
265	28 + 2	26 + 1	30 + 4

Dating is most accurate when carried out before 24 weeks. It should not be attempted after 28 weeks of gestation.

APPENDIX 6: GROWTH OF ABDOMINAL CIRCUMFERENCE (AC) DERIVED FROM TRANSVERSE ABDOMINAL DIAMETER (TAD) AND ANTEROPOSTERIOR ABDOMINAL DIAMETER (APAD) WITH GESTATIONAL AGE (AFTER CHITTY ET AL 1994B)

Weeks of gestation	Centile					
	3rd	10th	50th	90th	97th	SD
12	48.0	50.5	55.8	61.1	63.6	4.1
13	58.5	61.3	67.4	73.4	76.3	4.7
14	68.8	72.0	78.9	85.7	88.9	5.3
15	79.1	82.7	90.3	97.9	101.5	5.9
16	89.3	93.3	101.6	110.0	113.9	6.5
17	99.5	103.8	112.9	122.1	126.4	7.2
18	109.5	114.2	124.1	134.0	138.7	7.8
19	119.5	124.5	135.2	145.9	150.9	8.4
20	129.4	134.8	146.2	157.7	161.1	9.0
21	139.2	144.9	157.1	169.4	175.1	9.6
22	148.9	155.0	168.0	181.0	187.1	10.2
23	158.5	164.9	178.7	192.5	198.9	10.8
24	167.9	174.8	189.3	203.8	210.7	11.4
25	177.3	184.5	199.8	215.1	222.3	12.0
26	186.6	194.1	210.2	226.3	233.3	12.6
27	195.7	203.6	220.4	237.3	245.2	13.2
28	204.7	212.9	230.6	248.2	256.4	13.8
29	213.5	222.2	240.5	258.9	267.6	14.4
30	222.3	231.2	250.4	269.6	278.6	15.0
31	230.8	240.2	260.1	280.1	289.4	15.6
32	239.3	249.0	269.7	290.4	300.1	16.2
33	247.6	257.6	279.1	300.6	310.6	16.8
34	255.7	266.1	288.4	310.6	321.0	17.4
35	263.7	274.4	297.5	320.5	331.3	18.0
36	271.5	282.6	306.4	330.2	341.3	18.6
37	279.1	290.6	315.1	339.7	351.2	19.2
38	286.5	298.4	323.7	349.1	360.9	19.3
39	293.8	306.0	332.1	358.2	370.5	20.4
40	300.9	313.5	340.4	367.2	379.8	21.0
41	307.8	320.8	348.4	376.0	389.0	21.6
42	314.5	327.8	356.2	384.6	398.0	22.2

APPENDIX 7: ESTIMATION OF GESTATIONAL AGE (GA) FROM FEMUR LENGTH (AFTER ALTMAN & CHITTY 1997)

Femur (mm)	Estimated GA (weeks + days)	5th centile (weeks + days)	95th centile (weeks + days)
10	13 + 0	12 + 1	13 + 6
11	13 + 2	12 + 3	14 + 1
12	13 + 4	12 + 5	14 + 4
13	13 + 6	13 + 0	14 + 6
14	14 + 1	13 + 1	15 + 1
15	14 + 3	13 + 3	15 + 3
16	14 + 5	13 + 5	15 + 6
17	15 + 0	14 + 0	16 + 1
18	15 + 2	14 + 2	16 + 3
19	15 + 5	14 + 4	16 + 6
20	16 + 0	14 + 6	17 + 1
21	16 + 2	15 + 1	17 + 3
22	16 + 4	15 + 3	17 + 6
23	16 + 6	15 + 5	18 + 1
24	17 + 2	16 + 0	18 + 4
25	17 + 4	16 + 2	18 + 6
26	17 + 6	16 + 4	19 + 2
27	18 + 2	16 + 6	19 + 5
28	18 + 4	17 + 1	20 + 0
29	18 + 6	17 + 4	20 + 3
30	19 + 2	17 + 6	20 + 5
31	19 + 4	18 + 1	21 + 1
32	20 + 0	18 + 3	21 + 4
33	20 + 2	18 + 5	22 + 0
34	20 + 5	19 + 1	22 + 3
35	21 + 0	19 + 3	22 + 5
36	21 + 3	19 + 5	23 + 1
37	21 + 5	20 + 1	23 + 4
38	22 + 1	20 + 3	24 + 0
39	22 + 4	20 + 5	24 + 3
40	22 + 6	21 + 1	24 + 6
41	23 + 2	21 + 3	25 + 2
42	23 + 5	21 + 6	25 + 5
43	24 + 1	22 + 1	26 + 1
44	24 + 3	22 + 4	26 + 4
45	24 + 6	22 + 6	27 + 1
46	25 + 2	23 + 2	27 + 4
47	25 + 5	23 + 4	28 + 0
48	26 + 1	24 + 0	28 + 3
49	26 + 4	24 + 3	29 + 0
50	27 + 0	24 + 5	29 + 3
51	27 + 3	25 + 1	30 + 0
52	27 + 6	25 + 4	30 + 3
53	28 + 2	26 + 0	31 + 0

Dating is most accurate when carried out before 24 weeks. It should not be attempted after 28 weeks of gestation.

APPENDIX 8: GROWTH OF BIPARIETAL DIAMETER (BPD) (OUTER TO OUTER) WITH GESTATIONAL AGE (AFTER CHITTY ET AL 1994A)

Weeks of gestation	Centile				
	3rd	10th	50th	90th	97th
12	15.5	16.8	19.7	22.5	23.9
13	19.2	20.6	23.5	26.5	27.8
14	22.9	24.3	27.3	30.3	31.7
15	26.5	28.0	31.0	34.1	35.6
16	30.1	31.6	34.7	37.9	39.4
17	33.6	35.1	38.3	41.6	43.1
18	37.0	38.6	41.9	45.2	46.8
19	40.4	42.0	45.4	48.8	50.4
20	43.7	45.4	48.8	52.3	53.9
21	47.0	48.6	52.2	55.7	57.4
22	50.2	51.9	55.5	59.1	60.8
23	53.3	55.0	58.7	62.3	64.1
24	56.3	58.0	61.8	65.5	67.3
25	59.2	61.0	64.8	68.6	70.4
26	62.0	63.8	67.8	71.7	73.5
27	64.8	66.6	70.6	74.6	76.5
28	67.4	69.3	73.4	77.4	79.3
29	69.9	71.9	76.0	80.1	82.1
30	72.4	74.3	78.6	82.8	84.7
31	74.7	76.7	81.0	85.3	87.3
32	76.9	79.0	83.3	87.7	89.7
33	79.0	81.1	85.5	90.0	92.1
34	81.0	83.1	87.6	92.1	94.3
35	82.9	85.0	89.6	94.2	96.3
36	84.6	86.3	91.5	96.1	98.3
37	86.2	88.4	93.2	97.9	100.1
38	87.7	89.9	94.8	99.6	101.8
39	89.0	91.3	96.2	101.1	103.4
40	90.2	92.6	97.5	102.5	104.8
41	91.3	93.6	98.7	103.7	106.1
42	92.2	94.6	99.7	104.8	107.2

APPENDIX 9: GROWTH OF FEMUR LENGTH (FL) WITH GESTATIONAL AGE (AFTER CHITTY ET AL 1994C)

Weeks of gestation	Centile					SD
	3rd	10th	50th	90th	97th	
12	4.4	5.5	7.7	10.0	11.1	1.8
13	7.5	8.6	10.9	13.3	14.4	1.8
14	10.6	11.7	14.1	16.5	17.6	1.9
15	13.6	14.7	17.2	19.7	20.8	1.9
16	16.5	17.7	20.3	22.8	24.0	2.0
17	19.4	20.7	23.3	25.9	27.2	2.1
18	22.3	23.6	26.3	29.0	30.2	2.1
19	25.1	26.4	29.2	32.0	33.3	2.2
20	27.9	29.2	32.1	34.9	36.3	2.2
21	30.6	32.0	34.9	37.8	39.2	2.3
22	33.2	34.6	37.6	40.6	42.0	2.3
23	35.8	37.2	40.3	43.4	44.8	2.4
24	38.3	39.8	42.9	46.1	47.6	2.5
25	40.8	42.3	45.5	48.7	50.2	2.5
26	43.1	44.7	48.0	51.3	52.8	2.6
27	45.4	47.0	50.4	53.8	55.3	2.6
28	47.6	49.3	52.7	56.2	57.8	2.7
29	49.8	51.4	55.0	58.5	60.1	2.8
30	51.8	53.5	57.1	60.7	62.4	2.8
31	53.8	55.5	59.2	62.9	64.6	2.9
32	55.7	57.4	61.2	64.9	66.7	2.9
33	57.5	59.3	63.1	66.9	68.7	3.0
34	59.2	61.0	64.9	68.8	70.6	3.0
35	60.8	62.6	66.6	70.6	72.4	3.1
36	62.3	64.2	68.2	72.3	74.1	3.2
37	63.7	65.6	69.7	73.8	75.8	3.2
38	64.9	66.9	71.1	75.3	77.3	3.3
39	66.1	68.1	72.4	76.7	78.7	3.3
40	67.2	69.2	73.6	77.9	79.9	3.4
41	68.1	70.2	74.6	79.0	81.1	3.5
42	69.0	71.1	75.6	80.1	82.2	3.5

APPENDIX 10: GROWTH OF ANTEROPOSTERIOR DIAMETER, TRANSVERSE DIAMETER AND LONGITUDINAL DIAMETER OF THE KIDNEY WITH GESTATIONAL AGE (ADAPTED FROM CHITTY & ALTMAN 1993)

Antero-posterior diameter (mm)

Weeks of gestation	5th centile	50th centile	95th centile
14	4.1	6.7	9.8
15	4.8	7.6	10.9
16	5.6	8.5	12.0
17	6.4	9.5	13.2
18	7.2	10.4	14.3
19	8.0	11.4	15.5
20	8.8	12.4	16.6
21	9.6	13.4	17.7
22	10.5	14.3	18.8
23	11.3	15.3	19.9
24	12.1	16.2	21.0
25	12.9	17.1	22.0
26	13.6	18.0	23.0
27	14.4	18.9	24.0
28	15.1	19.7	24.9
29	15.8	20.5	25.8
30	16.5	21.3	26.7
31	17.1	22.0	27.5
32	17.7	22.7	28.2
33	18.2	23.3	28.9
34	18.8	23.8	29.5
35	19.2	24.4	30.1
36	19.6	24.8	30.6
37	20.0	25.2	31.1
38	20.3	25.6	31.5
39	20.6	25.9	31.8
40	20.8	26.1	32.1
41	21.0	26.3	32.3
42	21.1	26.4	32.4

Transverse diameter (mm)

Weeks of gestation	5th centile	50th centile	95th centile
14	4.4	7.1	10.4
15	5.1	8.0	11.6
16	6.0	9.0	12.8
17	6.8	10.0	14.0
18	7.6	11.1	15.2
19	8.5	12.1	16.4
20	9.3	13.1	17.5
21	10.2	14.1	18.7
22	11.0	15.1	19.9
23	11.9	16.1	21.0
24	12.7	17.1	22.1
25	13.5	18.0	23.1
26	14.3	18.9	24.1
27	15.0	19.7	25.1
28	15.7	20.5	26.0
29	16.4	21.3	26.8
30	17.0	22.0	27.6
31	17.6	22.7	28.4
32	18.1	23.3	29.0
33	18.6	23.8	29.6
34	19.0	24.3	30.2
35	19.4	24.7	30.7
36	19.7	25.1	31.1
37	20.0	25.4	31.4
38	20.2	25.6	31.6
39	20.3	25.8	31.8
40	20.4	25.8	31.9
41	20.4	25.9	31.9
42	20.4	25.8	31.9

Longitudinal diameter (mm)

Weeks of gestation	5th centile	50th centile	95th centile
14	8.0	9.8	11.8
15	9.3	11.4	13.7
16	10.6	13.1	15.8
17	12.0	14.8	17.9
18	13.4	16.5	20.0
19	14.8	18.3	22.2
20	16.2	20.1	24.4
21	17.6	21.8	26.5
22	19.0	23.6	28.7
23	20.4	25.3	30.8
24	21.8	27.0	32.8
25	23.2	28.7	34.8
26	24.5	30.3	36.8
27	25.8	31.9	38.6
28	27.0	33.4	40.4
29	28.2	34.8	42.1
30	29.4	36.2	43.6
31	30.5	37.4	45.1
32	31.5	38.6	46.4
33	32.4	39.7	47.6
34	33.3	40.6	48.7
35	34.1	41.5	49.7
36	34.9	42.3	50.5
37	35.5	43.0	51.1
38	36.1	43.5	51.6
39	36.6	43.9	52.0
40	36.9	44.2	52.2
41	37.3	44.4	52.3
42	37.5	44.5	52.2

APPENDIX 11: MARKERS OF CHROMOSOMAL ABNORMALITY

Marker	Karyotype	Probable risk of on of abnormal karyotypes listed in column 2.
Agenesis of corpus callosum	trisomy 13	5%
Cardiac abnormalities	trisomy 13, 18, 21	15%
Choroid plexus cysts	trisomy 18	low
Clasped or overlapping fingers	trisomy 18	nk
Clinodactyly	trisomy 21	nk
Cystic hygroma	45 XO, trisomy 21, 18, 13	90%
Diaphragmatic hernia	trisomy 18	15%
Dilated ureters	trisomy 18, 21	low
Duodenal atresia	trisomy 21	30%
Echogenic focus	trisomy 21	low
Echogenic bowel	trisomy 21	low
Holoprosencephaly	trisomy 13, 18	90%
Increased nuchal translucency	trisomy 21	75%
Increased nuchal fold	trisomy 21	30%
Severe IUGR	triploidy, trisomy 18	5%
Ventriculomegaly	trisomy 21	<1%
Lateral facial cleft	trisomy 18	<1%
Median facial cleft	trisomy 13	50%
Multicystic renal dysplasia	trisomy 18	low
Non-immune hydrops	45 XO	–
Cystic hygroma	45 XO	99%
Omphalocele	trisomy 13, 18	30%
Radial aplasia/thumb hypoplasia	trisomy 13	90%
Rocker bottom feet	trisomy 18	50%
Sandal gap	trisomy 21	10%
Short femur or humerus	trisomy 21	low
Single umbilical artery	trisomy 18, 21	5%
Syndactyly/polydactyly	trisomy 13	–

The figures are the best estimate that can be obtained from the prenatal diagnosis literature.

–, risk is not calculable in these markers; `low', these markers show a weak association with aneuploidy and on their own do not currently warrant karyotyping; nk, not known.

APPENDIX 12: DIFFERENTIAL DIAGNOSIS OF COMMON PROBLEMS

Causes of small for dates

- Wrong dates
- Constitutionally small baby
- Fetal death
- Intrauterine growth restriction
- Oligohydramnios
- Spontaneous rupture of membranes

Causes of bleeding

First trimester

- Miscarriage
  - incomplete
  - missed
  - threatened
- Hydatidiform mole
- Ectopic gestation

Second and third trimesters

- Placenta previa
- Abruption
- Hydatidiform mole
- Marginal sinus rupture

Causes of large for dates

- Incorrect dates
- Constitutionally large baby
- Multiple pregnancy
- Fetal macrosomia
- Uterine fibroids
- Ovarian cysts
- Polyhydramnios

Causes of lower abdominal pain

First and second trimester

- Ectopic gestation
- Corpus luteal cyst hemorrhage or rupture
- Miscarriage
- Fibroid degeneration

Third trimester

- Abruption
- Preterm labour
- Fibroid degeneration

APPENDIX 13: DIFFERENTIAL DIAGNOSIS OF ABNORMAL ULTRASOUND FINDINGS AND COMMONLY ASSOCIATED ABNORMALITIES

Causes of polyhydramnios

- Multiple pregnancy
- Twin–twin transfusion syndrome
- Maternal diabetes mellitus
- Fetal and placental tumours:
  - placental chorioangioma
  - sacrococcygeal teratoma
- Fetal upper intestinal abnormality:
  - esophageal or small bowel atresia
  - volvulus or meconium ileus
- Fetal neurological abnormality because of impaired fetal swallowing:
  - anencephaly or arthrogryposis
- Other fetal abnormalities:
  - fetal anemia
  - hydrops fetalis (any etiology)

Causes of oligohydramnios

- Spontaneous rupture of the membranes
- Intrauterine growth restriction
- Lesions of the fetal urinary tract:
  - bilateral renal agenesis or multicystic dysplasia
  - posterior urethral valves

Most common causes of fetal non-cystic mass

Head

- Encephalocele

Neck

- Increased skin fold thickness

Chest

- Diaphragmatic hernia containing liver or spleen
- Ectopia cordis, i.e. the heart being outside the chest cavity
- Congenital cystic adenomatoid malformation
- Pulmonary sequestration

Abdomen

- Echogenic bowel
- Multicystic renal dysplasia
- Infantile polycystic kidneys
- Omphalocele
- Gastroschisis

Spine

- Spina bifida
- Sacrococcygeal teratoma

Causes of echo-free areas within the fetus

Fetal head

- Ventriculomegaly
- Hydranencephaly
- Holoprosencephaly
- Porencephalic cyst
- Choroid plexus cyst
- Dandy–Walker malformation
- Arachnoid cyst

Chest

- Diaphragmatic hernia
- Lung cyst (congenital cystic adenomatoid malformation)
- Pleural effusion
- Pericardial effusion

Abdomen

Normal

- Structures – stomach, bladder, gallbladder and renal pelvis
- Vascular – umbilical vein, portal vein, aorta and inferior vena cava

Single
- Solitary cyst of the kidney, liver, ovary and mesentery
- Unilateral renal pelvic dilatation
- Bowel duplication cyst
- Enlarged bladder due to urethral atresia or stenosis

Double
- Duodenal atresia
- Bilateral renal pelvic dilatation
- Choledochal cyst

Triple
- Jejunal atresia
- Obstructive uropathy (bladder, dilated ureters and renal pelves)

Multiple
- Multicystic or polycystic kidneys
- Ascites

Common fetal abnormality associations

Abnormality	Associations
Achondroplasia	Spina bifida
	Microcephaly
	Infantile polycystic kidneys
Median cleft lip	Arrhinencephaly
Facial anomalies, e.g. cyclopia, proboscis	Holoprosencephaly
Cloacal extrophy	Spina bifida
	Omphalocele
Diaphragmatic hernia	Spina bifida
	Hydronephrosis
Duodenal atresia	Down's syndrome
Gastroschisis	Usually none
Ventriculomegaly	Spina bifida
Obstructive uropathy	Spina bifida
	Bowel abnormalities
Omphalocele	Cardiac anomalies
	Chromosome anomalies
	Neural tube defects
Renal dysplasia	Encephalocele*
	Ventriculomegaly*
	Microcephaly*
	Polydactyly*

*Any of the above with renal dysplasia is known as Meckel's syndrome.

REFERENCES AND FURTHER READING

Altman D G, Chitty L S 1997 New charts for ultrasound dating of pregnancy. Ultrasound in Obstetrics and Gynecology 10:174–191

Chitty L S, Altman D G 1993 Charts of fetal size. In: Dewbury K, Meire H, Cosgrove D (eds) Ultrasound in Obstetrics and Gynaecology. Churchill Livingstone, Edinburgh, p 550–553

Chitty L S, Altman D G, Henderson A, Campbell S 1994a Charts of fetal size: 2. Head measurements. British Journal of Obstetrics and Gynaecology 101:35–43

Chitty L S, Altman D G, Henderson A, Campbell S 1994b Charts of fetal size: 3. Abdominal measurements. British Journal of Obstetrics and Gynaecology 101:125–131

Chitty L S, Altman D G, Henderson A, Campbell S 1994c Charts of fetal size: 4. Femur length. British Journal of Obstetrics and Gynaecology 101:132–135

Robinson H P, Fleming J E E 1975 A critical evaluation of sonar crown–rump length measurements. British Journal of Obstetrics and Gynaecology 82:702–710

Index